Casebook of the Brief Psychotherapies

APPLIED CLINICAL PSYCHOLOGY

Series Editors:
Alan S. Bellack, *Medical College of Pennsylvania at EPPI, Philadelphia, Pennsylvania,*
and Michel Hersen, *Nova University School of Psychology, Fort Lauderdale, Florida*

Current Volumes in This Series

ACTIVITY MEASUREMENT IN PSYCHOLOGY AND MEDICINE
Warren W. Tryon

BEHAVIOR ANALYSIS AND TREATMENT
Edited by Ron Van Houten and Saul Axelrod

CASEBOOK OF THE BRIEF PSYCHOTHERAPIES
Edited by Richard A. Wells and Vincent J. Giannetti

CLINICAL PSYCHOLOGY
Historical and Research Foundations
Edited by C. Eugene Walker

CLINICAL PSYCHOLOGY SINCE 1917
Science, Practice, and Organization
Donald K. Routh

ETHNIC VALIDITY, ECOLOGY, AND PSYCHOTHERAPY
A Psychosocial Competence Model
Forrest B. Tyler, Deborah Ridley Brome, and Janice E. Williams

PERSPECTIVES AND PROMISES OF CLINICAL PSYCHOLOGY
Edited by Anke Ehlers, Wolfgang Fiegenbaum, Irmela Florin, and Jürgen Margraf

SEXUAL BEHAVIOR
Problems and Management
Nathaniel McConaghy

THERAPEUTIC CHANGE
An Object Relations Perspective
Sidney J. Blatt and Richard Q. Ford

USING RATIONAL-EMOTIVE THERAPY EFFECTIVELY
A Practitioner's Guide
Edited by Michael E. Bernard

Casebook of the Brief Psychotherapies

Edited by
RICHARD A. WELLS
University of Pittsburgh
Pittsburgh, Pennsylvania

and

VINCENT J. GIANNETTI
Duquesne University
Pittsburgh, Pennsylvania

PLENUM PRESS • NEW YORK AND LONDON

Library of Congress Cataloging-in-Publication Data

Casebook of the brief psychotherapies / edited by Richard A. Wells and Vincent J. Giannetti.
p. cm. -- (Applied clinical psychology)
Includes bibliographical references and index.
ISBN 0-306-44392-9 (hb.). -- ISBN 0-306-44393-7 (pbk.)
1. Brief psychotherapy--Case studies. I. Wells, Richard A. II. Giannetti, Vincent J. III. Series.
[DNLM: 1. Psychotherapy, Brief--case studies. WM 40 C3375 1993]
RC480.55.C36 1993
616.89'14--dc20
DNLM/DLC
for Library of Congress 93-28857
CIP

ISBN 0-306-44392-9 (hardcover)
ISBN 0-306-44393-7 (paperback)

A Division of Plenum Publishing Corporation
233 Spring Street, New York, N.Y. 10013

Printed in the United States of America

To our parents,

Frank and Angela
—V.G.

Charles and Myrtle
—R.W.

Contributors

BRAD A. ALFORD, Department of Psychology, University of Scranton, Scranton, Pennsylvania 18510

HAROLD S. BERNARD, Department of Psychiatry and Group Psychotherapy Program, Psychology Service, New York University Medical Center, New York, New York 10016

LAURA BLACK, State Hospital, Lanark, Scotland ML11 8RP

SIMON H. BUDMAN, Harvard Community Health Plan, Harvard Medical School, and Innovative Training Systems, 24 Loring Street, Newton, Massachusetts 02159

WILLIAM I. COHEN, Child Development Unit, Children's Hospital of Pittsburgh, 3705 Fifth Avenue, Pittsburgh, Pennsylvania 15213

CLEON CORNES, Western Psychiatric Institute and Clinic, 3811 O'Hara Street, Pittsburgh, Pennsylvania 15213

BARRY L. DUNCAN, Dayton Institute for Family Therapy, 65 West Franklin Street, Centerville, Ohio 45459

STUART FINE, Division of Child Psychiatry, University of British Columbia, Vancouver, British Columbia, Canada V5Z 1M9

STUART G. FISHER, Worcester Youth Guidance Center, 275 Belmont Avenue, Worcester, Massachusetts 01609

VINCENT J. GIANNETTI, School of Pharmacy, Duquesne University, Pittsburgh, Pennsylvania 15282

MERVYN GILBERT, Department of Psychology, Vancouver General Hospital, Vancouver, British Columbia, Canada V5Z 1M9

CAROL J. GOLDEN-SCADUTO, Department of Psychiatry, New York University Medical Center and Bellevue Hospital Center, New York, New York 10016

CARLOS J. GONSALVES, Institute for the Study of Psychopolitical Trauma, and Kaiser-Permanente Medical Center, Santa Clara, California 95120

MICHAEL A. GREENWALD, Program in Counseling Psychology, Department of Psychology in Education, University of Pittsburgh, Pittsburgh, Pennsylvania 15213

BERNARD G. GUERNEY, JR., Individual and Family Consultation Center, Department of Human Development and Family Studies, Pennsylvania State University, University Park, Pennsylvania 16802

MICHAEL F. HOYT, Department of Psychiatry, Kaiser-Permanente Medical Center, 27400 Hesperian Boulevard, Hayward, California 94545-4299

DANIEL J. HURLEY, Worcester Youth Guidance Center, 275 Belmont Avenue, Worcester, Massachusetts 01609

JOEL KATZ, Department of Psychology, Toronto Hospital, 200 Elizabeth Street, Toronto, Ontario, Canada M5G 2C4

JOSEPH LOPICCOLO, Department of Psychology, University of Missouri, Columbia, Missouri 65211

LAMBERT MAGUIRE, School of Social Work, University of Pittsburgh, Pittsburgh, Pennsylvania 15260

ALVIN R. MAHRER, School of Psychology, University of Ottawa, Ottawa, Ontario, Canada K1N 6N5

RAYMOND W. NOVACO, School of Social Ecology, University of California at Irvine, Irvine, California 92717

Elam Nunnally, School of Social Welfare, University of Wisconsin–Milwaukee, Milwaukee, Wisconsin 53201

Larry V. Pacoe, Departments of Psychiatry and Psychology, University of Pittsburgh, Pittsburgh, Pennsylvania 15213

Phillip A. Phelps, Child Development Unit, Children's Hospital of Pittsburgh, 3705 Fifth Avenue, Pittsburgh, Pennsylvania 15213

Gregory K. Popchak, Family and Personal Consultation Network, 117 Opal Boulevard, Steubenville, Ohio 43952

Cathryn G. Pridal, Department of Psychology, University of Missouri–Columbia, Columbia, Missouri 65211

Kathleen Reed, Pittsburgh Action Against Rape, 81 South 19th Street, Pittsburgh, Pensylvania 15203

Martine Roberge, School of Psychology, University of Ottawa, Ottawa, Ontario, Canada K1N 6N5

Robert Rosenbaum, California Institute for Integral Studies, 765 Ashbury St., San Francisco, California 94117

Jaime Ross, Institute for the Study of Psychopolitical Trauma, and Miramonte Mental Health Services, Palo Alto, California 94301

Brian F. Shaw, Department of Psychology, Toronto Hospital, 200 Elizabeth Street, Toronto, Ontario, Canada M5G 2C4

Elizabeth Siegel, New Directions, 837 South Fair Oaks, Suite 201, Pasadena, California 91105

Irene Siotis, Department of Psychiatry, McMaster University, Hamilton, Ontario, Canada L8N 3Z5

Maryhelen Snyder, New Mexico Relationship Enhancement Institute, 422 Camino del Bosque, Albuquerque, New Mexico 87114

Karen Subramanian, School of Social Work, University of Southern California, Los Angeles, California 90089-0411

RICHARD A. WELLS, School of Social Work, University of Pittsburgh, Pittsburgh, Pennsylvania 15260

JASON WORCHEL, 1020 East Jefferson Street, Charlottesville, Virginia 21901

Preface

Following the publication of the *Handbook of the Brief Psychotherapies* (Wells & Giannetti, 1990), the editors began to conceptualize the idea of a collection of case studies encompassing a number of the commonly encountered clinical problems that have been treated with such approaches. The *Casebook of the Brief Psychotherapies* is the result. The *Casebook* details clinical interventions with client populations as diverse as substance abusers, torture victims, the physically handicapped and other exceptional groups, and the economically disadvantaged with emotional and behavioral problems, as well as individuals experiencing sexual dysfunction or eating disorders. In addition, topics such as bereavement, depression, anger, and many crucial aspects of marital and family therapy are discussed by eminent clinical practitioners. Although the cases draw heavily upon cognitive behavioral and strategic structural formulations, psychodynamic, interpersonal, and experiential approaches are also included.

The *Casebook* is clinically oriented, with a minimum of theory. Ample case material and commentary allow the reader to experience directly the application of brief therapy to specific client problems. What emerges from this compendium of approaches and problems is a tapestry of action-oriented, problem-solving, skill-building, rational approaches to therapy that balance the client's ability to change with the demands and limits of time. The result is a bringing together of a variety of parsimonious, pragmatic, and *effective* methods for delivering psychotherapeutic services to diverse clients in this era of declining resources and cost-containment pressure on administrators and policymakers in the mental health field.

We agree with Garfield's (1989) summation and forecast:

> Most of the psychotherapy that is conducted in the United States, at least, is brief therapy, and there is no basis for expecting any change in the

> future. There are still opportunities for those individuals who want to enter psychoanalysis or receive some other type of long-term psychotherapy as a means of personal self-exploration in terms of a specific theory of personality. However, such therapy is clearly for the very few who desire such an experience and can afford to pay for it. For the rest of the population, brief psychotherapy remains the treatment of choice. (p. 156)

Thus, in the spirit of Garfield's injunction, the *Casebook* is devoted to clear explication of how time-limited interventions are actually carried out by expert practitioners. In addition, the editors hope that the volume will stimulate further interest and experimentation with brief psychotherapy for the purpose of benefiting clients and contributing to the continued development of efficacious and cost-effective psychotherapeutic services.

REFERENCES

Garfield, S. L. (1989). *The practice of brief psychotherapy.* New York: Pergamon Press.

Wells, R. A., & Giannetti, V. J. (Eds.). (1990). *Handbook of the brief psychotherapies.* New York: Plenum Press.

Contents

I

Introduction

1

Clinical Strategies in Brief Psychotherapy

RICHARD A. WELLS

INTRODUCTION

With the many works now appearing on the various forms of brief psychotherapy, this type of clinical intervention is long past the point where its use in clinical practice needs justification. Almost everyone, it seems, is doing at least some brief therapy, whereas others have adopted it as their major, if not exclusive method. An earlier paper (Wells & Phelps, 1990) reviewed the array of social, economic, ethical, and metaphilosophic factors that have contributed to this trend, and they will not be repeated here.

For the empirically minded in the field, a substantial body of research studies of the outcome of brief psychotherapy has accumulated, and comprehensive reviews of these findings are offered by Koss and Butcher (1986), Budman and Gurman (1988), and Bloom (1992). These reviews support the position that a quite reasonable case can be made for the overall efficacy of brief interventions across a wide range of client problems and populations and contend that in many instances of clinical practice it is the treatment of choice.

Beyond the realm of the scientific, in certain areas of the country some types of brief psychotherapies have assumed an almost cult di-

---

RICHARD A. WELLS • School of Social Work, University of Pittsburgh, Pittsburgh, Pennsylvania 15260.

Casebook of the Brief Psychotherapies, edited by Richard A. Wells and Vincent J. Giannetti. Plenum Press, New York, 1993.

mension with, for example, the blossoming of any number of institutes, foundations, and erstwhile training organizations dedicated to the memory of that most iconoclastic (and irreproducible) of brief therapists, Milton Erickson. Self-acclaimed experts and advocates tour the country offering workshops to new enthusiasts.

Despite these indications of growing acceptance, it is still difficult to accurately ascertain the amount of brief therapy actually conducted within current clinical practice. In a previous review (Wells & Phelps, 1990), brief psychotherapy was estimated to comprise a significant but minority position in the everyday practice of psychotherapy—it was utilized by perhaps 20% to 30% of practitioners in our estimate, based on extrapolations from data available at that time. A recent study by Bolter, Levenson, and Alvarez (1990) of a randomly selected sample of clinical psychologists practicing in California offers some confirmation of this view. They found that 34% of their sample of 550 practitioners favored the brief approaches, in contrast to 54% who favored long-term therapy. There was a small but meaningful group of clinicians—12%—who indicated no preference.

Although justification of its use may no longer be necessary, there is still a need for examination and explication of the clinical parameters of brief psychotherapy. As a prelude to the case studies of brief psychotherapy that will follow in this book, I will attempt to highlight the common factors running across the clinical implementation of a number of forms of brief therapies. My overall purpose will be to identify critical dimensions in the therapeutic interaction between clinician and client that stimulate the significant changes that can arise from brief episodes of therapy.

The 29 case studies appearing in the following 24 chapters of this book will serve as a source of raw material for this analysis as they represent the current clinical work of many brief therapists, drawn from all of the helping professions, practicing in a variety of outpatient clinics, mental health centers, hospitals, and private practice settings across this continent. Although they by no means constitute a representative sample of brief psychotherapy practice—and, indeed, were solicited for inclusion in this volume because of the clinical relevance and vitality of their work—they provide an instructive glimpse of brief therapy as it is actually practiced today and clearly illustrate many of its clinical parameters.

In relation to treatment focus, for instance, the problems experienced by the clients treated in these cases fall largely into three major areas:

1. Difficulties in managing important aspects of social, interpersonal and family relationships, the last including problems with children and adolescents.
2. Emergent or chronic marital dissatisfaction and conflict.
3. Moderate to severe problems with troublesome emotions such as anger, depression, and anxiety.

In consonance with the historical development of brief psychotherapy (Wells & Phelps, 1990), two theoretical frameworks predominate in the case studies. Thus, we find a little more than one-third of the cases based upon principles derived from cognitive or cognitive/behavioral formulations, another third are based on various permutations of strategic/structural family therapy, whereas a distinctly psychodynamic influence is apparent in only a small minority of the interventions.

Critical Dimensions of Brief Psycyhotherapy

In examining the key aspects of therapist and client activity that commonly characterize brief psychotherapy I will look at these factors across three main stages: (1) engagement processes, (2) intervention strategies, and (3) termination procedures. Within an explicitly time-limited context this division is, admittedly, somewhat arbitrary and artificial as, in actual practice, the brief therapist may compress and overlap these phases into the time duration of but a session or two. Despite this, examining the activity of the clinician across these three areas will help to illuminate the structure inherent in what might otherwise appear to be an entirely intuitive process. My contention throughout will be that although one must recognize the artistic elements of any form of psychotherapy, brief therapy is best understood as the deliberate use of a limited number of technical and conceptual principles, applied in a focused and purposeful manner.

Engagement: Teaching the Client about Therapy

Although most brief therapies do not call for a distinct and separate "diagnostic" phase, all recognize that there are a number of important considerations that must be dealt with in the initial contact with the client (or clients, in the case of couple, family, and group interventions).

These are importantly concerned, of course, with identifying and better understanding the problems the client wishes to deal with in treatment but, within this data-gathering context, the therapist moves quickly to create an optimal relationship base for the intervention that will follow (or that, in instances of very brief intervention, is already underway). Even if the client's concerns are not appropriate for brief treatment, the influence base established through an active engagement process can be helpful in connecting the individual to needed services elsewhere. Within this initial phase, a number of clinical strategies are evident:

1. *Accept (and refine) the client's problem statement.* For the most part, brief therapists are quite willing to work on the problems that the client presents in the first meeting and are not particularly concerned about whether this is the "real" problem. This willingness to work on the client's identified problems is both a key characteristic of time-limited intervention and an aspect of brief therapy that has led its critics to accusations of superficiality and simplicity. There is no doubt that brief psychotherapy is highly consumer-oriented—it is the client, the customer, who defines the problem to be worked on, and in most episodes of brief therapy the clinician takes this definition literally and seriously (Bolter et al., 1990). Much of the effectiveness of brief therapy, in my opinion, lies in just this concentrated focus on the concerns of the client, and it is this emphasis, along with the explicit time limits, that account for its markedly lower dropout rates (Sledge et al., 1990).

Such an emphasis, however, does not mean that the client who is vague or scattered in the initial interview will not be assisted, through supportive questioning, in expressing his or her concerns more clearly. This is clearly illustrated in the second case in Hoyt's chapter where he encourages Sue, a depressed and demoralized woman, to identify her desire to be reunited with her husband and children. Nor does it mean that the therapist may not have a different view than the client about what constitutes the most effective way of *solving* a specific problem. Thus, in Snyder and Guerney's description of work with a troubled marital couple who see only separation and divorce ahead of them, the therapist agrees with their description of the painful state of their marriage but offers the powerful structure of Relationship Enhancement training as a way out of their dilemma.

2. *Start working on the problem immediately.* In that most exquisite form of brief therapy, the single-session intervention (Rosenbaum, Hoyt, & Talmon, 1990; Talmon, 1990), the clinician literally has no time to lose. This is most dramatically illustrated in Hoyt's work in an HMO setting with a 67-year-old man who was afraid to walk following a stroke. Meet-

ing his client in the waiting room, Hoyt asks him whether he prefers to walk, or ride in his wheelchair, to his (Hoyt's) office. The man chooses to ride but, a moment or so later, Hoyt persuades him (on the grounds that it is too bulky) to leave the wheelchair at the office door and walk the remaining few feet to a chair. Within the span of a moment or two, the therapist has clearly established that the man *can* walk and that the crux of his problem is his fear of doing so on his own initiative. The remainder of the single-session intervention can then assume a meaningful focus on this key issue.

3. *"Diagnose" through action.* Salvatore Minuchin is reported to have said that "diagnosis is what a family does when I tell them to do something." Hoyt's brilliant use of action in establishing the essential nature of his client's difficulties has already been described in the preceding section. In a similar vein, in his exposition of a single-session intervention with a client concerned with weight control, Rosenbaum speaks of how, from the very beginning of contact, the brief therapist "makes small interventions, monitors the client's response to the intervention, makes adjustments, and intervenes again." In both instances, assessment is not viewed as a static process, or the affixing of a particular diagnostic label on the client, but as the product of a dynamic interaction between therapist and client and, most significantly, has a direct relevance to better understanding of the difficulties the client wishes to resolve.

4. *Educate clients in their role.* A neglected area of psychotherapy research is the work done on the effect of the so-called role-induction interview in eliciting a positive client set toward therapy and, importantly, lowering dropout rates (Heitler, 1976; Orlinsky & Howard, 1978). In this earlier research, clients were given a separate interview that provided factual information on the nature of therapy and explained the expected role of the client but, as a number of the case studies illustrate, similar considerations can be easily incorporated into the engagement process.

For example, in the brief treatment of depression, both cognitive therapy (Shaw et al., Chapter 6) and interpersonal psychotherapy (Cornes, Chapter 4) directly inform their clients about the nature of depression and provide clear information on the expectations and demands that therapy will place on them. In his account of very brief therapy with panic disorder, Alston devotes much of his first session to explaining to his client the nature of the cognitive treatment of anxiety. Similarly, Pacoe and Greenwald (Chapter 9) begin by carefully instructing their highly anxious client about the nature of anxiety and how it can be aroused and mediated by automatic thoughts. It is significant, I believe, that the case studies where this kind of factual information giving particularly stands out are those concerned with treatment of such powerful, pervasive emotions as depression and anxiety where the need to demystify and normalize is especially important.

Finally, in their case study of the brief treatment of vaginismus, Pridal and LoPiccolo (Chapter 22) spend significant portions of the first two sessions explaining the nature of the dysfunction and its treatment. They additionally reinforce these explanations by having the client view a videotape illustrating the entire treatment process. Their approach is particularly consonant, of course, with the metaphilosophy of brief sexual therapy which, since its inception, has always placed a strong emphasis on client education (Masters & Johnson, 1970).

5. *Set up a collaborative relationship with the client.* Alford, in his chapter on the brief treatment of a panic disorder, suggests that the collaborative, empirical relationship of cognitive therapy may well be a model for the client/therapist relationship across all of the brief psychotherapies. Certainly many of the case studies in the following chapters describe direct and open efforts to set up an equalitarian working alliance. It is interesting to note that this spirit of cooperation appears to exist in comfortable conjunction with the directive therapist role that characterizes much of brief psychotherapy. In this regard, both solution focused brief therapy and Guerney's Relationship Enhancement approach to marital conflict tend to characterize the therapist as a *coach*, a term that, in its commonly understood meaning, incorporates both of these qualities of direction and cooperation.

It is also worth noting that the emphasis on collaboration has both philosophical and practical meaning in its application in brief psychotherapy. Ross and Gonsalves's chapter, for example, emphasizes the importance of the survivor of torture being in control of the treatment process, in contrast to the feelings of helplessness and lack of control suffered by such individuals in their experiences with being tortured. This is similar to Subramanian and Siegel's characterization of their group approach with chronic pain patients as involving "a partnership between patient and group leader with the patient taking responsibility for learning, practicing, and incorporating the skills into his/her own life."

INTERVENTION: SETTING THE CLIENT TO WORK

However structured and directive the immediate process of brief therapy may be, it is a predominant belief among brief therapists that the most important changes take place outside the therapy session through the client's own efforts (Bolter et al., 1990). This belief is operationalized through the frequent employment of reality-based tasks, as well as by the positive pressures exerted by the setting of a time limit. Both of these strategies implicitly convey to clients that they themselves have the responsibility—and the capability—of dealing with their problems.

Once engaged in brief psychotherapy, clients are typically set to work upon their problems in an active and purposeful way. Indeed, conveying this expectation of direct and immediate activity on the client's part is an essential aspect of the engagement process itself and, in this respect, it is difficult to separate engagement from intervention. Allowing, therefore, for the fact that in the often-rapid process of brief therapy the stages of engagement and intervention may significantly overlap, the case studies suggest and illustrate a number of guidelines for promoting and directing the client's problem-solving and solution-seeking activities.

1. *Persistently present alternative views of reality.* As Jerome Frank (Frank & Frank, 1991) has long pointed out, troubled people are demoralized and, consequently, negative in their view of their world. The cognitive therapy of Aaron Beck and his associates (1979) has emphasized a similar skewing of the assumptive world. Thus, it becomes a primary responsibility of the therapist, and a key function of therapy, to provide clients with what will be more functional beliefs and attitudes toward themselves and their world. Working from a constructivist viewpoint that posits that meaning and reality are constructed rather than discovered, Duncan, in Chapter 21, calls these "meaning revision opportunities" and utilizes both conjoint and individual sessions to alter the distressed marital couple's views of each other and of their relationship.

On the other hand, solution focused brief therapy, described by Nunnally in Chapter 18, involves a radically different therapeutic process in which the client is directed to examine past, present, and future instances in which the problem *did not* occur, and is encouraged to expand on and strengthen these. The very notion of concentrating solely on solutions (rather than the conventional therapeutic procedure of examining problems) is, in itself, a tour de force of positive reframing.

Finally, in Popchak and Wells's description of family intervention with a low-SES family, perhaps the major theme of the intervention was the therapist's consistent presentation of a more positive viewpoint through the persistent use of reframing. This was especially important with a disadvantaged family in which the key members saw themselves as powerless and out of control, but such a strategy has profound implications for many of our distressed clients, whatever their socioeconomic status.

2. *Rearrange or remove obstacles through task assignments.* In many instances, the main result of the client's own problem-solving efforts has been to create an even more unworkable situation. This is particularly evident in Cohen and Reed's case where the family's efforts to have the elderly Mrs. A. live at home with her husband resulted only in acrimonious disputes and her being returned to the nursing home. Certainly these difficulties stemmed from Mrs. A.'s belief that her food was being poisoned, but neither medication nor rational disputing seemed likely to change her viewpoint. Cohen and Reed deftly played around this issue by, first, removing the oversolicitious family members from the situation and, second, restructuring the couple's living arrangements so that Mrs. A. was placed in sole charge of ordering and preparing her own food. One can regard these therapeutic strategies as ignoring a "pathological" belief or, more profoundly, as a way of empowering an elderly person to lead a more satisfying life, whatever the nature or accuracy of her or his beliefs.

3. *Challenge the client from a novel perspective.* There are times when the therapist must find a way of intensifying the impact of a particular experience, or a means of detouring around client reluctance to change. In his chapter on HMO therapy, Hoyt does this most dramatically when he throws himself on the floor in front of his elderly patient and asks the patient to coach him in how to get up after having fallen. In my own practice I have used a somewhat less dramatic variant of the same device:

> Mr. B., a 55-year-old, working-class man, rather dour and nonverbal in manner, was referred for stress-management training after suffering two heart attacks. I followed the usual procedure of guiding him through a series of relaxation exercises but, after a session or two, it was obvious that he was only making the most minimal gains in tension reduction, even in the office setting. Rather than trying to explore his apparent "resistance," I praised his quickness at learning and suggested that it was now time for *him* to lead both of us through the relaxation exercises. In this, and a subsequent session, Mr. B. did a credible job of leading the exercise and, for his own part, made quite satisfactory progress in developing relaxation skills.

In both Hoyt's case and my own example, the issue might have been characterized as one of client resistance, but the brief therapist doesn't have the luxury of time necessary to explore this in any depth, nor can the therapist simply "wait out" the block, as one can do in open-ended therapy. In both instances, control was placed in the patient's hands, clearly demonstrating his competence, and making him change his own responsibility.

Perhaps one of the most intriguing (and puzzling) of the case studies presented in this volume is Budman and Hoyt's work with a young man with a socially distressing tic. Their intervention, in effect, called for him to adopt a "blemish," other than the one being expressed through his current tic, that would be less obvious and intrusive. They base their intervention on theoretical considerations drawn from Control Mastery theory (Engel & Ferguson, 1990; Weiss & Sampson, 1986), but it is interesting to note that there is a distinct resemblance between their intervention and the cognitive behavioral intervention described by Azrin and Nunn (1973) in their work with over 400 individuals suffering from a variety of tics and habits. Along with stress-management training, the latter therapists coached their clients in the use of a "competing" gesture that was designed to substitute for the tic in a less visible and distracting manner. Although Budman and Hoyt's intervention is quite brief (six sessions), Azrin and Nunn's work (1973) was even briefer, with most of their clients being seen for only a single session.

4. *Provide the simplest, most immediate intervention.* There are a number of instances, in the chapters that follow, where a brief, focused treatment was all that was needed to resolve seemingly complex difficulties—the single-session cases described by Rosenbaum, or Hoyt, are clear examples of this kind of therapeutic impact. Cohen and Reed offer yet another example.

In the cases noted above the therapist's interventions were conducted within the extremely brief time durations of one or two sessions, and certainly simplicity was of the essence. Yet although a number of the case studies based on a cognitive/behavioral framework—Alford's chapter, for example, or the chapters by Pacoe and Greenwald, and Shaw and his colleagues—involve somewhat greater treatment durations, they still center around an essentially simple idea. Their major theoretical theme that such troublesome emotions as depression or anxiety are stimulated and maintained by the client's faulty perception and interpretation of her or his interpersonal world has proven to be of immense clinical utility but cannot be regarded as an especially complicated notion. Most clients grasp it readily, although they may well need careful training in its application.

Bloom (1981), in his seminal writing on single-session intervention, sums up most succinctly:

> I try not to do too much. If I can find just one issue, just one idea, just a teaspoonful, that is useful to the client, the intervention can be a successful one. . . . My personal rule of thumb is that if I cannot express a fundamental

> issue of concern to the client in ten words—ten *short* words—or less, I do not understand the issue. (pp. 187–188, italics in original)

5. *Look for opportunities to teach life skills.* Yet another simple explanation for client difficulty is that important social skills are either deficient or poorly utilized. This is not a new idea by any means nor one that derives only from a behavioral perspective. A neglected article by Ian Stevenson (1959), a psychodynamically oriented psychiatrist, described his focus on helping his patients directly deal with problems in assertion, affiliation, and communication. A similar direct emphasis on the development or refinement of needed social skills appears in case after case in the following chapters.

Thus, training in assertive skills is utilized in several case studies. For example, it is a component in the package of skills taught in Subramanian and Siegel's (Chapter 23) short-term group training with chronic pain patients. They view it as providing the patient with a more effective way of managing interpersonal and social relationships that may be circumscribed by the effects of chronic pain. Similarly, Pacoe and Greenwald, in the second phase of their work with a highly anxious client, coach him in assertive skills. Their focus in this stage of treatment is on their client's self-critical attitudes, and need to please other people, and the development of assertive skills are designed to give him an alternative to dealing with others only through compliance.

In at least two of the chapters—Popchak and Wells's work with a low-SES family, and Black and Novaco's description of anger-control training with a mentally retarded man—explicit emphasis is placed on teaching problem-solving skills. Although Black and Novaco's case is strongly influenced by a cognitive behavioral framework, whereas the Popchak and Wells chapter is predominantly strategic/structural family therapy, in either instance the structured problem solving is easily integrated into the approach and usefully supplements the other interventions.

Finally, training in relaxation skills appears in both Subramanian and Siegel's short-term group treatment of chronic pain patients as well as in the chapter describing Ross and Gonsalves's work with exiled survivors of torture. In both instances, instructing clients in the coping skills of relaxation empowers them in self-managing the emotional and physical sequelae of their difficulties.

6. *Work flexibly across modalities.* For too long, the field of psychotherapy has been hampered by not only an unthinking adherence to theoretical frameworks but by an equally unreflective utilization of the individual, group, and family modalities. Therapists tend to develop a favored way of working with their clients and stick to this modality

tenaciously. Yet although there is much to be said for seeing troubled marital couples in conjoint interviews, for example, or interviewing parents and children together, these are not the only ways of stimulating needed change in family relationships (Szapocznik et al., 1990). Similarly, individual and group modalities have been too often seen as mutually exclusive, if not directly competitive.

Golden-Scaduto and Bernard's chapter on short-term group intervention with a herpes patient is a clear illustration of the power inherent in combining modalities. In this instance, the group treatment not only offered a supportive and educative focus but allowed for the raising of social norms (related, of course, to the patient's infecting her sexual partners) in a way that individual therapy could not. In addition, they found that powerful transference feelings were aroused in the interplay between the two modalities—the individual therapist also colead the short-term group—that were highly significant material in the continuing long-term therapy.

Duncan, on the other hand, combines conjoint and individual sessions in working with marital couples in a manner that is reminiscent in certain of his strategies with the One-Person Family therapy methodology pioneered by Jose Szapocznik and his colleagues at the Spanish Family Guidance Clinic in Miami (Szapocznik et al., 1990). Thus, in Duncan's work, conjoint interviews are followed by individual sessions in which the therapeutic alliance is strengthened and, most importantly, tasks are devised and assigned that will impact upon the relationship difficulties the couple are experiencing.

Termination: Releasing the Client

Knowing when—and how—to stop treatment is one of the most important but least discussed aspects of brief psychotherapy. Most brief therapists explicitly set a specific time limit for treatment during the initial interview and, at the least, as Sledge and his colleagues (1990) determined, this has a significant effect in reducing premature dropout. They found a 32% dropout in time-specific brief therapy, in contrast to 61% to 67% dropout when no time limits were given. This research underscores the importance of the time limit, and the case studies highlight a number of clinical guidelines for managing the termination stage of the brief treatment process.

1. *Let clients know they can return for further help.* Several of the chapters in this volume describe cases in which the intervention was com-

plete within a single helping episode, yet an increasingly persuasive viewpoint is one that conceptualizes short-term treatment as (at least potentially) intermittent. In this model, the relationship between client and therapist is assumed to be a continuing one, over time, although actual face-to-face contact is intermittent, and each episode of therapy has distinct time boundaries.

From this perspective, a given client problem is seen as responsive to a suitable brief intervention, but the individual is also encouraged to return at a later time if the difficulty needs further work, or if a new problem has arisen. This is clearly illustrated in Phelps's description of his work with the parents of an oppositional child. There is no doubt that Phelps's first intervention with the Boston family, in which he trained the parents in behavioral child management, was both appropriate and genuinely helpful. However, a year later, changed family circumstances brought about their return for another time-limited intervention. It is interesting to note that once a few sessions of family therapy had resolved the systemic imbalance, the parents were able to reinstitute the behavioral child management strategies that had previously been successful.

2. *Avoid attractive detours that can prolong therapy.* This guideline was one of the key facets of very brief intervention identified by Bernard Bloom (1981) in his work on single-session intervention. As he points out, the prolonging of therapy duration can be as much a product of therapist curiosity as a question of client need:

> There are numerous occasions in every intervention when I find myself wishing I could explore some little phrase for just a few minutes, but such diversions have nearly always turned out to be technical errors. . . . I try to narrow the domain of inquiry in proportion to what I am learning about the client, and I do not single out a particular issue or conflict to concentrate on until I have every reason to believe it is an appropriate target for investigation and clarification. (Bloom, 1981, p. 189)

It is difficult to point out examples of this aspect of brief intervention in the case studies as most simply don't report on what they didn't do. However, the issue was an acute one for Phelps in his work with the Boston family and their oppositional youngster, and he speaks of his discomfort toward the end of the family intervention about whether further work was needed on the parent's marital issues.

3. *Connect people to needed resources.* A good way of ending therapy is to make the therapist unnecessary. This can be most readily accomplished by encouraging the client, following a suitable brief intervention, to make fuller use of the formal and informal sources of help that are available within his or her natural environment. From this perspec-

tive, the time-limited work of the brief therapist can be seen as directed toward assisting the client in moving past (or around) a troublesome impasse and is successful when this has been accomplished.

In this regard, although Hoyt's immediate work was largely complete within a single session—his 67-year-old client had resumed walking by the time of the follow-up interview—Hoyt used this positive change to refer his client to an older adult's therapy group to deal with other life issues facing him. Both Black and Novaco, after training their client in anger-control skills, and Cohen and Reed, following their family intervention, arranged for community-based agencies to monitor the client's continued progress. In all of these instances, it should be noted, the brief therapy made these further connections possible (and meaningful), but the brief therapists limited their therapeutic ambitions to a single, critical issue.

4. *Let go but in a positive way.* In a much earlier commentary on Milton Erickson's work, Haley (1969) spoke of Erickson's ability to allow his patients to find their own solutions and his willingness to release the patient after a brief episode of help. Similarly, working in the interpersonal framework, Cornes (Chapter 4) finds his patient expressing concern in the final interview about some unresolved but minor areas, although her depression is much relieved. He responds to this by suggesting that she could continue to work on some of these issues on her own in the future. This firm ending avoids a needless prolonging of therapy but implicitly conveys the therapist's confidence in the patient's capability to manage her own life. Phelps's discussion of ending brief therapy sums up this viewpoint when he says that "there is always unfinished business when people leave therapy, and it can be difficult to let go of the felt responsibility to make it all better."

A common and helpful device in this final stage of brief therapy lies in the use of follow-up interviews (Wells, 1982). In two of the chapters describing single-session intervention, both Hoyt and Rosenbaum arrange for follow-up sessions as a way of positively releasing their clients but also maintaining a meaningful contact that will allow for further intervention, if needed.

Conclusion: Is Brief Therapy Really Brief?

This introductory chapter has looked at a wide variety of brief psychotherapy cases, conducted by practitioners expert in this mode of intervention, and used their work to draw out a number of the key strategies employed in time-limited therapy. It may now seem odd to question whether brief therapy is really brief, and the literal (and accurate) response is *that it is relatively short in duration of therapist/client contact, sometimes radically so.* The great majority of the cases described in this volume were in the 8- to 12-session range, a very few were longer, whereas there were eight cases involving 1 to 6 sessions of therapeutic contact.

However, although each instance of brief therapy can be viewed, in its time-limited and action-oriented focus, as complete in itself, this is by no means the whole picture. Beyond the specific strategies that I have identified, we must keep in mind that therapy does not occur in an interpersonal or social vacuum. This is especially so in brief psychotherapy where the emphasis, albeit within explicit time boundaries, is on the client's ongoing and current coping with his or her immediate life problems. Therapists and their clients together create an interpersonal context that can have meaning beyond the time duration of their actual work together. In addition, with the emphasis in many instances of brief therapy on task assignments involving the client's current family and social relationships, direct changes are instigated that can continue to reverberate within the client's life.

In a similar vein, therapists often practice within sponsoring agencies and institutions that can provide supporting services that augment and amplify the changes stimulated by a specific episode of brief intervention. Whether functioning within an agency setting or in private practice, the effective therapist must be continually aware of the framework of helping resources available from the client's family, friends, and social networks. This emphasis is quite explicit, of course, in Maguire's chapter on brief social support system intervention but appears implicitly in many of the other chapters. Thus, the effective brief practitioner will not regard a particular therapeutic episode as an isolated happening, or even a truly time-limited event, but as occurring within one or all of these contexts, and as a means of stimulating and encouraging clients to more fully use the entire fabric of personal, interpersonal, and social resources available to them.

REFERENCES

Azrin, N. J., & Nunn, R. G. (1973). Habit reversal: A method of eliminating nervous habits and tics. *Behavior Research and Therapy, 11,* 619–628.

Beck, A. T., Rush, A. J., Shaw, B. F., & Emergy, G. (1979). *Cognitive therapy of depression.* New York: Guilford.

Bloom, B. L. (1981). Focused single-session therapy: Initial development and evaluation. In S. H. Budman (Ed.), *Forms of brief therapy* (pp. 167–218). New York: Guilford.

Bloom, B. L. (1992). *Planned short-term psychotherapy: A clinical handbook.* Boston: Allyn and Bacon.

Bolter, K., Levenson, H., & Alvarez, W. (1990). Differences in values between short-term and long-term therapists. *Professional Psychology, 21,* 285–290.

Budman, S. H., & Gurman, A. S. (1988). *The practice of brief therapy.* New York: Guilford.

Engel, L., & Ferguson, T. (1990). *Imaginary crimes.* Boston: Houghton Mifflin.

Frank, J., & Frank, J. (1991). *Persuasion and healing* (3rd ed.). Baltimore, MD: Johns Hopkins University Press.

Haley, J. (Ed.). (1969). *Advanced techniques of hypnosis and psychotherapy: Selected papers of Milton F. Erickson, M.D.* New York: Grune & Stratton.

Heitler, J. B. (1976). Preparatory techniques in initiating expressive psychotherapy with lower-class, unsophisticated patients. *Psychological Bulletin, 83,* 339–352.

Koss, M. P., & Butcher, J. N. (1986). Research in brief and crisis-oriented therapy. In S. L. Garfield & A. E. Bergin (Eds.), *Handbook of psychotherapy and behavior change* (3rd ed., pp. 627–670). New York: Wiley.

Masters, W. H., & Johnson, V. E. (1970). *Human sexual inadequacy.* Boston: Little, Brown.

Orlinsky, D. E., & Howard, K. I. (1978). The relationship of process to outcome in psychotherapy. In S. L. Garfield & A. E. Bergin (Eds.), *Handbook of psychotherapy and behavior change* (2nd ed., pp. 283–329). New York: Wiley.

Rosenbaum, R., Hoyt, M. F., & Talmon, M. (1990). The challenge of single-session therapies: Creating pivotal moments. In R. A. Wells & V. J. Giannetti (Eds.), *Handbook of the brief psychotherapies* (pp. 165–189). New York: Plenum Press.

Sledge, W. H., Moras, K., Hartley, D., & Levine, M. (1990). Effect of time-limited therapy on patient dropout rates. *American Journal of Psychiatry, 147,* 1341–1347.

Stevenson, I. (1959). Direct instigation of behavioral changes in psychotherapy. *Archives of General Psychiatry, 61,* 99–117.

Szapocznik, J., Kurtines, W. M., Perez-Vidal, A., Hervis, O. E., & Foote, F. H. (1990). One person family therapy. In R. A. Wells & V. J. Giannetti (Eds.), *Handbook of the brief psychotherapies* (pp. 493–510). New York: Plenum Press.

Talmon, M. (1990). *Single-session therapy.* San Francisco: Jossey-Bass.

Weiss, J., & Sampson, H. (1986). *The psychoanalytic process.* New York: Guilford.

Wells, R. A. (1982). *Planned short-term treatment.* New York: Free Press.

Wells, R. A., & Phelps, P. A. (1990). The brief psychotherapies: A selective overview. In R. A. Wells & V. J. Giannetti (Eds.), *Handbook of the brief psychotherapies* (pp. 3–26). New York: Plenum Press.

II

Individual Intervention

2

Active Interventions in Brief Therapy and Control Mastery Theory

A Case Study

SIMON H. BUDMAN AND MICHAEL F. HOYT

INTRODUCTION

Control Mastery Theory (Engel & Ferguson, 1990; Weiss & Sampson, 1986) is a recent modification of more traditional psychoanalytic thinking. There are a number of technical and theoretical ways in which the Control Mastery model differs from classical Freudian thinking. Three important features of the Control Mastery model are particularly relevant to this case. First is the idea that people do not just act in their own self-interest but often act in ways that are prosocial and altruistic, sometimes doing harm to themselves, in an attempt to deal with guilt over what Engel and Ferguson (1990) called "imaginary crimes." Second is the idea that patients have an unconscious "plan" regarding what they need to grow and deal with their problems. Therapeutic interventions will be useful if they are "proplan" and will be ineffective or even coun-

SIMON H. BUDMAN • Harvard Community Health Plan, Harvard Medical School, and Innovative Training Systems, 24 Loring Street, Newton, Massachusetts 02159. MICHAEL F. HOYT • Department of Psychiatry, Kaiser-Permanente Medical Center, 27400 Hesperian Boulevard, Hayward, California 94545-4299.

Casebook of the Brief Psychotherapies, edited by Richard A. Wells and Vincent J. Giannetti. Plenum Press, New York, 1993.

terproductive if they run counter to the patient's plan. Third is the idea of "passing the test," the notion that patients will create situations in therapy to see if the therapist will retraumatize them or will instead provide a safe and salutary response different from that which they experienced earlier in their lives.

Although Control Mastery conceptualizations have been utilized to understand various psychoanalytic cases (e.g., Weiss, 1990) and have been applied to one case that might be described as cognitive/behavioral (Persons et al., 1991), there are no published reports of Control Mastery thinking being used in treatments that are more eclectic or strategic (Ericksonian) in nature. This chapter is an attempt to do just that. The man who is described in this case was treated by the senior author (S. H. B.). The overall theoretical model that is used is the Interpersonal-Developmental-Existential (I-D-E) brief treatment model developed by Budman and Gurman (1988). This model subsumes a broad array of therapeutic possibilities as it identifies and integrates answers to the question, "Why now does the patient seek therapy?" Elements of Control Mastery Theory have recently been incorporated into the I-D-E model, even though this approach is far from analytic in nature (Budman & Gurman, 1992). In the case to be described, Control Mastery concepts proved to be critical in gaining a clearer understanding of the patient and thereby developing a useful intervention strategy.

THE CASE

Tom, a 30-year-old medical resident, was referred by his primary-care physician for hypnotherapy. He had suffered for the past 8 years with an unusual tic. Between 60 and 80 times per minute, throughout the day, Tom would make a strange clicking sound in the back of his throat. It was loud enough to be quite distracting to those with whom he interacted. Still in his residency, Tom's supervisors had urged him to get some type of help for this problem before he completed his training.

Tom had undergone two short courses of nonspecific, insight-oriented psychotherapy. These treatments had no discernable impact upon his symptom. He entered therapy with the focal goal of ridding himself of his tic.

The I-D-E model recommends that when a patient is primarily seeking symptomatic improvement the focus for the treatment should be the symptom itself (Budman & Gurman, 1988). It may certainly be the case that the symptom is simply a "cover-up" for another underlying issue. However, it has been our experience that for patients who are seeking symptomatic amelioration, when the therapist ignores or bypasses these issues in favor of an "underlying" problem, the patient feels that he or she is not being heard, and a cycle of frustration and disappointment often ensues. After the symptom is addressed, other issues or concerns may surface, but first taking the symptom seriously and trying to address it is critical.

The Treatment

Tom was the first of three children. He had a younger brother who was morbidly obese, being 5'3" tall and weighing more than 350 pounds! (Tom himself was a muscular man, about 6' tall.) He also had a younger sister who was born with severe brain damage. This sister had spent much of her life in an institution, near the city where Tom's parents lived. Tom described his parents as "very unhappily married." They would have left one another long ago, if they were not "both too frightened to do so." Tom's mother was described as feeling great disgust for both of her younger children.

Tom perceived his mother as a rather controlling and dominant woman, while his father was a "wimp," who was unable to "stand up" to his mother. His mother had also been quite controlling toward Tom in a variety of ways. He felt that both of his parents were quite depressed and unable to function very well within the family, although they both had high-level and responsible professional positions.

In initiating the therapy, the therapist began by taking a direct hypnotic approach (Hammond, 1990). The patient was hypnotized and offered a suggestion for relaxation, since he had reported that anxiety exacerbated the symptom. An audiotape was made that described a relaxing scene. It was requested that Tom use the tape twice each day for 15 minutes at a time.

Upon returning for his next session, 2 weeks later, Tom reported that although he had had some initial, minor improvement, the symptom was now about as bad as it had ever been, and additional use of the hypnotic tape was proving fruitless. We decided to approach the problem using a different tact. This time, Tom was told that the problem could be understood as relating to his need to "discharge the tension, sadness, and pain that you feel about your family situation." (He had indicated that even thinking about his family problems made him feel very depressed and upset.) He was also told that if he could find a time early in the day and/or late in the evening to discharge these sad feelings, he could possibly feel better during the rest of the day. In taking this paradoxical approach, it was hoped that Tom would produce the symptom and thereby gain control over it.

This approach seemed also to lead to little gain for Tom. After using this technique for several weeks without benefit, it was discontinued.

At this point, the therapist began to think more about Tom's problem in Control Mastery terms. If his sibs were so "defective," perhaps he felt a sense of survivor guilt and responsibility that he had been able to do as well as he had. The possibility was posed to him that the reason for his symptom was that he needed a way to himself feel "blemished and defective, like your siblings."

Tom's response to this interpretation was extremely positive. He indicated that he did have a sense of being "the only hope in the family" and at the same time felt that it was merely a "trick of fate" that he was not more severely impaired. It was suggested to him that since his symptom served such a useful purpose, it would be important for him to maintain some type of blemish, although different from the current one. Several possible blemishes (e.g., shaving a small section of one of his eyebrows, drawing a little scar on his face, and so on) were suggested to him, and he was asked to think about what it was that he would like to use as a flaw.

After the session, the therapist mailed him the following letter (for an extensive discussion of the use of letter writing in brief psychotherapy, see White and Epston [1990]):

> Dear Tom:
>
> I hope that you found our last meeting helpful to you. It became very clear to me at that time that your tic represents a "blemish." You have (fortunately) been spared some of the problems which your brother and sister seem to have. A solution has been to find a way to blemish yourself.
>
> I hope that you are thinking about other possible defects which may be used as substitutes for or alternating with the current one.

When Tom returned the next session, he excitedly reported that he had found the perfect blemish. Several days after our session, he had purchased the ugliest eyeglass frames (with clear, nonprescription lenses) he could find. Since the time that he had first worn these glasses, 3 weeks before, his symptom had disappeared.

Tom displayed the glasses and wore them for the remainder of the session. The therapist indicated to Tom that it was likely that he could, at some point, have a relapse. If this were to occur, he was instructed to obtain band-aids and to wear the glasses with several band-aids wrapped around the bridge. He found this suggestion quite amusing and assured the therapist that he would follow these were the symptom to return.

Follow Up

Six months after the treatment, Tom remains completely free of his tic. He feels that the treatment was tremendously useful to him. This is the first time in 8 years that he has had any extended (more than several hours) period of being without his symptom. Whenever he is feeling tense, he wears his glasses and feels that this has worked to prevent any reoccurrence. He had one brief and minor relapse several months after the symptom was resolved. This took place during a period in which his sister had to be hospitalized because of a severe deterioration in her condition. He had followed the therapist's advice regarding relapse and wrapped the bridge of his glasses in band-aids. This method served to temporarily increase Tom's own "blemish" and the symptom had disappeared.

Discussion

Tom was successfully treated for a severe and chronic tic, in six sessions (most were half-hours) over a 12-week period. He has the option to meet with the therapist, as needed, in the future.

The turning point in the therapy seemed to come when the therapist understood the symptom as the patient's way of expressing and expiating his guilt about and concern for his siblings. Tom was then able to himself devise a useful substitute symptom and to rid himself of the debilitating tic that had plagued him for many years.

It is hard to identify for certain the most important element of this therapy. Was it the interpretation of the guilt? Would he have overcome the problem with only this interpretation and without the task of looking for another substitute? Did requiring a proplan *action* potentiate insight? Was there some other element of the relationship between him and the therapist that lead to the change? Perhaps the therapist's sticking with him, even after his "failure" to improve, was central since this would run counter to his parent's "giving up on" his sibs.

In any case, this is a case where a strategic (Ericksonian) symptom-oriented technique was applied while at the same time Control Mastery Theory helped the therapist in clarifying and contextualizing the meaning of the specific method and technique to be used. An accurate case formulation, one that helps tailor interventions to the psychology of the particular patient, may be key to therapeutic effectiveness (Persons et al., 1992; Silberschatz, Fretter, & Curtis, 1986).

Rather than viewing these treatment models as inherently in opposition to one another (Haley, 1989) or eschewing the use of any theoretical models at all when taking a solution-oriented approach (O'Hanlon & Weiner-Davis, 1989), it may be that much cross-pollination is possible when both psychoanalytic and strategic or Ericksonian approaches are applied together.

REFERENCES

Budman, S. H., & Gurman, A. S. (1988). *Theory and practice of brief therapy.* New York: Guilford Press.

Budman, S. H., & Gurman, A. S. (1992). A time-sensitive model of brief therapy: The I-D-E approach. In S. H. Budman, M. F. Hoyt, & S. Friedman (Eds.), *The first session of brief therapy: A book of cases* (pp. 111–134). New York: Guilford Press.

Engel, L., & Ferguson, T. (1990). *Imaginary crimes.* Boston: Houghton Mifflin Company.

Haley, J. (1990). Why not long-term therapy? In J. K. Zeig & S. G. Gilligan (Eds.), *Brief therapy: Myths, methods and metaphors* (pp. 3–17). New York: Brunner/Mazel.

Hammond, D. C. (1990). *Handbook of hypnotic suggestions and metaphors.* New York: W. W. Norton.

O'Hanlon, W. H., & Weiner-Davis, M. (1989). *In search of solutions: A new direction in psychotherapy.* New York: W. W. Norton.

Persons, J. B., Curtis, J. T., & Silberschatz, G. (1991). Psychodynamic and cognitive-behavioral formulations of a single case. *Psychotherapy, 28,* 608–617.

Silberschatz, G., Fretter, P. B., & Curtis, J. T. (1986). How do interpretations influence the process of psychotherapy? *Journal of Consulting and Clinical Psychology, 54,* 646–652.

Weiss, J. (1990). Unconscious mental functioning. *Scientific American,* 103–109.

Weiss, J., & Sampson, H. (1986). *The psychoanalytic process.* New York: Guilford Press.

White, M., & Epston, D. (1990). *Narrative means to therapeutic ends.* New York: Norton.

3

Brief Treatment of a Torture Survivor

JAIME ROSS AND CARLOS J. GONSALVES

INTRODUCTION

Survivors of massive trauma such as torture require a comprehensive form of psychotherapy. The assault of torture upon individuals and their familial and social systems is profound. Therefore, therapeutic interventions need to address individual, couple, and family issues, stressing the connection between the traumatic experience and the sociopolitical environment in which it occurred (Fischman & Ross, 1990; Gonsalves, Torres, Fischman, Ross, & Vargas, in press). Furthermore, the psychological and physical sequelae of torture are usually compounded by the multiple difficulties associated with exile and acculturation (Gonsalves, 1990). Accordingly, treatment requires a flexible approach on the part of the clinician, as well as the use of a wide variety of techniques to address the multiple symptoms that survivors present.

The multiple needs of this patient population stand in sharp contrast with the shrinking availability of health care resources, making shorter forms of treatment necessary. However, many of the standard criteria for inclusion in brief therapy cannot be applied to torture sur-

---

JAIME ROSS • Institute for the Study of Psychopolitical Trauma, P.O. Box 959, Palo Alto, California. 94301, and Miramonte Mental Health Services, Palo Alto, California 94301. Carlos J. Gonsalves • Institute for the Study of Psychopolitical Trauma, and Kaiser-Permanente Medical Center, Santa Clara, California 95120.

Casebook of the Brief Psychotherapies, edited by Richard A. Wells and Vincent J. Giannetti. Plenum Press, New York, 1993.

vivors. Other authors (e.g., Ortmann, Genefke, Jakobsen, & Lunde, 1987; Somnier & Genefke, 1986) have pointed out the limitations of conventional therapeutic procedures in the treatment of survivors of this form of trauma.

The work presented here describes an attempt to do brief therapy with an adult torture survivor from Guatemala.[1] The client's torture experiences were preceded by childhood trauma of emotional and physical abuse and aggravated by the losses associated with exile. The main therapeutic goal was to ameliorate the client's most distressing symptoms and not to promote characterologic change. Significant progress was observed in several major symptoms during the 15-session duration of the treatment.

The treatment approach selected for this client is Wolberg's eclectic short-term psychotherapy (1980). This author's methodology is characterized by its use of various modalities of treatment, ranging from behavior therapy techniques to dream analysis. Wolberg emphasizes the importance of symptom removal through techniques adjusted to the needs of the individual patient, as well as enhancing the client's self-observation and self-understanding.

CASE IDENTIFICATION AND PRESENTING COMPLAINTS

The client, Nicolás, is a 42-year-old married Latino man, unemployed, and living with his wife (the family's sole breadwinner) and their only child, a 13-year-old boy. He was referred for treatment by the director of a halfway house in the San Francisco Bay Area. Nicolás stayed in that program for 2 weeks after being hospitalized due to suicidal ideation.

Eight months earlier, in September 1990, Nicolás had arrived in the Bay Area to reunite with his family. He had lived in France for 6 years, where he attended a special treatment program for refugees. During his stay in France, he had thoughts of killing himself and made one suicide attempt. Shortly after relocating to the Bay Area, he again experienced suicidal ideation but did not act on it. At the time of referral he was not considered a suicide risk.

Nicolás was described as being highly motivated for treatment and having a solid educational background. He had been placed on a waiting

[1]Some identifying information has been changed in order to protect the identity of the client.

list and, when offered the opportunity of being treated in his own native language by a male Latino therapist, he readily agreed.

Nicolás's chief presenting complaint was dissatisfaction with his wife. He felt demeaned because he was unemployed and, as a result, financially dependent on her. He admitted also to feelings of loneliness and isolation as well as anxiety and depression. He had a history of alcohol abuse dating back to age 20, although he minimized its severity during the assessment.

Background Information

Nicolás and his wife had originally come to the Bay Area 13 years ago from Guatemala. He was seeking refuge from political persecution and torture. Shortly before their son was born, Nicolás was deported back to his homeland because he had entered the United States illegally. Once in Guatemala, he was again imprisoned for 3 months, unbeknownst to his wife. He was tortured for the first 2 weeks of his detention and released after 10 more weeks in a common jail. He then fled to Costa Rica, where he lived for 3 months. In spite of supportive offers from newly encountered friends, he decided to move to France, attracted by a special assistance program for torture survivors and exiles.

Throughout the years of separation from his wife and son, the little contact he made was directed mostly to the latter. He talked to his wife only occasionally to seek financial support. Finally, Nicolás abruptly decided to move to the San Francisco Bay Area so he could live with his son.

Family of Origin

Nicolás was born in Guatemala, the third child in a family of six siblings. His parents' first child, a son, died at the age of 2 months. The client described his mother as a harsh and authoritarian person who, together with her own father, despised her husband and often abused her only son, physically and emotionally. He was unable to explain why she singled him out for that kind of treatment. Nicolás's father, on the other hand, was more supportive but would remain passive even while his wife insulted him or physically abused their son. In spite of his father's passivity, Nicolás remembers him with fondness and as someone who provided some respite from mother's harshness.

Two events from his childhood stand out as particularly significant for him. They both happened around age 10 or 11 and involved intense humiliation from being beaten by his mother in front of other people.

During these late childhood years, while attending a community center, Nicolás had developed strong ties to a social worker who became a loving maternal figure for him. Just as he began to feel that he was her favorite pupil, she was captured, tortured, and killed by the army. This was the first shock in a long chain of critical losses that the client has suffered throughout the years.

At age 18, Nicolás became involved in political activities in his native country. He combined social action with his work as an elementary-school teacher by providing assistance for peasants, an activity for which he was considered subversive.

Detention and Torture

Shortly after starting his teaching career and political involvement, he was caught in possession of political leaflets and incarcerated for a year. During this and other incommunicado detentions, he was subjected to several forms of torture. While naked and blindfolded, electric shocks were applied to sensitive parts of the body, such as gums and genitals; his head was forced under water until he nearly asphyxiated; he was subjected to prolonged and at times daily beatings, including what his torturers mockingly called the "airplane." This consisted of two soldiers grabbing the bound prisoner by his hands and feet in a hammocklike fashion, balancing him sideways several times before thrusting him several feet into the air. Psychological torture included sham executions, threats, verbal abuse, and humiliations. None of his incarcerations was preceded by a trial. He was often deprived of food and water while locked in cold and humid cells, sometimes in solitary confinement and other times in overcrowded cells where space and newspaper "blankets" became precious commodities.

All of his incarcerations started in a detention center where torture was applied daily, for up to 4 months in the case of his longest detention. These were followed, without any sentencing, by transfers to common prisons, where torture was discontinued.

Upon his release, Nicolás resumed his political involvement. In order to alleviate the intense aftereffects of torture, he began using alcohol occasionally. Two years later, he was imprisoned again and confined to an overcrowded jail. Every night for 3 months the prisoners were picked randomly for severe beatings and/or electric shocks. He was then transferred to a common jail for another $3\frac{1}{2}$ years.

Over the next 12 years, his main source of support came from his consistent involvement in educational, artistic, and consciousness-raising activities. This may have lowered his need for alcohol as an anxiety-reducing device, while paradoxically making him the target of persecution by the army.

Those activities, however, were continuously interrupted by eight or nine other imprisonments of 2 to 12 weeks duration, as well as frequent forced trips (sometimes on foot) to neighboring countries, attempting to flee from the army. After his last incarceration at age 36, he fled to Costa Rica and, 3 months later, to France. Shortly after moving to that country, he increased his intake of beer as a way of alleviating an exacerbated insomnia.

Diagnostic and Assessment Interview

Nicolás was punctual at the first interview, after mistakenly showing up the day before and waiting for an hour before realizing the actual appointment time. A handsome man, he was dressed neatly and casually, although he wore a heavy jacket in spite of the hot weather. His responses were consistent with emotional numbing. Nicolás spoke in a guarded way, sat rigidly, and showed constricted affect. He seemed confused and in need of guidance, but no thought derailments or delusions were noted. He denied any current self-destructive ideas. He stated that he used alcohol occasionally, only when his depression intensified, and was not presently using it.

Nicolás was aware that, as part of the referral process, the therapist knew already about his traumatic experiences as a political prisoner. However, as expected, he pointedly avoided any reference to this material in our first session. We discussed nonthreatening subjects such as his newly found relationship with his son, his living arrangements, current activities (soccer, drawing, and cooking), and his forced migrations over the last 13 years.

A preliminary family history and an initial sketch of his present symptoms were also obtained. It was explained to him then that we would meet for 15 sessions of individual therapy, in addition to couple and family sessions.

Treatment Process

The process of therapy will be described session by session, with a brief comment following the description of each session.

Treatment Plan

Since trust is a crucial issue for survivors of torture (Fischman & Ross, 1990), no attempt was made in the first session to direct the client's discourse into torture-related material. Thus, except for a few assessment questions, only his presenting concerns were addressed, so that he could begin to develop a sense of trust and control over his own treatment. In light of his presenting complaints, the therapist suggested a few preliminary therapeutic and behavioral goals: to diminish anxiety by learning relaxation skills, to work toward strengthening the relationship with his son, and to bring resolution into his marital relationship.

When the client's symptoms became more overt, the immediate focus (Wolberg, 1980) selected for treatment consisted of the symptoms presented by Nicolás as the most distressing to him, that is, anxiety, insomnia, nightmares, and intrusive thoughts. When the client's substance abuse became evident, its control was added as another focus of treatment. Also, since the inclusion of the family in the treatment of torture victims is of vital importance (Torres, 1989), the client's wife and son would be included for couple and family counseling.

First session. Another salient aspect of the initial session was Nicolás's resentment about being unemployed and financially dependent on his wife. He complained that her jealousy was driving him away, but that he could not leave his son. He seemed perplexed by his elevated anxiety level, inability to feel, isolation, and confusion. He longed for his previous self, which he described as happy, outgoing, and sensitive.

The therapist, for his part, informed Nicolás about the process of therapy and what would take place during the sessions. He was told that he was not expected to pay for treatment, but that his consistent attendance to all 15 weekly therapy sessions was a fundamental condition for treatment. It was emphasized to him that treatment would be focused on his most distressing symptoms and that traumatic events would be dealt with only as they influenced his present symptoms.

Comments. The client's presentation and demeanor are common to most trauma survivors when they initiate treatment. Since discussing the trauma elicits fears of reenactment, considerable energy goes into its denial and suppression (Allodi, 1991). Verbalizing the traumatic experience means making it real. Therefore, the survivor does not put it into words, in an attempt to deprive it of reality (Lira & Weinstein, 1984). Denial of the trauma may also be an attempt to go back to the former (pretorture) idealized self.

Second session. Nicolás presented a state of extreme anxiety, which was triggered by an abrupt attempt to recount three recent nightmares. He revealed that he had experienced suicidal impulses over the previous 2 days. As he launched into a fragmentary description of one of the nightmares, he muttered disconnected phrases in complete obliviousness to the therapist's interventions. Suddenly he stopped talking, took several sheets of paper, and started drawing. The therapist remained silent as Nicolás produced two more drawings, which he later said were sketches of his nightmares. He refused to elaborate, stating that they were very frightening. Nicolás began pacing and sobbing, complaining that intense nightmares troubled him every night and saying that killing himself would make things so much easier.

After several minutes, he sat down and described one of his nightmares. An old woman dressed in black invited him to the center of a lake. Another woman, dressed in white was also there, but remained silent. As he approached the lake, he saw two seagulls, one of which was peacefully eating crabs, and the other one was trying to release itself because it was chained. When Nicolás attempted to help, the seagull jumped at him and started pecking at his eyes. Shortly after this session, the client's high anxiety level and suicidal thoughts led to a 1-week hospitalization, during which time treatment was interrupted.

While waiting to be assessed by hospital staff, Nicolás revealed, in a confessionlike way, that he hears internal "voices" when his anxiety rises. With considerable difficulty and embarrassment, he said he heard the "voice" of his close friend Anibal, whose death by a point-blank shot to the head he was forced to witness. (Seconds after Anibal's killing, another soldier had fired two shots into the air while holding his gun right next to Nicolás ear. He still suffers from ringing in his ears.) Nicolás stated that he occasionally "talks" with his dead friend, who gently encourages him to kill himself "when things get rough."

Comments. The overcontrolling defenses (emotional numbing, confusion, rigidity) shown by the client in the first session were rather tenuous. After an indirect approximation to the trauma, its magnitude weakened his denial. The client's defenses gave way to a massive reexperiencing of the trauma through nightmares, involuntary recollections of the event, self-destructive ideas, auditory hallucinations, and heightened anxiety. The repression used against conscious memories of torture is absent in the nightmare, where defense mechanisms usually subside (Somnier & Genefke, 1986). The above nightmare, though frightening for the client, reveals dualities in which one of the elements (e.g., woman in white, the peaceful seagull) may represent a healthier, hopeful element, an attempt to resolve the traumatic (black, threatening) elements.

Third session. Nicolás admitted that he had stopped taking the medication prescribed for him when he was discharged from the hospital because he was "afraid of getting addicted to medications and they didn't stop the nightmares anyway." His level of anxiety rose once again to the point that it became difficult for him to remain seated during this session. He complained that a confined space reminded him of the torture chambers. Thus, part of this session was spent walking outdoors, which noticeably alleviated his anxiety. He was then instructed in the use of Wolpe's (1982) tensing-relaxation technique.

At this point, the therapist's interventions were directed at fostering Nicolás's sense of self-control through explaining the nature of his symptoms and experiences. Scurfield's (1985) suggestions were employed to clarify the characteristics of posttraumatic stress disorder (PTSD) and to trace the recovery process. Nicolás was advised that: (1) Traumatic events such as torture and childhood physical abuse can produce symptoms similar to his (nightmares, insomnia, rage, depression) in almost anyone. These symptoms can be intense and long-lasting, but are responsive to treatment. Although some of the symptoms may not disappear completely, he can at least understand and come to manage them better. (2) Feelings of losing control over certain emotions are not uncommon and do not mean that he is "going crazy." These feelings, as well as his nightmares and intrusive thoughts, often point to unresolved issues that need to be worked through (Torres, 1986). (3) Once he starts discussing his symptoms in therapy, they usually get worse before getting better. This early regression is a temporary and necessary step to work through his unresolved issues. He was reassured that he would not have to go through this by himself. The therapist made himself available at all times and encouraged Nicolás to call whenever he felt the need to do so. In addition, his family's support would be enlisted by facilitating a more open communication about the traumatic events that led to his present symptoms.

Comments. One of the primary goals of treatment with traumatized individuals is to reempower them by helping them develop a sense of control over their lives (Fischman & Ross, 1990; van der Kolk, 1988). In Nicolás's case, his persistent anxiety is largely due to a lack of control over his symptoms. Therefore, attempts at developing mastery began with an educational approach to help him understand the connections between symptoms and past history. In addition to learning relaxation techniques, he was encouraged to attend meetings of Alcoholics Anonymous and to enroll in an alcoholism program.

The treatment of torture survivors often requires the involvement of other health professionals. Unfortunately, as in the present case, the different components of health care do not always unify therapy goals, resulting in a fragmentation of services and further confusion for the client. Nicolás added to this fragmentation by refusing medications and missing referrals for aftercare.

Fourth session. A week later, Nicolás reported that the relaxation technique he learned had allowed him to "get up to 2 hours of sleep and then rise without wanting to kill myself." During these brief periods of sleep, however, he experienced nightmares, intensified by the recent, sudden death of a close friend, in which he vividly saw skulls and scenes from his first imprisonment. He tearfully recalled the intense feelings of powerlessness elicited by his inability to defend himself from the actual beatings.

Another nightmare involved "a woman who was cooking in two large pots. In one of them, an angry pig was staring at me; in the other one, the gentle eyes of a cow were looking at me." In a separate dream, "there were two young pretty girls: One of them, with long hair and tattoos on her arms and legs, looked angry, ran after my friend, and threw a bottle at him. The other one, gentle and smiling, tapped me on the back and smiled at me." One of his associations was to his mother's angry face, staring at him just before a beating.

Nicolás now identified his nightmares and insomnia as his most distressing symptoms. His intense fear of the night was a reaction to his dread of sleep and its harrowing nightmares. This triad (fear of the night, insomnia, and nightmares) was added to the goals of treatment and agreed upon with the client. We traced the origins of these symptoms to his first imprisonment, where he had felt compelled to remain alert at night in dreadful anticipation of another torture session.

At this point, the therapist advised Nicolás not to equate improvement with absence of symptoms but to look for and observe any changes in the intensity and frequency of nightmares, insomnia, and related feelings of fear and depression. As an assignment, he was also instructed to look for and identify his "triggers," that is, events or behaviors that are in some way related to the trauma and therefore increase his anxiety and nightmares. An example of a nightmare trigger might be reading highly charged political material before sleep. In a rather spontaneous way, Nicolás indicates a wish to "strengthen our relationship; I believe you [therapist] can help me."

Comments. Trauma survivors show an inability to modulate arousal. In response to stress, such as the loss of a loved one, they often show an all-or-nothing response (van der Kolk, 1988). Any strong feeling is experienced as indistinguishable from the effects triggered by the traumatic memories (Krystal, 1978).

The above nightmares were subsequent to an important loss and depict the two traumas affecting this client. In two of the dreams, the dualities may be symbolizing the presence of splitting, a defense mechanism often developed by physically abused children. Two of the dreams reveal the early abuse and depict the angry, punishing mother versus the loving, idealized one.

Fifth session. Nicolás showed considerable resistance to elaborate on his torture experiences. He claimed that, since the therapist had never been imprisoned, he would not be able to understand what Nicolás had gone through. As the therapist acknowledged Nicolás's need for self-protection by distancing himself from the therapist and torture-related material, Nicolás's resistance decreased, and he was able to begin recounting scattered memories of his torture and exile.

Nicolás then identified two events that he feels changed him in a permanent way. During his first imprisonment, a strong kick to the back of his head left him unconscious for an undetermined period of time. When he awoke in his cell, he vomited continuously for several hours. According to his own appraisal, after this event, "I was never myself again; I had lost something."

The second event took place when he was forced to flee from his native country. He felt that "something had been taken away from me and lost forever." He had been tortured by his own people and now felt rejected by his own country. His trust and well-being were under attack. This longing for his country and the loss he experienced had triggered a severe episode of depression and even a suicidal attempt while living in France. A few days after relating this, Nicolás began drinking as a way of alleviating intense feelings of loss. Treatment was interrupted for 2 weeks, and Nicolás was referred to a detoxification program. Upon discharge from detoxification, the client made a decision to stop drinking and to enroll in college.

During that time, and with the client's consent, a home visit was held to learn more about his environment and family situation. In a conversation with his wife, the therapist learned that both she and her son feel anxious and frustrated over Nicolás's behavior, and that they do not know anything about his imprisonments and torture.

Comments. Loss of aspects of the self (trust, control) is one of the universal themes common to trauma survivors (Horowitz, 1976; Scurfield, 1985; Torres, 1986). Blitz and Greenberg (1984) have found the same subjective experience of losing something of oneself among combat veterans. Mollica (1988) refers to this dimension of trauma as "losing the world," that is, as the total subjective loss of one's reality. Also, the massive losses involved in exile have been documented elsewhere: A group of torture survivors emphasized that "exile is the worst form of torture" (Fischman & Ross, 1990); 32 Chilean refugees saw their forced uprooting as a continuation of their suffering (Gonsalves, 1990).

Alcohol is often used as self-medication for many PTSD symptoms and for alleviating intense feelings of loss, anger, sadness, and guilt. However, its repeated consumption leads to tolerance and a consequent increase in drinking to achieve the desired effects. When chronic consumption is discontinued, symptoms similar to PTSD emerge, which in turn promote more alcohol intake (Lacoursiere, Godfrey, & Ruby, 1980).

Sixth and seventh sessions. At this stage of treatment, given the intensity of Nicolás's symptoms, some of his traumatic memories and nightmares were treated using EMDR (Shapiro, 1989).[2] He was able to process several memories, ranging from physical abuse by his mother to his capture by the secret police and first day of imprisonment. While processing his detention, his anxiety rose considerably. He began sobbing but was able to focus on the instructions and gradually brought his SUDs down to a zero.[3] However, Nicolás chose not to deal with specific incidents of torture. Furthermore, when an attempt was made to process the vivid memories of his friend Anibal's killing, he pointedly and somewhat angrily refused to continue. He demanded to know whether the consultant and therapist were trying to take the memory of his friend away from him.

Comments. EMDR involves the desensitization of traumatic affects and cognitions through reciprocal eye movements. It is still in its early stages of development, and its mechanism of success is still a mystery. Promising reports of its effectiveness are still anecdotal, but some studies are gradually emerging. For example, Marquis (1991) reports on the outcome of 78 clients and 530 themes treated with eye movement desensitization. Though "scientifically blemished in several ways," results showed that the highest effectiveness of this technique was with past trauma and isolated sources of distress.

[2]*Eye Movement Desensitization and Reprocessing.* When consulted on the use of systematic desensitization with nightmares, John Marquis, PhD, volunteered that he had obtained better and quicker results using EMDR with traumatized people. Because the therapist in the present case lacked experience in the use of this new technique, Marquis offered to treat, on a pro-bono basis, Nicolás's traumatic memories using EMDR. A total of two 120-minute sessions were conducted mostly in English (which Nicolás had mastered well enough to communicate), with the regular therapist present to suggest possible foci of intervention. A more in-depth description of this part of the treatment is beyond the scope of this chapter and will be published in a future paper.

[3]This technique relies on Wolpe's (1982) concept of SUDs (Subjective Units of Discomfort), a scale from 0 to 10 that serves as a numerical self-rating of the client's anxiety.

Nicolás's own report after the first EMDR session was that "it's like magic; I feel no anxiety; I don't feel like leaving home and not knowing where to go. [Two days ago] I was laughing so much." His determined refusal to desensitize the traumatic memory of his dead friend's killing might be understood as a sense of loyalty to his friend (Torres, 1986, personal communication) and as a need to "bear witness" (Bettelheim, 1980). Also, the memory of his dead friend served as a safety device. As stated by Horowitz (1986), "[w]hen others have been injured or killed, it is a relief to realize that one has been spared. . . . If one has eluded the Fates, it may seem to have been unfairly at the expense of other victims."

Eighth session. Following the use of EMDR, Nicolás reported an ability to sleep every night, as well as a marked decrease in the frequency and intensity of his nightmares. From an incidence of up to two or three intense daily nightmares prior to the use of this technique, Nicolás was now reporting three nightmares in a week. He rated the intensity of post-EMDR nightmares as a 3, adding that he was not concerned about them and could barely remember their contents. Nicolás was able to recall only the presence of a black bird in a dream disturbing enough to wake him up. However, he stated that this time he resolved to block the dream and managed to regain an anxiety-free sleep.

He began daily attendance to an Alcoholics Anonymous group, spoke very highly of their doctrines, and attributed to them his renewed self-confidence and his absence of insomnia and self-destructiveness. For the first time, he fully admitted he was an alcoholic and emphasized his determination to remain abstinent.

Comments. Nicolás had overestimated his family's (and especially his son's) ability to provide emotional gratification. Disappointed at his own family, Nicolás is now transferring his idealization to a new element. In Nicolás's eyes, Alcoholics Anonymous has become a new and gratifying group. He has now shifted to the structure and predictability of AA groups, accepted its precepts, and changed part of his self-concept possibly in order to belong to this new "family."

Self-help organizations such as AA provide a traumatized individual such as Nicolás with opportunities for building attachments with others, as well as developing trust within a support system.

Ninth session. The relief he obtained from the alleviation of his nightmares and his involvement in AA did not quell other depressive symptoms. He reported some progress but also noted that over the previous 3 days he had been feeling very sad, bored, and irritable, particularly when home in the evenings. Nicolás bitterly complained about what he called his wife's smothering care of him, her persistent attempts to turn him into the "man of the house," as well as her increasing displays of affection and emotional dependence on him. At the same time, he continued to resent his own financial dependence on his wife. He felt trapped and obligated to reciprocate with sex and affection to his wife's kindness.

Nicolás reported early morning awakening, as well as three nightmares since the previous session. He assigned an intensity of one SUDs to two of them, while the other one he rated as a 5. In the latter dream, an old man with a thin mustache, unknown to him, was ahead of him. Somehow the man got behind Nicolás and started chasing him with a knife, threatening to kill him.

Comments. The intensity of the trauma-related symptoms has subsided to a point where the client is now focusing less on individual issues and more on interpersonal ones. The disturbance produced by the trauma is so global that the client focuses on family conflicts as a way of controlling and reducing its impact. Furthermore, this emphasis on family issues may also be an attempt to deny the trauma by focusing on other issues. The nightmare was interpreted as transferential. Though initially hesitant, Nicolás was able to recognize that he sometimes feels pursued by the therapist, who "chases" him into facing his traumas.

A few days later, upon the reoccurrence of a sudden episode of depression triggered by the death of another close friend, Nicolás started abusing alcohol again. A day-and-night alcohol binge continued for 3 weeks, forcing the interruption of treatment.

Tenth session. Upon resuming treatment, Nicolás complained bitterly that he suffers from frequent and pronounced mood swings, for no apparent cause, and in unexpected circumstances. He explained that he started drinking "almost inadvertently, without really realizing" what he was doing; and because he had suddenly felt lonesome and sad, and wished to die. Initially, he was able to identify the sources of these feelings but later realized that his friend's death had had a strong impact on him. Another anxiety-provoking event, subsequent to his friend's death and leading to his relapse, was a severe nightmare in which a group of men were threatening to kill him. He had a few other mild nightmares, the intensity of which he rated as two or three SUDs. In them, he was alone in his home country, without any relatives and just a few acquaintances.

Comments. Trauma survivors often lose the ability to differentiate and express emotions and to establish connections between the stressful stimulus and their emotional response. Their reaction to a stressor may go from an initial numbing in which no feelings are identified, to severe emotional outbursts similar to those triggered by the original trauma, that is, the "all-or-nothing" response (van der Kolk, 1988). These overreactions in turn cloud the survivor's cognitive abilities, prompting them into impulsive action (e.g., substance abuse) instead of rational thinking. Vulnerability to subsequent losses may be heightened by a history of childhood trauma, that is, physical abuse from the primary caregiver, as well as early losses, such as the death of the social worker to whom Nicolás had been so close.

Eleventh and twelfth sessions. An increasing focus on family conflicts and a concurrent avoidance of traumatic issues are now prominent. Talkative and less guarded, Nicolás resents his wife's complaints about his withdrawal. She reacts to his silence with jealous accusations and criticizes Nicolás's harsh methods of disciplining their son when he arrives late from school. Nicolás imposes severe restrictions over his son's freedom to leave the house. The latter's noncompliance enhances Nicolás's feelings of powerlessness vis-à-vis what he perceives as an alliance between wife and son.

Sudden bouts of depression are still present, but Nicolás now realizes that they often occur during periods of inactivity. As a way of dealing with these feelings, he has increased attendance to AA meetings, which he highly praises.

Nicolás has now identified some of his "triggers," that is, anxiety-provoking behaviors. They include reading political material or about experiences of other torture survivors; seeing the police arresting someone or parents beating a child. He immediately thinks of the past and gets sad, but it does not last very long. "I tell myself that it's all in the past and that I can't do anything about it."

It was brought to his attention that three more treatment sessions are left, to which he responded with a dry, monosyllabic agreement. Attempts at exploring his reactions to termination were met with an emphatic denial of its impact.

Dreams of being persecuted, which he associates to abuse both by the military and his mother, are still frequent but much less intense. In one such dream (SUDs 3), "a fat man with a swollen face is running after me and throwing rocks at me. I ran and came to a place where a [unidentifiable] friend was forcing a young woman to embrace him. She was resisting, finally broke herself away from his arms and ran to mine, cuddling up to me and feeling very comfortable."

He reports no longer being afraid of the night, as well as a marked improvement in his insomnia and anxiety. However, he minimizes this progress and continues to ascribe it to AA.

Comments. Changes in dream intensity and content (e.g., a loving woman protected by him as opposed to threatening ones who render him powerless) point to an improvement in Nicolás's emotional status and possibly a growing mastery of the trauma. A significant change in self-perception is symbolized in his transformation from a helpless escapee to a protector of others.

The autonomy strivings of Nicolás's adolescent son are experienced by the client as a violation of his attempts to build a predictable, secure environment. By attempting to control the actions of others, Nicolás seems to be trying to regain a sense of self-control. Since his son has failed to fulfill Nicolás's unconscious expectations of showing the self-control that Nicolás lacks, the client's former idealization of his son has turned into rage, even over the latter's minor failures. Nicolás's poor empathy with his son's and wife's needs is reported commonly in traumatized people (Steele, 1970). Furthermore, like other severely traumatized people, Nicolás "doesn't discriminate between appropriate and inappropriate demands and gets enraged about minor disappointments coming from others" (van der Kolk, 1988).

Thirteenth session. Although no nightmares or sleep problems have occurred, Nicolás states that "if my depression does not change, nothing has really changed." He reports that these depressive episodes are still pronounced; for example, he felt quite dejected for a 2-hour period prior to a recent soccer game, without knowing why. While in a sad mood, he tells himself that "everything is lost; there's no hope or reason to live." His initial reaction is "to let depression take over, but then I pull myself through by asking myself what can be so wrong, looking at what I have and remembering some of the things we have discussed in therapy."

In the absence of further progress, he has been "getting bored." Nicolás admitted that this feeling often results from many of his activities, except politics, "where things changed daily." As a result, he has repeatedly told his wife and son, in a rather casual way, that he would soon go back to Guatemala by himself. He admitted to the therapist that he has detached himself from his son's behavioral problems and from his wife's jealousy and demands. In fact, he refused to incorporate them into the family sessions originally agreed upon.

The client was confronted with a lack of reciprocity often present in his relationships with others; how he remains receptive while others (wife, therapists, friends) take care of him, until he gets bored and leaves home or even the country. He said he did not like this aspect of his personality and appeared surprised at the therapist's observation that help seems to come to him in a rather effortless way.

In recent dreams, he appears in a country resembling his own, often with friendly smiling strangers. According to the client, these dreams now prevail over dreams of persecution.

Comments. As termination draws nearer, issues of abandonment associated with early maternal abuse begin to emerge. Nicolás defends against the ensuing depression by constricting his involvement in activities and relationships. He has withdrawn from his family after they failed to provide emotional gratification, showing what Krystal (1978) describes as a "giving up of hope for satisfactory human contact, which is the result of the destruction of basic trust." He is also distancing from the therapist by devaluing the process and gains of therapy. According to Krystal, people who have suffered severe abuse as children fear their own emotions (which are often experienced as trauma screens) and are unable to tolerate affects. Together with their constant efforts to avoid pain, they show a lifelong anhedonia, that is, an inability to experience pleasure, which Nicolás persistently reports as boredom.

Nicolás failed to attend a couple's therapy session that had been scheduled the previous week, and he did not notify the therapist. However, his wife did attend. It became apparent that she deeply resents Nicolás's emotional and sexual withdrawal and feels strongly rejected by him. She promptly dismisses as false the few sketchy allusions to torture experiences that Nicolás has made over the last several weeks. She is convinced that her husband's symptoms are the result of frustrated love affairs. The therapist encouraged her to try to find the facts from Nicolás, which would be discussed in a marital session.

Fourteenth session. Initially detached and guarded, Nicolás rejected the therapist's offer to have another couple's session. Later, as part of a long monologue, Nicolás spontaneously talks about imprisonments and torture experiences, without any noticeable anxiety. In fact, he appears surprised when this is pointed out to him. Involuntary recollections of his torture experiences have decreased in frequency and, above all, intensity. He reports feeling better. Nicolás expressed a wish to be self-sufficient and not have to rely on mental health professionals for his well-being, adding that he has difficulties coming to therapy. Again, he attributes his improvement to time, claiming that "talking doesn't help that much; only talking to friends who have also been tortured. When I talk in therapy, I feel a lot of heat in my body, as well as an urge to smoke."

Nicolás said he did not believe his former French therapist's claims that he cared about him and remarked that "in the same way my torturers didn't give a damn about me, I generalized to thinking that nobody cared about me."

Comments. The client's avoidance of the traumatic material has decreased. He is now acknowledging it, discusses it in detail, and puts it together spontaneously. However, he mentions mostly facts and hardly any emotions. The therapist's attempts to explore the underlying affects further are met with defensive statements devaluing the process of therapy. These statements, together with his wish to leave and failure to show up for a couple's session, may be reactions to the termination of therapy, an attempt to abandon the therapist before being "rejected" by him.

Like other traumatized individuals, Nicolás experiences some emotions as physical states (Krystal, 1978); namely, anxiety is felt as body heat, with little awareness of the sources of that anxiety.

The family's complaints about Nicolás's withdrawal constitute another source of stress. As stated by Allodi (1991):

> Traumatized refugees are frequently depressed and, therefore, unable to cope with family or other problems unrelated to the original trauma, but these problems become by themselves a new source of strain and depression. (p. 8)

Fifteenth session. Again, Nicolás initiated the session by giving short affectless responses. He reported "not feeling any emotions" over the termination of therapy. His guardedness, as well as his unwillingness to present any dreams, were interpreted as possible indications of resentment over termination. He flatly denied this assertion.

His evaluation of the treatment process was that it allowed him "to stabilize a little; [therapy] opened new ways of handling my depression and other problems. I think more and am less impulsive. I want to put into practice what I learned here. I feel quite confident." Nicolás stated that he now looks for things to do or tries to change his thoughts when he is in the middle of a depressive episode. "My depressions happen less frequently and are not as overwhelming as they used to be; I don't feel defeated."

He reiterated that he is now able to get up to 8 or 9 hours of uninterrupted sleep and that he has not had any nightmares in the past 2 weeks. Nicolás has not felt any urge to use alcohol and continues to attend AA meetings at least three times per week. He was instructed about the circumstances under which symptoms are likely to reappear, but he only skeptically accepted there was any need for continued self-observation. With the end of a school term only a few days away, he scarcely showed any pride in his academic achievements.

Comments. The symptoms that formed the immediate focus of treatment continue to be in remission. After devaluing treatment and expressing anger at the therapist in previous sessions, Nicolás is now doing a more realistic assessment of the outcome of therapy. In addition, Nicolás's feelings of helplessness have decreased significantly. He is now showing a regained sense of being able to influence his life, as well as an improved self-concept. However, he appears overconfident about his stability and lack of symptoms.

Several factors seem to have contributed to Nicolás's detachment. First, the evaluation of progress, with its concomitant reminder of the client's conflicts, may have strengthened his distancing maneuvers. Furthermore, he withdrew from the task of dealing with termination and instead acted out the separation through emotional and physical detachment. This suggests that this client could have benefited from a longer treatment.

Second, the link that Nicolás was able to establish between his torture experiences and present symptoms should have also been incorporated into the new three-member family's view of itself. Instead, the traumatic antecedents of the client's symptoms remained unavailable to his wife and son, leaving a large vacuum in the developing "script" of the newly formed family. When Nicolás refused to reveal that link to his family, the latter withdrew in frustration and bewilderment over his disturbed behaviors. The resulting emotional distance between the client and his family was transferred to the therapeutic relationship (Fischman, 1991).

Finally, after the recent deaths of two close friends, the threat of abandonment is perhaps intensified again by the termination of treatment. Nicolás reacts to the latter by distancing from the therapist with an alleged indifference, while firmly disavowing any feelings of rejection or abandonment. He pretends to have no needs and guards against showing any effects.

CLINICAL ISSUES

Torture survivors such as Nicolás illustrate the multiple layers of trauma that psychotherapy may need to address. Four areas of trauma and its effects are discussed now. First, torture may be compounded by preexisting problems such as the early physical and emotional abuse experienced by Nicolás. Second, PTSD symptoms often complicate the treatment process because of the intensity and unpredictability of their onset. Nicolás's vivid nightmares and heightened anxiety reflected some of the psychological sequelae. Third, exile or refugee status adds a frequently underestimated pain to the trauma of torture. Nicolás has migrated through three countries and two continents and demonstrates the vulnerability of the sojourner. Fourth, the treatment outcome demonstrates the potential need for modified criteria for inclusion of severely traumatized clients in brief therapy.

Preexisting Problems

Torture survivors may present a variety of problems. Some may suffer from alcohol or drug problems even before torture. Others lived in desperate poverty and grew up without formal education. We limit ourselves here to the physical and emotional abuse Nicolás sustained during childhood and reflect on its added impact to his torture experience.

Physically abused children show disrupted attachment relationships. They tend to form fewer friends, behave in a more aggressive fashion, and misperceive many social situations (Cicchetti, 1984; Egeland & Stroufe, 1981; Shirk, 1988). When an early trauma of physical abuse is added later on to that of torture, these symptoms become exacerbated.

Trauma by its very nature overwhelms the coping ability of the survivor (van der Kolk, 1988). A history of early repeated trauma would suggest that even minor stress would engender a response appropriate to an emergency. In other words, the survivor of multiple traumas lives in a state of continual arousal such that ordinary problem-solving and common sense are compromised (Horowitz, 1986). Thus, Nicolás was unable to relate on an equal footing with his wife, remained highly irritable for days after a report of misbehavior from his son's school, abused alcohol possibly as a way to diminish or manage his aggressiveness, and vacillated from session to session because his social sensitivity was poor (Frodi & Smetann, 1984).

Posttraumatic Stress Disorder Symptoms

This case demonstrates the need to help clients control their inner life. PTSD responses usually include a physiological reaction. As a result, the typical tendency for PTSD survivors is to "fight, flight, or freeze" (van der Kolk, 1988, p. 171). Nicolás's accusations toward his wife and son (fight), drinking (flight), and inability to move beyond his nightmares (freeze) exemplify these responses. PTSD reactions have such demand quality because emotions tend to be experienced as physical states and result purely in bodily reactions (Krystal, 1984; van der Kolk, 1988). In other words, emotions are not experienced as cognitive modes that are open to verbal and symbolic access. Thus, Nicolás's nightmares and anxiety, as well as his depression and alcohol use, are not accessible to the control of words or symbols. EMDR became a critical treatment mode precisely because its healing mechanism is hypothesized to lie partially at the physiological level (Shapiro, 1989).

Refugee Status

Social and psychological stress is considerably higher in exiled torture victims than in immigrants who have not been persecuted or tortured (Allodi & Rojas, 1985). For torture survivors, flight from their homeland is experienced more and more as a psychological equivalent to the trauma of torture. The statement can be made this boldly because their migration is forced, their loss of social and cultural support systems is almost total, and their sense of rejection by their homeland heightened. Thus, particular focus should be placed on the refugee experience.

Nicolás has fled to the United States, then Costa Rica, followed by France, and now back to the United States. He appears to be rootless. This sense of being a sojourner and lacking psychological belonging is common to most refugees but has become magnified in Nicolás. In order to alleviate the stress of exile and acculturation, the client needs to develop linkages both with people from his homeland who live here and with people and causes in Central America with whom he can identify. Torture aims to break the human spirit. Forced flight has as its goal the creation of a rootless people. For Nicolás's spirit to be restored, a sense of his roots, of who he is as a Central American, and a continued commitment to his country must be reestablished.

Criteria for Inclusion

Brief therapy has traditionally been considered useful for people who function generally well but have experienced a recent and specific crisis. With the continuing tendency toward eclecticism and integrative models in brief therapy (Reid, 1990), the criteria for patient selection have broadened, particularly in the nonpsychodynamic approaches (Budman & Stone, 1983). Even so, disorders such as chronic psychosis, chronic alcohol or drug abuse, chronic physical symptoms that lack a physical basis, and symptoms consistent with a severe personality disorder would exclude many individuals from a variety of brief therapy approaches. Nicolás indeed met two of the criteria for exclusion, but the data were unknown to the therapist at the time of referral. One limitation of work with torture survivors is that they frequently speak a language other than English. Few bilingual and bicultural mental health professionals are to be found in acute psychiatric hospitals, crisis centers, or outpatient clinics. As a result, many torture survivors will lack a complete psychosocial history. Because cases such as Nicolás's are prevalent, it may be necessary to broaden the criteria for inclusion of this client population in short-term therapy.

OVERALL EVALUATION

This case exemplifies many of the characteristic symptoms of PTSD, such as the arousal-numbing cycle, reenactment of the trauma, physiological correlates, and so forth. It also illustrates how alcohol is used frequently by PTSD patients, especially torture victims (Torres, personal communication) and combat veterans, as a means of avoiding the negative and highly charged memories of the trauma (Boudewyns & Hyer, 1990; Kolb, 1987; Lacoursier, Godfrey, & Ruby, 1980). As Boudewyns et al. (1991) observed, "there is a strong connection between substance abuse/use and the stressor that resulted in PTSD, regardless of any predisposition." Thus Nicolás's alcohol abuse seems to be a defensive measure to avoid the memories of the terror and stress of his torture experience.

Some issues present in the treatment of torture survivors, however, may present a unique case of PTSD symptoms. As Allodi (1991) states:

> What is so unique in torture victims . . . is the sense of personal humiliation and shame, the mistrust of friends, neighbors, authorities, or institutions, and, at times, the confusion of values and of self at a most intimate level. Those after-effects are related to the circumstances and the very objectives of the torture: to regress, humiliate, and devastate the self-esteem of the victims and to confuse their values and philosophy of life, using techniques that take advantage of the most basic needs of any human being under conditions of total dependence. (p. 7)

Allodi (1991) further states that "PTSD, as a model for the study of victims of torture, political violence, and other abuse of state power, has been criticized as narrow insofar as it reduces what is often a complex politicohistorical problem to the individual psychological level."

The process of Nicolás's treatment touched on three other topics that have not been discussed widely in the literature: the torture of an individual traumatized previously in childhood; the inclusion during the process of brief therapy of an outside consultant contributing to the treatment; and finally, the complications for torture survivors of treatment outside their homeland.

Nicolás's early physical and emotional abuse followed by his subsequent multiple detentions and torture would seem to call into question his ability to establish trust. Parental abuse as well as governmental abuse arise from social systems meant to protect rather than to punish individuals. Nicolás continued to dream about his angry mother staring malevolently at him. He mocked the assertion of the therapist who said people cared about him. Yet, in spite of his many assaults, Nicolás was able to establish trust in the therapist and move to some resolution of his symptoms. Thus, even preexisting conditions of abuse do not rule out the possibility of forming a mutual relationship of trust with survivors of torture in a brief therapy model.

Second, treatment of severely traumatized individuals such as torture survivors may stretch the clinical resources of many psychotherapists. Intervention with this population implies knowledge of the theory and praxis of torture, awareness of the cultural behaviors and beliefs of the survivors, and a familiarity with a wide range of strategies to be applied to individual, couple, and family systems. Thus, work with torture survivors may push the psychotherapist to function as a case manager during certain stages of the therapeutic process. Such a role puts the resources of the entire community at hand for the psychotherapist. However, several important considerations are in order before involving other professionals: (a) A solid therapeutic alliance should precede the introduction of other professionals. (b) The client needs to understand the reasons for introducing another clinician before consenting to this approach. (c) The presence of the primary psychotherapist whenever a second expert is involved contributes to maintain the therapeutic links with the client. The use of a particular expert needs to be confined to two or three sessions so that the primary transference with the original therapist not be diluted. (d) Several experts theoretically could be utilized when needed, as long as these considerations are kept in mind. However, in practice, our limited state of knowledge would caution us to use consultants only in truly critical psychotherapeutic issues.

Third, Nicolás's situation leads us to reemphasize the difficulties for torture survivors who are outside their homeland. Previous history is often difficult to obtain because mental health professionals able to speak Spanish or other foreign languages are in short supply. As a result, a meager or even inaccurate history may accompany the client and may not include salient facts necessary for accurate diagnosis and treatment planning. Additionally, the culture of the survivor may not be understood well, and well-meaning but monolingual and monocultural intervenors may have distorted information or misinterpreted cultural cues due to ignorance of proper behavior on how to address the client.

Added to these problems is the very real tendency in professionals who treat torture survivors to minimize or even to overlook the full impact of their experience of torture and exile from their homeland (Fischman, 1991). Survivors outside their homeland feel often estranged, and outside their world of meaning. Thus, symptom-focused brief therapy by itself may not be sufficient for the task of making self-management possible for torture survivors.

Existential psychotherapists emphasize the inclusion of themes such as finitude, freedom, meaning, and time with clients. For those subjected to wanton pain inflicted deliberately by fellow human beings and threatened arbitrarily with death as a constant undercurrent, such themes can resonate. Torture survivors have conveyed that at times they wished for their own death (Fischman, Torres, personal communications). Their ability to choose has been turned against them such that they "are exposed to a pseudochoice between alternatives whereby they must either submit to additional torture or cooperate with the torturers' demands and suffer the pain of losing values and integrity" (Fischman & Ross, 1990).

Former certainties have evaporated because one's meaning context has been shredded. Even time seems to trap the survivor. The past tends to be avoided at all costs due to its intrusive memories of horror and suffering. The present tends to be experienced as empty, damaged, and even as continuing the torture. A future tends to be lacking because torture teaches that one's life ends once torture begins. Thus, psychotherapy for survivors of torture may be incomplete unless their future is opened up to them.

Nicolás seemed to have grasped unconsciously his absence of himself as flowing through time. So he moved once more to the United States to reunite with some of his family of origin (his past), while seeking at the same time to establish at last a relationship with his son (his future). A therapist fluent in his native language (his world of meaning) addresses the memories of his past, appreciates the magnitude of the loss of his homeland, and in this way makes possible some peace for his present mode of being. Now he may be able to project himself into the future and continue undoing the past ravages.

References

Allodi, F. (1991). Assessment and treatment of torture victims: A critical review. *The Journal of Nervous and Mental Disease, 179*(1), 4–11.

Allodi, F., & Rojas, A. (1985). The health and adaptation of victims of political violence in Latin America. In P. Pichot, P. Berner, R. Wolfe et al. (Eds.), *Psychiatry, the state of the art. Vol. 6. Drug dependency and alcoholism, forensic psychiatry, military psychiatry* (pp. 243–248). New York: Plenum Press.

Bettelheim, B. (1980). *Surviving and other essays.* New York: Vintage Books.

Blitz, R., & Greenberg, R. (1984). Nightmares of the traumatic neuroses: Implications for theory and treatment. In H. J. Schwartz (Ed.), *Psychotherapy of the combat veteran* (pp. 103–124). New York: Spectrum Publications.

Boudewyns, P., & Hyer, L. (1990). Physiological response to combat memories and preliminary treatment outcome in Vietnam veteran PTSD patients treated with direct therapeutic exposure. *Behavior Therapy, 21,* 63–87.

Boudewyns, P., Woods, M., Hyer, L., & Albrecht, J. (1991). Chronic combat-related PTSD and concurrent substance abuse: Implications for treatment of this frequent "dual diagnosis." *Journal of Traumatic Stress, 4,* 549–560.

Budman, S., & Stone, J. (1983). Advances in brief psychotherapy: A review of recent literature. *Hospital and Community Psychiatry, 34,* 939–946.

Cicchetti, D. (1984). The emergence of developmental psychopathology. *Child Development, 55,* 1–7.

Cienfuegos, A. J., & Monelli, C. (1983). The testimony of political repression as a therapeutic instrument. *American Journal of Orthopsychiatry, 53,* 43–51.

Cowgill, G., & Doupe, G. (1985). Recognizing and helping victims of torture. *Canadian Nurse, 12,* 19–22.

Egeland, B., & Stroufe, A. (1981). Developmental sequelae of maltreatment in infancy. In R. Rizly & D. Cicchetti (Eds.), *New directions for child development: Developmental perspectives in child maltreatment* (pp. 225–239). San Francisco: Jossey-Bass.

Erickson, E. (1968). *Identity: Youth and crisis.* New York: Norton.

Fischman, Y. (1991). Interacting with trauma: Clinicians' responses to treating psychological aftereffects of political repression. *American Journal of Orthopsychiatry, 61,* 179–185.

Fischman, Y., & Ross, J. (1990). Group treatment of exiled survivors of torture. *American Journal of Orthopsychiatry, 60,* 135–142.

Frodi, S., & Smetann, M. (1984). Abused, neglected and normal preschoolers' ability to discriminate emotions in others. *Child Abuse and Neglect, 8,* 459–465.

Gonsalves, C. (1990). The psychological effects of political repression on Chilean exiles in the U.S. *American Journal of Orthopsychiatry, 60,* 143–153.

Gonsalves, C., Torres, T., Fischman, Y., Ross, J., & Vargas, M. (in press). The theory of torture and the treatment of its survivors: An intervention model. *Journal of Traumatic Stress.*

Horowitz, M. (1986). *Stress response syndromes* (2nd ed.). Northvale, NJ: Jason Aronson.

Horowitz, M. et al. (1984). *Personality styles and brief psychotherapy.* New York: Basic Books.

Kolb, L. (1987). A neuropsychological hypothesis explaining posttraumatic stress disorders. *American Journal of Psychiatry, 144,* 989–995.

Krystal, H. (1978). Trauma and effects. *The Psychoanalytic Study of the Child, 33,* 81–116.

Krystal, H. (1984). Psychoanalytic views on human emotional damages. In B. van der Kolk (Ed.), *Post-traumatic stress disorder: Psychological and biological sequelae* (pp. 1–28). Washington, DC: American Psychiatric Association Press.

Lacoursiere, R., Godfrey, K., & Ruby, L. (1980). Traumatic neurosis in the etiology of alcoholism: Viet Nam combat and other trauma. *American Journal of Psychiatry, 137*(8), 966–968.

Lira, E., & Weinstein, E. (1984). El testimonio de experiencias politicas traumáticas como instrumento terapéutico [The testimony of traumatic political experiences as a therapeutic instrument]. In E. Lira, E. Weinstein, R. Domínguez, J. Kovalskys, A. Maggi, E. Morales, & F. Pollarolo (Eds.), *Psicoterapia y represión politica* [Psychotherapy and political repression] (pp. 17–36). Mexico, DF: Siglo Veintiuno Editores.

Marquis, J. (1991). A report on seventy-eight cases treated by eye movement desensitization. *Journal of Behavior Therapy and Experimental Psychiatry, 22,* 187–192.

Mollica, R. (1988). The trauma story: The psychiatric care of refugee survivors of violence and torture. In F. Ochberg (Ed.), *Post-traumatic therapy and victims of violence* (pp. 295–314). New York: Brunner/Mazel.

Ortmann, J., Genefke, I., Jakobsen, L., & Lunde, I. (1987). Rehabilitation of torture victims: An interdisciplinary treatment model. *American Journal of Social Psychiatry, 4*, 161–167.

Reid, W. (1990). An integrative model for short-term treatment: In R. Wells & V. Giannetti (Eds.), *Handbook of the brief psychotherapies* (pp. 55–77). New York: Plenum Press.

Scurfield, R. (1985). Post-trauma stress assessment and treatment. Overview and formulations. In C. Figley (Ed.), *Trauma and its wake* (pp. 209–231). New York: Brunner/Mazel.

Shapiro, F. (1989). Eye movement desensitization: A new treatment for Post-Traumatic Stress Disorder. *Journal of Behavior Therapy and Experimental Psychiatry, 20*(3), 211–217.

Shirk, S. (1988). The interpersonal legacy of physical abuse of children. In M. Straus (Ed.), *Abuse and victimization across the life span* (pp. 57–81). Baltimore: Johns Hopkins University Press.

Somnier, F., & Genefke, I. (1986). Psychotherapy for victims of torture. *British Journal of Psychiatry, 149*, 323–329.

Steele, B. (1970). Parental abuse of infants and small children. In R. Anthony & T. Benedict (Eds.), *Parenthood: Its psychology and psychopathology* (pp. 449–478). Boston: Little, Brown.

Torres, T. (1986, April). Treatment of survivors of torture. Lecture presented at Peninsula Hospital, Burlingame, CA.

Torres, T. (1989, October). *Torture as a social practice*. Paper presented at the annual meeting of the Society for Traumatic Stress Studies, San Francisco.

Van der Kolk, B. (1988). Trauma in men: Effects on family life. In M. Strauss (Ed.), *Abuse and victimization across the life span* (pp. 170–187). Baltimore: Johns Hopkins University Press.

Wolberg, L. (1980). *Handbook of short-term psychotherapy*. New York: Thieme-Stratton.

Wolpe, J. (1982). *The practice of behavior therapy* (3rd ed.). New York: Pergamon Press.

4

Interpersonal Psychotherapy of Depression

A Case Study

CLEON CORNES

INTRODUCTION

Interpersonal psychotherapy of depression (IPT) has been developed over the past 20 years, initially in the New Haven–Boston Collaborative Depression Research Project by Gerald Klerman, Myrna Weissman, and colleagues. It has been described in detail in a training manual and subsequently in a textbook (Klerman et al., 1984). I have summarized the development and application of IPT, including illustrative case examples, in the *Handbook of the Brief Psychotherapies* (Cornes, 1990).

In this case,[1] I will be using IPT to treat a 36-year-old white married social worker and mother of four children who is suffering from a second episode of major depression. The treatment consisted of 16 weekly sessions lasting approximately 50 minutes each. The patient was seen individually, and there was no contact with family members or other persons in her life.

[1]To ensure confidentiality, descriptive details about the patient have been modified in ways that should protect her identity but not interfere with the value of the case as an example of IPT.

CLEON CORNES • Western Psychiatric Institute and Clinic, 3811 O'Hara Street, Pittsburgh, Pennsylvania 15213.

Casebook of the Brief Psychotherapies, edited by Richard A. Wells and Vincent J. Giannetti. Plenum Press, New York, 1993.

THE INITIAL SESSIONS: FOCUS AND PLAN

She began the first session by telling me that her depression began approximately a year ago when her husband was placed in a nursing home. He was suffering from cancer and had become so debilitated she was no longer able to care for him at home. He had several previous hospitalizations and was not expected to live much longer. She stated, "when he went into the home I looked around and my house was a mess and my life was in shreds." She went to see her family doctor when she began vomiting frequently. He told her she was depressed, but she did not seek further treatment at that time. Over the past year her symptoms have increased, including decreased energy, fluctuating appetite, depressed mood, irritability, frequent crying, feelings of emptiness and loneliness, anhedonia, decreased interest in activities including sex, poor concentration and memory, trouble sleeping, increased social isolation, poor performance at work, and thoughts about "giving up." She said concerns about losing her job had prompted her to seek treatment at this time.

She talked about a drastic change in her life after her husband went into the nursing home: "it seemed like everything crumbled . . . everybody's relationships have changed . . . we all struggled to be king of the mountain." The patient has been married for 15 years and has four children: two daughters age 14 and 13, and two sons age 12 and 10. She is Caucasian and her husband is Oriental. They were married when she was a college student and he was working as a bank teller. She phoned her parents to tell them she was married, and they attempted unsuccessfully to have her committed to a psychiatric hospital. Her interracial marriage and her parents' reaction have led to continuing dissension in the family, but she feels her parents are treating her quite differently since her husband's illness: "Now that he's out of the picture they are trying to be helpful to the point of choking me." She describes her mother as "domineering, intrusive and controlling, aggressive and mouthy." Her father was described as "quiet, German, avoiding conflict and sneaky." She has a younger sister who also has an interracial marriage and lives out of the country. Her youngest sibling, a brother, was recently married and is described as "mother's favorite." Her parents and brother live about 300 miles from the patient, but they rarely visited after her marriage. None of her family members has been treated for psychiatric illness.

The patient describes her marriage as fairly good except for the last 2 years since his illness, and one period of time 10 years ago. After the birth of her youngest son, her husband had an affair, they separated for several months, she became depressed and made a suicide attempt. She saw a psychiatrist briefly who "helped me put things in perspective, and I went back to my husband." Since his illness, the husband has been "more angry, critical, and demanding." He wants her to take him home more often for visits and blames her for his deteriorating health. After visits with him "I just sit and cry." She also describes a lot of conflict with her children which has emerged in the past year: "I feel guilty that I haven't managed them well; they are very outspoken, very selfish, not doing well in school."

Near the end of the first session I outlined some aspects of IPT for the patient. I suggested that we plan to meet weekly for about 16 weeks, that we continue to try to understand some of the factors that have contributed to her depression, and that we develop a plan to work on the major problem areas in her life. I indicated that IPT has been quite effective in reducing the symptoms of depression and that one goal of treatment would be to get over the current episode of depression and to learn ways of preventing depression in the future. She said, "that's what I'm concerned about . . . getting depressed again." We discussed the course of recurrent depression, comparing it to diabetes, arthritis, or other persistent illnesses, and agreed to work toward reducing her vulnerability to depression.

In sessions 2 and 3, we continued to review the symptoms of depression and the life events associated with the onset and course of her illness over the past year. We also continued to conduct an inventory of the important interpersonal relationships in her life currently and in the past. I suggested that we might try to identify one or two major problems to focus on that seem to be contributing to her depression. She talked about trying to accomplish more at work but still feels depressed, angry, and irritable. She related an incident in which her daughter was refusing to go to school, and they screamed and shouted at each other. She stated: "I wonder how good my judgment is . . . I know teenagers are difficult, but we seem to be constantly struggling for authority . . . I really feel drained . . . before my husband went to the nursing home they listened to him . . . now I'm the authority figure."

I said, "it sounds like there was a big change in all your relationships after he went to the nursing home." She agreed. I asked about any supportive relationships now, and she mentioned a female friend at work and a male friend of her husband's. She continued to describe recent conflicts with the children about school, boyfriends, and visits with their father. She talked about the difficulty all of them are having dealing with their feelings about his illness and imminent death, stating, "knowing that someone is going to die is a weird thing . . . I've gone through different stages from being angry to accepting it . . . and then he didn't die which was very confusing . . . and I got angry at him for leaving me with the kids. Now I feel I have to get on with my life in spite of what happens to him." I pointed out that she has been anticipating his death and going through a normal process of grief and mourning.

She described her mother's recent interest in her welfare, buying new furniture for the house and clothes for the children. She has mixed feelings about her mother's activities and talked about how hard it is to experience pleasure when you're depressed: "even from things that would ordinarily make you feel good." She expressed concern about her judgment, and I pointed out that it is difficult to make decisions when depressed, and suggested that she would be better able to use good judgment when her depression has improved. She described a recent discussion with her children about their father's illness. "They don't like to admit that he is dying and it hurts me when they cry. It makes me cry too [she is tearful]. They struggle with the changes they see in him." I said, "yes, you are all trying to cope with many changes in the best way you can." She then seemed to feel more empathic toward the children, talking about them struggling with their biracial identity, and how that gets played out in their relationships with their parents and grandparents.

The theoretical and empirical bases of IPT (Klerman et al., 1984) suggest that there are four major problem areas associated with the onset of depression. These are delayed grief, role disputes, role transitions, and interpersonal deficit. It is important in the first few sessions of IPT to try to select one or two of these problem areas to focus on throughout the course of treatment. It seemed to me that the patient was appropriately grieving the loss of a closer relationship with her husband and anticipating his death. Also, she was not living an isolated, lonely lifestyle characteristic of interpersonal deficit. I therefore thought that role transition and/or role dispute would be the most useful areas to focus on in the therapy. Since her depression began around the time her husband went into a nursing home, causing many changes in her life and close relationships, I chose to focus on role transition initially. Also it is often easier for patients to talk about struggling to cope with changes in their life than with disputes in important relationships, which may be more effectively worked on later in the therapy when the patient is more comfortable and the alliance is stronger.

Near the end of the third session I expressed my opinion to the patient that she was suffering from a major depressive illness that seemed to be related to the important changes that had taken place in her life in relation to her husband's illness, and particularly to his going into a nursing home. I suggested that we try to understand more about those changes in her role as a wife and mother, as well as other important areas of her life, with the goals of alleviating her depression and improving the quality of her interpersonal relationships. We agreed to that plan for our work together. I also pointed out that depression could be treated with medication as well as psychotherapy, but that in her case I believed that we could accomplish our goals without medication, and she agreed. We therefore embarked on the middle phase of IPT, which would last about 10 weeks.

Middle Phase: Facing Transition and Conflict

The patient began session 4 by stating she was feeling better. "I had more energy this week, which was nice." She described bringing her husband home for a visit over the Christmas holiday, and even though it was difficult, she didn't get so upset. Also he was rehospitalized after falling out of bed, and "I felt like screaming at first, but then I calmed down and was able to handle it." She described friends visiting them over the holiday, her husband participating in conversations . . . "probably the closest thing to normal we've had in the past year. That gave me some pleasure." She talked with sadness about how they had struggled together for 15 years saying, "death may pull us apart . . . even now he has his own world and I have mine . . . he couldn't live with us anymore." I suggested it must have been very painful and difficult for her to come to that conclusion. She replied, "I realized after Christmas how final our separation is . . . it was more like a good friend coming to visit for the holiday." I said it must be hard for her and the children to know how to fit into these two separate worlds. She agreed and said, "I'm not sure how to help them . . . I don't know how to soften the reality for them . . . sometimes they blame me for the fact that he's in a nursing home . . . but they seemed more understanding after his visit . . . they realized how sick he is and how much care he needs."

We continued to talk about the many changes that had taken place in the family in relation to her husband's illness, and I said it was interesting that she had not gotten depressed before he went into the nursing home. She responded: "I had all kinds of things to deal with . . . he was in and out of the hospital . . . it was like being in a tornado . . . then he went to the nursing home, and the tornado was over. I looked around at the devastation in my life . . . it felt like my kids had been ignored for a year while I was trying to take care of him . . . there's only so much you can do." She went on to talk about feeling disappointed and angry at her husband and children for not appreciating all her efforts. We discussed the fact that all of them had been hurting, were under tremendous stress, and might find it harder to be sympathetic toward each other's needs. She said, "I've tried not to let these experiences destroy me," and talked about feeling guilty and sad while "trying to keep a happy face." I suggested she was struggling with a lot of feelings such as fear, resentment, guilt, anger, sadness, and disappointment that may be contributing to her depression. We discussed how expressing those feelings here in our sessions might allow for some relief of the stress and tension and might lead to some reduction of her depressive symptoms.

Throughout the next several sessions we continued to focus on the theme of her attempts to cope with major changes in her life in the face of painful conflicting feelings, and her depression continued to improve. She said, "things seem to be falling into place . . . I'm dealing with the children better, sleeping better, not so anxious, have more energy, and the kids seem more reasonable." I pointed out the interactive process: "As you become less depressed, less irritable, have more energy, they respond in more positive ways." She went on to talk about how the children were expressing fear that they might lose their mother, too. We agreed that was a typical reaction after the loss of one parent through death or divorce. She continued to struggle with feelings of guilt and said that "probably guilt delayed my decision to place him in a nursing home. I'm getting chest pains thinking about doing that . . . I feel very anxious now . . . like until death do us part . . . I probably feel guilty about hurting my parents, too, by getting married to someone they can't accept."

I suggested that a pattern of not accepting and dealing with painful realities had been prominent in her family, and learning that pattern had made it more difficult for her to deal with her husband's illness. She described what it was like to go back for her brother's wedding, and for the first time in 15 years had to deal with all the feelings and reactions of her whole family. Her anxiety about that also contributed to her decision to seek help.

As her depression improved, she noted that her work was going better, and in fact she was promoted to a more responsible position. "I still feel nervous at times, but my anger is subsiding, I'm concentrating better, and I don't worry so much about losing my mind." I agreed that she was making progress and began to shift the focus more toward interpersonal dispute, especially with her husband. "He is complaining about me not visiting him enough . . . I feel sad about that, but he's so selfish . . . much more since he got sick. We loved each other a lot . . .

had a nice, easy relationship . . . now it's all gone." She also expressed a lot of anger toward her mother who "always managed to keep me under control . . . until I got married." She informed me that her mother was planning to visit her in several weeks. "It will be a real shock for her . . . she hasn't seen the kids for 4 years." I suggested we continue to talk about her relationship with her mother in anticipation of her visit.

By the midpoint of the therapy (session 8) she was "feeling much better . . . doing okay at work . . . settling in with the children . . . the flat feeling [depression] has just about completely gone." I reminded her that we were halfway through the treatment, and we spent some time reviewing the past 8 weeks. We agreed that there has been considerable improvement in her depression and the impact it was having on her life. She is communicating better with her children and is working out some of the conflicts in her relationships with them. She is functioning much better at work and is no longer fearful of losing her job. She has become aware of many painful feelings about the changes in her life and is expressing those feelings in her work with me. We agreed to spend some of our remaining time together focusing on the continuing conflicts, especially with her husband and mother.

In session 9, the patient talked about her mother's recent visit. "She did pretty well while she was here . . . wasn't very patient with some of the teenager behavior, but she seemed to like the kids . . . and it was nice to have someone else in the house." She said her mother did try to control her behavior at times, rearranged the furniture and drapes, "but I didn't make a big issue out of it . . . in fact I missed her after she left." She also talked to her husband's social worker and doctor and got a better understanding of his condition. "He's responding to treatment . . . might be able to live for quite a while."

We talked about how their relationship has changed over the past 2 years. He is much more dependent on her, can't help her with problems or meet her needs, and she is angry about that. When I asked how she was dealing with her anger, she said "I try to ignore it . . . I've done everything I can, and he's given me very little comfort." I asked how that was affecting her, and she responded "if he wasn't so sick I would probably divorce him . . . but I can't do that . . . and I feel trapped and angry and think if he would just die . . . then I feel guilty about that . . . I'll be 37 next month . . . don't I have the right to some pleasure in the rest of my life [tearful] . . . I don't really have a husband any more." I said her feelings were understandable, and it might be useful for us to continue to talk about how she is trying to deal with him and also trying to put her life back together. "It's like I'm married, but I'm not married . . . maybe that is the hardest thing for me to talk about."

In the next session she continued to talk about conflicts with her husband in the past, describing how he moved from one job to another, didn't want to buy a house, had several affairs, etc. "I was often disappointed and angry with him." I asked if she had been able to let him know how she felt [she wasn't sure], because "I've noticed that you tell me about these very painful incidents with a big smile on your face." She replied, "If I don't I would just cry . . . have to detach myself. I was very disappointed with him . . . it affected our relationship." I indicated that I understood what she was struggling with but suggested that she might be able to express some of her feelings more directly here. She was somewhat resistant, saying "I don't want to think about it . . . it would upset me too much . . . I don't want to talk about how sad and angry I feel . . . especially at him for getting sick . . . it's too painful." I responded, "I agree that it's very painful, and you will have to decide what you can talk about. But it's been my experience that keeping feelings like that bottled up can lead to depression and anxiety, and it might be helpful to express some of them as directly as you can." She remained reluctant, saying "I don't know . . . so ugly . . . we had a lot of crappy times . . . still don't understand him . . . he hurts me so much even now . . . we have four or five bad times for every good time together." I asked if she could think of any ways to increase the good times. "I don't know . . . it might help to visit him more often . . . he would be happier . . . that would make things better for me." We ended the session talking about the possibility of negotiating some things with him and getting more control over how things go in their relationship.

In session 11 the patient talked about feeling better and being able to handle some difficult things. Her husband has been rehospitalized, and she has been discussing the issue with his doctors of using extreme measures to prolong his life. She also said she only had an occasional dispute with her children and has been able to continue to work "when other people are crumbling under the stress." I agreed that she seemed stronger, less depressed and better able to cope with many difficult situations in her life. "I'm beginning to think about what will happen when I stop coming here . . . will I begin to break under the stress . . . I wonder how well I actually am." I stated those were reasonable questions, that we still had five sessions to address them, but that I had no reason to think that her improvement would not continue. She went on to talk about her mixed feelings about seeing a psychiatrist, the stigma that still exists, and the fact that she had told her coworkers about coming here. I asked how she was feeling about coming here, and she replied, "at first I didn't think anybody could help me . . . but I was desperate . . . knew I had to do something . . . now I feel better . . . more realistic about things . . . the future won't be great, but I can handle it." She went on to talk about raising the children herself, about the possibility of remarrying . . . "I think I can have a good life."

In the next couple of sessions we continued to work on conflicts with her husband. She described her efforts to help him celebrate his birthday, which didn't go well. I was able to help her see that some of the problem centers around a battle for control and that his illness has deprived him of so much control of his life that he may resent her efforts to make decisions "in his interest." She continued to express a lot of anger at him "for not caring about the children" and "for abusing me." We talked about how she is trying to cope with her anger in ways that are less disruptive to her life.

Termination: Reinforcing Progress

In the last three sessions we continued to review the course of therapy, talk about progress that was made, deal with feelings about stopping and make plans for the future. She described how she is trying to avoid getting into battles over control with her husband and with the children. She continued to mourn the loss of the kind of life they had before he got so sick. We discussed how difficult it had been for her to express her feelings more directly in the past, and she expressed some anger at her husband for getting sick, and at God for letting that happen. She described sitting down with the children, talking about their father's situation, and crying together. She also said she stopped having anxiety attacks on the job, was doing better, and was being considered for a supervisory position. I pointed out that she was doing well in several areas that we had decided to focus on: Her depressive symptoms have improved, her comfort and performance on the job improved, and her relationships with the children and her mother were a lot better. She has made some progress in improving her relationship with her husband, but that was still the most difficult area. "Yes, but the future seems better to me . . . I realize now that there are pleasant things in addition to the painful ones . . . and life goes on."

We talked more about the stigma surrounding mental illness and its treatment, and how that made it difficult for her to seek help. "It's a shame more people can't get help . . . I'm very pleased . . . I've learned to face some things about myself . . . one example is the issue of getting into the middle of things . . . I would have spent my whole life doing that . . . it's a tremendous relief not to have to do it." I agreed that she had been able to extricate herself from some of the conflicts with the children, between her mother and the children, her husband and the children, her husband and his doctors, etc. "We've done a lot . . . I no longer have that ugly, flat, depressed feeling . . . I would have been happy just with that, and I think we've accomplished a lot more . . . I've expelled a lot of the bitterness I had when I came in here . . . I didn't even realize how angry I was . . . I'm beginning to put my relationship with my husband in perspective . . . it wasn't the worst, it wasn't the best . . . it's nice to begin to feel that things are good again."

I asked if there were things we hadn't been able to accomplish or things about our work together that she was disappointed with. "We've accomplished more than I thought we would . . . I didn't expect too much . . . my mother has a much better relationship with the kids, but my father hasn't changed much . . . and I still don't handle money too well . . . I get anxious about the bills, and I hate it." I suggested that she could continue to work on some of those issues in the future. I also asked if she had found any ways to enjoy herself more—to experience more pleasure. "Yes, I have more fun with the kids, and even my husband occasionally . . . I've started sewing and reading again . . . using my time better."

In the last session she described a return of some symptoms, feeling more anxious and having difficulty sleeping. We discussed them as a transient reaction to the end of therapy and some apprehension about the future. She described having another conversation with the children about what would happen when their father dies. They discussed the issue of dying versus continuing to suffer, possible funeral arrangements, her husband's wish to have his friend sing at the funeral, etc. She became tearful and continued to mourn as we talked about the expectation that her feelings of grief will return on holidays, birthdays, and times of loss, like the end of therapy. She said, "We've been discussing that for the last 3 or 4 weeks, and I feel better about stopping . . . I think we've covered the major things . . . once a week for 4 months isn't a lot, but we've done very well . . . I really feel good about things . . . now I have a future." I asked about the areas she would like to continue to work on in the future. "I'd like to be more realistic . . . see things the way they are, which is sometimes painful . . . I need to be less controlling of my children, and in other relationships, too." I said I had enjoyed the opportunity of getting to know her and working with her and indicated I felt comfortable stopping for now. "I do, too . . . I can call and get more help if I need it . . . I'm glad I came . . . thank you."

DISCUSSION

This case illustrates the successful and rather typical use of IPT to treat a patient with major depression. Careful research has demonstrated that IPT is effective in treating approximately 70% of patients with depression (Elkin et al., 1989; Frank et al., 1990; Frank et al., 1991). The patient maintained a positive transference and good therapeutic alliance throughout the course of therapy, so I was able to follow the recommendation (Klerman *et. al.*, 1984) to avoid focusing on or interpreting the transference unless it begins to interfere in a major way with the therapeutic work. She did not manifest much resistance except in relation to her angry feelings and death wishes toward her husband which with gentle encouragement from me she was eventually able to express, leading to considerable improvement in her depressive symptoms. I admired the rather heroic struggle in which she was engaged as she attempted to cope with the major losses and changes in her life, and maintained empathic feelings toward her during our work together.

She manifested some histrionic personality traits, which did not interfere in any major way with the ongoing work and did not become a focus of the therapeutic interventions. One dynamic factor that seemed important was her strong need to be a caretaker, illustrated by her efforts to care for a very sick husband at home while raising four children and maintaining a full-time demanding job as a social worker. Her depression began when she gave up some of those caretaking responsibilities and placed her husband in a nursing home. That role transition, as well as the subsequent changes and disputes in her interpersonal relationships became the focus of therapy. She was able to recognize her pattern of attempting to control other people's behavior and putting herself in the middle of other people's conflicts. As the treatment progressed, she was able to change some of that controlling and intrusive behavior, leading to a decrease in tension and anxiety and more satisfaction and enjoyment in those relationships.

Typically, the patient experienced apprehension, increased anxiety, and a transient recurrence of some of the presenting symptoms as we approached the end of our work together. We were able to focus on her concerns and feelings during the process of termination, and we both felt comfortable about stopping after 16 sessions. She was seen for follow-up evaluations at 6, 12, and 18 months. Her depression did not recur, she did not seek further treatment, and was continuing to do well in her professional activities and interpersonal relationships.

REFERENCES

Cornes, C. L. (1990). Interpersonal psychotherapy of depression (IPT). In R. Wells & V. Giannetti (Eds.), *Handbook of the Brief Psychotherapies* (pp. 261–276). New York: Plenum Press.

Elkin, J., Shea, J. T., Watkins, S. D., Imber, S. M., Sotsky, J. F., Collins, D. R., Glass, D. R., Pilkonis, P. A., Leber, W. R., Docherty, J. P., Fiester, S. P., & Parloff, M. B. (1989). National Institute of Mental Health Treatment of Depression Collaborative Research Program: General effectiveness of treatments. *Archives of General Psychiatry, 46*, 971–982.

Frank, E., Kupfer, D. J., Perel, J. M., Cornes, C., Jarrett, D. B., Mallinger, A. G., Thase, M. E., McEachran, A. B., & Grochocinski, V. J. (1990). Three-year outcomes for maintenance therapies in recurrent depression. *Archives General Psychiatry, 47*, 1093–1099.

Frank, E., Kupfer, D. J., Wagner, E. F., McEachran, A. B., Cornes, C. L. (1991). Efficacy of interpersonal psychotherapy as a maintenance treatment of recurrent depression: Contributing factors. *Archives General Psychiatry, 48*, 1053–1059.

Klerman, G. L., Weissman, M. M., Rounsaville, B. J., & Chevron, E. S. (1984). *Interpersonal psychotherapy of depression*. New York: Basic Books.

5

Brief Cognitive Psychotherapy of Panic Disorder

BRAD A. ALFORD

INTRODUCTION

In the clinical treatment of panic disorder, the standard course of cognitive therapy has been shown to be an effective alternative to psychopharmacotherapy (Beck & Greenberg, 1988). Further, outcome studies have shown response to treatment to often be quite rapid, with reported panic attacks significantly reduced—and sometimes eliminated altogether—after only a few sessions (Sokol, Beck, Greenberg, Berchick, & Wright, 1989). Consistent with these findings, brief, focused cognitive psychotherapy may be the treatment of choice for certain uncomplicated panic disorder cases where agoraphobia is not severe (Alford, Beck, Freeman, & Wright, 1990).

Cognitive therapy of panic disorder is designed to enhance awareness and realistic interpretation of normal physiological responses or sensations associated with anxiety. If misperceived, such symptoms can escalate via catastrophic misinterpretation in a "vicious cycle" leading to panic. For example, often (as in the case described in this chapter)

BRAD A. ALFORD • Department of Psychology, University of Scranton, Scranton, Pennsylvania 18510.

Casebook of the Brief Psychotherapies, edited by Richard A. Wells and Vincent J. Giannetti. Plenum Press, New York, 1993.

pounding heartbeat is misinterpreted as impending "heart attack," which results in increased fear and, consequently, further increases in heart rate. Further increases in heart rate may then be mistakenly taken as evidence for the initial misinterpretation, thereby increasing the errant belief.

In the treatment approach presented in this chapter, the primary focus is to correct the panic patient's view of the nature of the sensations and symptoms associated with panic attacks. Thus, treatment focuses on the patient's subjective, frequently idiosyncratic beliefs regarding what it means to experience anxiety phenomena. Through use of guided discovery and other cognitive correction techniques, patients learn to intervene to disrupt the escalation of symptoms.

In a recent theoretical paper, Lazarus (1991) argues the necessity to take the private meaning of events into account to understand emotional responses, as follows:

> It is not the physical properties of the environment that count in the emotion process, but its subjective meanings. Therefore, the objective environment, physically speaking, is often irrelevant, and it is subjective meanings that we need to understand. (p. 831)

This theoretical formulation is consistent with Beck's cognitive theory of psychopathology and is *applied* in the practice of cognitive therapy. The following case explicates a brief, focused cognitive treatment of the specific distorted private meanings and misinterpretations typically found in panic disorder.

Case Identification, Background Information, and Presenting Complaints

The case used to illustrate brief, focused cognitive psychotherapy of panic was an 18-year-old female evaluated by use of the Structured Clinical Interview (SCID) (Spitzer, Williams, & Gibbons, 1987) for DSM-III-R. Axis I diagnosis was found to be Panic Disorder with Mild Agoraphobia (DSM-III-R 300.21). An interview by a consultant psychologist independently confirmed this diagnosis. The patient's panic symptoms had begun 8 months prior to therapy. Average frequency of panic attacks was reported to be approximately four per month. Symptom intensity had become increasingly more severe over the previous 2 months.

Treatment for panic had first been sought 3 days prior to referral. At that time the patient had rated panic attacks as "4–Extremely Severe" on the 1- to 5-point scale of severity on Lazarus's Life History Questionnaire. Prior to the current presenting problems, there was no history of psychiatric disorder. The patient had never taken medications for emotional disorder.

The Beck Anxiety Inventory (BAI) (Beck, Epstein, Brown, & Steer, 1988) and the Beck Depression Inventory (BDI) were administered prior to each therapy session. The Beck Hopelessness Scale (BHS) was administered prior to the first and last sessions. Symptoms obtained on these measures were judged during clinical evaluation and SCID assessment to be associated with or entirely secondary to panic disorder.

In order to ascertain "baseline" frequency of panic, the patient recorded—based on recall—all past panic attacks that had occurred during the preceding 30 days. At least three distinct major attacks had occurred in restaurants over the previous 30 days, during each of which she left the situation due to panic. Over the same period, she had experienced three additional milder attacks. One of these less severe attacks occurred on a subway, one in a psychologist's office during testing 3 days prior to her referral, and one in a theater the day before treatment began.

Treatment Process

In order to monitor continuously the impact of treatment, panic attack frequency was recorded daily by the patient during treatment. A "Panic Log" was used for this purpose and included the following six points of information: (1) date, time, and duration of the panic attack; (2) situation in which the panic attack occurred and severity of the attack (1–10); (3) description of the panic attack symptoms and sensations experienced; (4) interpretation of the sensations and accompanying thoughts and images; (5) whether the attack was a "full-blown" attack or not, and, if not, an explanation why; and (6) the patient's response to the panic—"What did you do?"

A total of four consecutive daily individual therapy sessions, approximately 50 minutes each, were conducted. The first treatment session focused on presentation of the cognitive model of treatment for panic. Consistent with the model developed for treatment of depression, this didactic presentation was as much as possible based on Socratic dialogue, with elicitation of patient feedback throughout. The therapist discussed with the patient the nature and symptoms of anxiety and panic, suggesting that she observe how degree of anxiety is a function of her perception of threat in relation to her personal perception of resources available to cope with the threat. This was described as the "risk/resources ratio," and was presented as one way to explain how anxiety is a normal response to the sense of vulnerability.

The nature of the autonomic nervous system was explained, and further discussion focused on the manner in which autonomic nervous system responses relate to the catastrophic misinterpretation model. Throughout this educative process, an emphasis was placed on the relationship between physiological sensations, misinterpretation, and panic. In presenting this model, the patient was in effect "socialized" to the cognitive conceptualization of panic disorder.

By communicating explicitly the theoretical perspective of the therapist, collaboration was facilitated. Additionally, this conceptualization served to set the stage for subsequent observation by the patient, during completion of homework assignments, to support (or refute) empirically the presented formulation. Seen from this perspective, the central clinical intervention was sharing with the patient the Beckian cognitive theoretical view of panic and encouraging the patient to test it on herself.

During the initial evaluation, the patient had described subjective experience of panic attacks as follows: "It's like when you're playing dodgeball when you're a kid, you know, that panic, like when there's that second when you're not sure whether that ball's going to hit you or not." Prior to treatment, she appeared aware only of what she called "fear" during the panic attacks. Consistent with cognitive therapy principles generally, the goal of therapy was first to recover automatic thoughts underlying this affect. A precise description of the patient's typical panic attack was therefore obtained, and the following panic scenario was identified: (1) nausea in stomach, (2) heart racing, (3) shaky, (4) muscle tension, (5) difficulty breathing, and (6) leave the situation.

When asked, "Before you leave [panic situations], do you notice any images or thoughts?," she replied, "I never really thought about that." At this point in treatment, the patient was entirely unconscious of the catastrophizing process. However, when directly questioned, "Do the symptoms themselves scare you?", she replied emphatically, "Oh, yeah!" (Note here the rapidity with which specific panicogenic unconscious material may be brought to the patient's attention.) The following dialogue demonstrates how subsequent discussion in this area assisted in orienting the patient to the catastrophic misinterpretation model:

PT: I've felt a couple of times like I was going to have a heart attack.
TH: Tell me about that.

PT: It's just like, it starts to beat so hard, and so fast, that, I mean, it *hurts*, and you just think, you're just like sitting there going (breathes rapidly to demonstrate how she hyperventilates).
TH: What was the effect, do you think, of that particular image or idea on the symptoms themselves?
PT: Oh, well, they get worse, as soon as you think . . . (pause).
TH: They get worse?
PT: Yeah.
TH: All right. Now, let's say that this is part of the process that's happening with you, that the symptoms are responding to these negative automatic thoughts or images, O.K.? Is that a possibility, that they are?
PT: I guess so.
TH: You'll have to notice in the situations that come up whether that happens or not, O.K.?
PT: If I get worse when I think about what's happening?
TH: If the image itself, when you have the thought of a heart attack—I guess it's obvious that that would be frightening.
PT: (laughing) Yeah.
TH: So you have a bodily sensation here at this point in the spiral of anxiety (pointing to diagram). The next step, thoughts that the sensation is a sign of catastrophe, that you're going to have a heart attack. What do you think happens to your thoughts when your heart rate does in fact go up? Because you said it would increase when you had this fear . . .
PT: Uh-huh.
TH: What would you think then?
PT: I just get really scared, and I have to get out of the situation that I'm in. I mean, I *have* to.
TH: O.K. So you see what's happening there. You perceive a danger, which would lead to more anxiety; the anxiety would make the symptoms worse, would make the heart rate even faster; and, you interpret that, then, as "I really *am* going to have a heart attack." Right?
PT: Yeah, but only fleetingly, you know, and then I go "I'm not going to have a heart attack, but I've got to get out of here!"
TH: O.K.
PT: But, I mean, *fleetingly,* I've also thought all kinds of, you know, I'm sure . . .

In addition to panic disorder, assessment showed this patient to have clinically significant levels of hopelessness and depression. As noted above, these symptoms were judged during clinical evaluation and SCID assessment to be associated with or entirely secondary to panic disorder. More specifically, because the patient could see objectively (when not experiencing panic) that her behavior was unrealistic, she had additional negative interpretations that her panic response meant she must be a "weak and pathetic" person.

To treat this psychopathological process, reattribution was used as a strategy to challenge these negative views of self. Reattribution focused on the explanation that misinterpretation of physiological sensations and the subsequent vicious cycle could better account for her panic experiences. That is to say, the anxiety/panic conceptualization—as originally presented—was once again invoked as a reasonable and sufficient explanation for the panic, thereby making alternative "theorizing" unnecessary (i.e., her own "theory" that the panic was due to her being a "weak and pathetic" person was no longer necessary as an explanation). To further enhance self-confidence, strategies of distraction and "rational response" were introduced as resources to be used against the panic symptoms. These strategies were discussed as techniques she could learn in order to interrupt the catastrophic interpretation, and, therefore, the panic itself.

In-office "panic inductions" were used to create immediate experience of panic sensations during the second and third therapy sessions. (Naturally, it is essential to make certain the patient has received a recent complete physical examination to rule out medical conditions that would be adversely affected by such a procedure.) The patient was instructed to hyperventilate, and this produced the following report of specific sensations: (1) feelings of unreality, (2) heart racing, (3) shakiness, (4) heart pounding, (5) tension, (6) tight muscles, and (7) breathlessness. In comparing these sensations to those associated with a typical panic attack, the patient found them to be highly similar. This exercise demonstrated to her satisfaction that normal physiological and psychological response to hyperventilation could create sensations like those experienced during spontaneous panic attacks. (Alternative methods of inducing paniclike symptoms may be employed for this purpose, such as strenuous exercises or presentation of disturbing visual patterns; see Beck & Greenberg, 1988).

From this point in treatment, the patient was encouraged to continue to evaluate further the meaning of this discovery. Consistent with cognitive theory regarding panic disorder etiology, in-office panic induction was followed by guided discovery to facilitate decatastrophizing of specific physiological sensations misinterpreted by the patient as dangerous. Collaborative exploration of sensations and thoughts following panic induction found the core cognitive component of this patient's panic disorder to be interpretation of rapid, pounding heartbeat as signaling possible "heart attack."

Hyperventilation was used to induce panic during sessions 2 and 3, but not the fourth (final) session. Rather, session 4 focused on review of the cognitive model of panic and rehearsal of realistic cognitive response

TABLE 1. Client Change on Key Clinical Measures

Measure	Session 1	Session 2	Session 3	Session 4
BAI[a]	23	7	11	5
BDI[b]	19	12	13	8
HS[c]	12	—	—	6
PA[d]	1	0	0	0

[a]Beck Anxiety Inventory.
[b]Beck Depression Inventory.
[c]Hopelessness Scale.
[d]Panic Attacks.

to automatic thoughts associated with sensations previously misinterpreted in the manner delineated above. Another focus of session 4 was discussion of success the patient had experienced the day before (following session 3) in returning to eat in a restaurant where she had previously experienced severe panic, a place that she had previously been avoiding.

Although she identified previous cognitive response to pounding heartbeat in that restaurant as "I'm going to die," she reported that, this time, "Everytime my heart rate increased I'd say, it's O.K., it's no big deal, I'm just sitting here in the restaurant, it's O.K." When asked, "How strongly did you believe the rational response?", she replied, categorically, "I believed it." It was clear that the course of brief, focused cognitive therapy administered to this particular patient had eliminated the panicogenic meaning she attributed to rapid pounding heartbeat associated with anxiety. Consequently, she reported an anxiety level in that situation of only "2" on a scale of intensity from 0 (none) to 10 (most severe). By interrupting the "vicious cycle" through realistic cognitive response, anxiety level did not escalate to the point of panic in this previously feared situation. Table 1 shows symptom report throughout treatment.

CLINICAL ISSUES

One of the central clinical issues in brief treatment of panic is the question of when one should deviate to shorten the usual standard course of cognitive therapy. Two obvious considerations include the presence of other disorders and patient response to treatment.

Treatment response was highly positive in this case. Following the fourth session, the patient did not feel the need for subsequent sessions.

(Consistent with the principle that cognitive psychotherapy promotes a *collaborative* therapy process, the patient should be allowed to play a role in determining the length of treatment.) The usual course of 12 to 20 weekly sessions was, therefore, not conducted.

Pinkerton and Rockwell (1990) have advanced an "eclectic" approach to the determination of when to end brief therapy, suggesting termination should be consistent with the goals of treatment and the nature and focus of the therapeutic relationship. Consistent with their observations, in the case described here, termination was considered to be appropriate because (1) the development of a "therapeutic relationship" had not been a central focus during the 4-day course of treatment; rather, treatment of this specific Axis I disorder had been highly problem-centered; (2) the patient had obtained what she wanted from therapy and felt ready to terminate; (3) the door was left open, so to speak, for a return to treatment as needed (cf. Pinkerton & Rockwell, 1990). (Point 3 is consistent, incidently, with N. Cummings's model of brief intermittent psychotherapy throughout the life span.) Given these considerations, patient and therapist concurred that treatment be terminated following the four consecutive daily sessions. Follow-up results supported this decision.

FOLLOW-UP

The patient was contacted by telephone for follow-up 1 month and 5 months after treatment. At 1 month, she reported no panic attacks. She admitted some mild worry of having another attack but felt she was working on this by making sure she did not avoid situations where she feared she might become anxious and have an attack. At 5 months, she again stated she had experienced no panic attacks since treatment and that she continued to approach situations that had previously been associated with panic.

OVERALL EVALUATION

A cognitive perspective on the brief psychotherapy of panic disorder was demonstrated in the described case. Initially being neither able to identify nor to correct misinterpretation of somatic sensations associated with anxiety, the patient had experienced an average of four panic attacks per month for the past 8 months. Upon identification of physiological sensations and negative automatic thoughts associated with the sensations, the patient was able to rapidly obtain some distance from her fearful thoughts. Armed with this new conceptual as well as experiential awareness of what was happening to her, panic attacks no longer occurred.

Specific observations support treatment integrity. The patient demonstrated her understanding of the cognitive model of panic during treatment sessions, and she reported using specific cognitive techniques, taught during therapy, in panic situations outside the therapist's office. For example, she reported at the beginning of the second session that she "tried rational responding last night, whenever I had a negative automatic thought." She spontaneously reported during the third session that she had used distraction when panic sensations began while she was on a bus, stating she had focused her attention on a man's shoes to distract herself from symptoms in that situation. During the fourth and final daily session, as was noted above, the patient reported utilizing what she had learned in cognitive therapy to prevent onset of panic in the restaurant where she had previously experienced her most severe panic attacks prior to treatment.

As treatment progressed over the four daily sessions, the patient reported a clinically significant decrease in symptoms of anxiety, depression, and hopelessness judged during previous clinical evaluation to be secondary to panic disorder. There was one panic attack reported the day prior to the first session, but none on days following the first, second, third, or fourth sessions. Additionally, the patient reported that she was not avoiding situations where she had previously experienced panic but rather was using cognitive skills learned in treatment to manage panic symptoms in these situations. Furthermore, during 1-month and 5-month follow-up interviews, the patient stated that she had experienced no panic attacks since treatment and that she continued to approach situations that had previously been associated with panic attacks. These results are certainly comparable to the best outcomes of standard cognitive therapy of panic disorder.

Finally, on an admittedly speculative, theoretical note, what aspects of this treatment may be responsible for facilitating rapid improvement? I will suggest one of several possibilities. Readers will observe that the content of the panic log (described in the treatment process section above) contains much in common with the "Daily Record of Dysfunctional Thoughts" used in the cognitive therapy of depression (see Beck, Rush, Shaw, & Emery, 1979). Such recordings serve to focus the patient's attention to specific problem symptoms, elicit conscious articulation of cognitions, and provide for evaluation of the veracity or accuracy of the interpretations or automatic thoughts that have been recorded. Use of such highly structured information-gathering devices designed to obtain symptom reports *as cognitive distortion occurs* may be one of the most active ingredients in successful brief cognitive therapy of depression, panic, as well as in the successful treatment of other disorders found to respond to this treatment approach.

It could be speculated that by rapidly encouraging the patient to monitor and evaluate cognitive, behavioral, and affective responses *outside* the formal therapy sessions, cognitive self-therapy extends the amount of constructive attention devoted to problem solving, thus resolving disorders in fewer formal therapy sessions. Such recording devices and noetic homework exercises emphasize awareness of relationships among cognitive, emotional, and behavioral aspects of human existence (the focus of cognitive therapy is not limited to thoughts alone), and may be found to play a special role in brief psychotherapy. In this manner, the collaborative and empirical nature of cognitive therapy—and its integrative potential—may provide a model for the brief psychotherapies generally (cf. Alford, 1991; Alford & Norcross, 1991; Beck, 1991). Along these same lines (i.e., the desirability of integration), Beck (1985) has noted:

> No one perspective is likely to provide an adequate explanation of clinical anxiety but a combination of different approaches can help fit together the various pieces of the puzzle. It is essential that investigators recognize the limitations and nonexclusivity of their own perspectives as well as recognize the contributions emerging from other vantage points. . . . A variety of research studies using a number of different models is most likely to advance our knowledge of the causes and treatment of clinical anxiety. (pp. 195–196)

This observation may be applied as well to the effectiveness of the various brief psychotherapies.

ACKNOWLEDGMENTS

Portions of this chapter are based on an article by Brad A. Alford, Aaron T. Beck, Arthur Freeman, and Fred D. Wright entitled "Brief Focused Cognitive Therapy of Panic Disorder," *Psychotherapy* (1990), *27*(3), 230–234. Correspondence should be addressed to Brad A. Alford, Department of Psychology, University of Scranton, Scranton, PA 18510.

REFERENCES

Alford, B. A. (1991). Integration of scientific criteria into the psychotherapy integration movement. *Journal of Behavior Therapy and Experimental Psychiatry, 22,* 211–216.

Alford, B. A., & Norcross, J. C. (1991). Cognitive therapy as integrative therapy. *Journal of Psychotherapy Integration, 1*(3), 175–190.

Alford, B. A., Beck, A. T., Freeman, A., & Wright, F. D. (1990). Brief focused cognitive therapy of panic disorder. *Psychotherapy, 27*(2), 230–234.

Beck, A. T. (1985). Theoretical perspectives on clinical anxiety. In A. H. Tuma & J. Maser (Eds.), *Anxiety and the anxiety disorders* (pp. 183–196). Hillsdale, NJ: Lawrence Erlbaum.

Beck, A. T. (1991). Cognitive therapy as *the* integrative therapy: Comments on Alford and Norcross. *Journal of Psychotherapy Integration, 1*(3), 191–198.

Beck, A. T., & Greenberg, R. L. (1988). Cognitive therapy of panic disorders. In R. E. Hales & A. J. Frances (Eds.), *American Psychiatric Press Review of Psychiatry* (Vol. 7, pp. 571–583). Washington, DC: American Psychiatric Press.

Beck, A. T., Epstein, N., Brown, G., & Steer, R. A. (1988). An inventory for measuring clinical anxiety: Psychometric properties. *Journal of Consulting and Clinical Psychology, 56*(6), 893–897.

Beck, A. T., Rush, A. J., Shaw, B. F., & Emery, G. (1979). *Cognitive therapy of depression.* New York: Guilford.

Lazarus, R. S. (1991). Progress on a cognitive-motivational-relational theory of emotion. *American Psychologist, 46*(8), 819–834.

Pinkerton, R. S., & Rockwell, W. J. K. (1990). Termination in brief psychotherapy: The Case for an eclectic approach. *Psychotherapy, 27*(3), 362–365.

Sokol, L., Beck, A. T., Greenberg, R. L., Berchick, R. J., & Wright, F. D. (1989). Cognitive therapy of panic disorder: A non-pharmacological alternative. *Journal of Nervous and Mental Disease, 177,* 711–716.

Spitzer, R. L., Williams, J. B. W., & Gibbons, M. (1987). *Instruction manual for the Structured Clinical Interview for DSM-III-R* (3/1/87 Revision). New York: Biometrics Research Department, New York State Psychiatric Institute.

6

Cognitive Therapy of Unipolar Depression

Brian F. Shaw, Joel Katz, and Irene Siotis

Introduction

For more than a decade, cognitive therapy (or cognitive/behavior therapy, CBT) has been considered as one of the standard treatments for unipolar depression. With the recognition that this approach is an efficacious treatment for depression and has considerable empirical support (see Dobson, 1989), clinicians began to test the limits of the conceptual framework of CBT with other populations (e.g., Freeman, Simon, Beutler, & Arkowitz, 1989).

This chapter will utilize the case-presentation format to illustrate several conceptual and practical issues relevant to the CB treatment of depressed patients. The clinician will be initially challenged to identify individuals who are likely to benefit from a short-term (approximately 20 sessions) CBT approach. Furthermore, he/she will want to manage meaningful problems, to address symptom changes, and to alter the propensity for future depressive episodes. The chapter will address the following issues associated with these challenges: selection criteria for short-term CBT, the ongoing assessment of depressive symptoms, and formulation of appropriate interventions. Following a case presentation,

---

Brian F. Shaw and Joel Katz • Department of Psychology, Toronto Hospital, 200 Elizabeth Street, Toronto, Ontario, Canada M5G 2C4. Irene Siotis • Department of Psychiatry, McMaster University, Hamilton, Ontario, Canada L8N 3Z5.

Casebook of the Brief Psychotherapies, edited by Richard A. Wells and Vincent J. Giannetti. Plenum Press, New York, 1993.

two treatment issues frequently encountered by CBT therapists will be discussed: managing the depressed patients with a combination of CBT and drug therapy and selecting specific interventions that are most likely to produce positive CBT change.

SELECTION CRITERIA FOR CBT

Considerable attention has been devoted to identifying the factors associated with positive outcome in various schools of psychotherapy. Psychotherapy research has demonstrated that the patients most likely to benefit from CBT respond positively to the treatment rationale, comply with homework assignments, and exhibit relatively fewer symptoms of depression and dysfunctional attitudes at the start of therapy (Fennell & Teasdale, 1987; Persons, Burns, & Perloff, 1988; Sotsky et al., 1991).

Safran, Segal, Shaw, and Vallis (1990) developed an interview-based assessment of nine criteria designed to (1) evaluate the patient's perception of the relevance/importance of the goals and tasks of cognitive therapy (as described by the interviewer), and (2) judge the patient's ability to engage in these tasks. The nine suitability items are as follows:

1. *Accessibility of automatic thoughts.* Can the patient report thoughts/images associated with feeling states related to his/her problems?
2. *Awareness and differentiation of emotions.* Can the patient identify and discriminate between different emotions (e.g., sadness, guilt, fear, anger)?
3. *Assuming personal responsibility for changes.* Does the patient view himself/herself as the agent of change (positive) or the passive recipient of treatment (negative)?
4. *Compatibility with cognitive therapy rationale.* Does the patient view the tasks and goals of CBT as relevant?
5. *Alliance potential: In-session evidence.* Does the patient form a working alliance with the interviewer?
6. *Alliance potential: Out-of-session evidence.* Is the patient able to form a relatively trusting relationship within a short time period using past relationships as the basis for judgment?
7. *Chronicity of problems.* Does the patient present with several chronic personal problems (this item is a negative indicator for a short-term intervention)?
8. *Security operations.* Does the patient present with significant defensive information processing strategies or interpersonal interactions designed to minimize anxiety.
9. *Focality.* Is the patient able to maintain a problem-oriented focus?

These suitability criteria are utilized to evaluate the likelihood that significant gains will be made in the usual 20-session, 16-week CBT protocol. A metric using 9-point rating scales may be used to obtain a numeric value that summarizes the patient's overall suitability for CBT.

Measurement of Depression

There are many methods of assessing depressive symptoms (see Shaw, Vallis, & McCabe, 1985), but for CBT it is important to use a standard instrument to identify target symptoms and to measure severity as well as change. One of the early practical decisions to be negotiated with the patient concerns his/her target symptoms (e.g., sadness, anhedonia, sleep disturbance) and most distressing life problems (e.g., changing relationship, employment, finances). CBT is designed to meet the following goals:

1. To provide patients with education and information about depression and its effects on thinking, feeling, behavior and physical functioning.
2. To increase activity; specifically, mastery and pleasurable activities.
3. To reappraise automatic thoughts.
4. To challenge dysfunctional attitudes.

In our clinic, we routinely use the SCL-90 (Derogatis, 1977), the Beck Depression Inventory (Beck et al., 1979) and the Hamilton Rating Scale For Depression (Hamilton, 1960) to identify the key target *symptoms*. Life problems are determined by interview. The goal of cognitive therapy is *not* to minimize or debate the patient's perception of his/her problems (or their apparent insolubility) but to address the target symptoms and the cognitive triad (a sense of worthlessness, helplessness, and hopelessness) before addressing the extent and meaning of the problem.

CBT Formulation

The formulation may be thought of as a series of hypotheses generated on an ongoing basis from the time of assessment to termination. As the formulation is likely to change with the progression of therapy, it is important to retain some flexibility in the formulating process particularly if new problems arise. In CBT, the formulation is discussed with the patient. Interventions are chosen based on both the formulation and the problems brought by the patient. Poor collaboration, unattended homework, poor feedback, or missed sessions may indicate among other explanations, an inaccurate formulation.

It may be useful to think of the formulation in terms of a hierarchy of cognitive accessibility that includes automatic thoughts, attitudes and assumptions, and self-schemata. Automatic thoughts (ATs) are usually accessible to the patient and may be spontaneously articulated by the patient at the first session. ATs provide the therapist with information about the patient's view of himself/herself, the world, and the future. Along with the patient's choice of words, cognitive distortions, and automatic thoughts provide starting material for the formulation. For example, a 25-year-old mother reported at the first interview:

> "There must be something wrong with me. My 2-year-old is driving me crazy, she never stays quiet, and I should be able to control her behavior. She never listens to me, but she always listens to her father. He only sees her 1 hour a day, and I spent all my time with her." The therapist can identify the cognitive distortions personalizing (something wrong with me) and all-or-nothing thinking (never stays quiet). Upon questioning, her automatic thoughts were: "There is something wrong with me." "I am not a good mother." She also viewed herself as failing as a wife. Her assumption was: "If I can't control my daughter's behavior, then I'm a failure."

At the level of attitudes and assumptions, information is less easily accessed. These assumptions reflect the values that guide an individual's thinking and behavior. Understanding the patient's dysfunctional attitudes early in the course of therapy guides the therapist's interventions. For example, subsequent inquiry revealed the aforementioned patient held dysfunctional attitudes that included a sense of self-worth based on how she evaluates her performance as a mother (i.e., a perfectionistic standard for motherhood against which she compared her performance). It is possible to hypothesize about this woman's self-schemata. With these dysfunctional attitudes about her role as a mother, she is likely to process information about her role as a mother, in a distorted manner. A self-schemata (bad mother) is *automatically* activated, and influences incoming information relating to the mother–child relationship.

How does this information help the process of therapy? One of the goals of the formulation is to guide the therapist in his/her choice of interventions. In this particular example, the therapist may teach the patient to recognize her cognitive distortions and recommend that she learn more about the behavior and development of 2-year-olds in an attempt to correct her unrealistic expectations. The reattribution of "failure" (i.e., looking for other explanations) and the use of imagery to identify successful coping (inconsistent with her negative self-schemata) are other possible interventions. As therapy progresses, the patient's vulnerability to future episodes of depression becomes understandable in terms of the relationship between her high standards of motherhood and her selective attention to problems with her child.

In summary, the formulation in CBT is an ongoing process. It is problem-based, and subsequent interventions are attempts to counter the patient's negative perceptions, to build coping skills, and maintain a problem-solving attitude. The hypotheses generated by the formulation are derived from the patient's thinking and behavior. If possible, the patient's automatic thoughts, dysfunctional attitudes, and self-schemata should be part of the final formulation.

Other Pretherapy Considerations

In general, the process of conceptualization or formulation involves an assessment of the patient's functioning in several domains. The cognitive therapist dealing with the depressed patient evaluates:

1. The cognitive triad—what thoughts/images does the patient have of him/herself, world, and future? From this point of view, symptoms such as self-criticism, helplessness, and hopelessness will be apparent.
2. Aspects of life that are most important to the patient and his/her self-concept usually expressed as an attitude reflecting relationships and/or aspirations and achievements (e.g., If people don't like me, then I'm worthless).
3. Target symptoms (i.e., symptoms of depression) and their relationship to automatic thoughts.
4. Life problems. Depression often stems from and/or causes real difficulties. These problems need to be resolved/addressed.
5. The patient's cognitive style including both biases in information processing (overgeneralization, selective abstraction) and attributional biases (i.e., blaming failures/problems on stable, internal characteristics while ignoring other salient and often contradictory information).

As a general rule CB therapists work on the patient's sense of hopelessness first and then address other target symptoms to facilitate change. A problem-solving approach is employed followed by a serious reappraisal of the patient's attitude/goals in life. These guidelines are illustrated in the next section.

CASE HISTORY

Mr. D. is a 31-year-old single man who referred himself to the Clinic because of difficulty finding work and past problems with relationships. Eighteen months earlier he had received dynamically oriented psychotherapy to address his interpersonal difficulties, but dropped out of therapy. At that time, he was engaged to a woman he had been seeing for 5 years, but suddenly cancelled the wedding plans. He was ambivalent about marriage and decided to seek help. Around the same time, he quit his job as a salesman after being bypassed for a promotion. To retaliate, he went to work for his company's major competitor but was soon fired. Although initially he viewed himself as having been "exploited" and "used," with time he came to the conclusion that he had been "disloyal and dishonest" for having retaliated against his employer by seeking employment with a competitor.

At the time of the initial assessment, he had been unemployed for 9 months, had ended his relationship with his former fiancée, and had not dated anyone since. He reported having felt depressed for approximately 2½ years with his symptoms increasing in severity over the past 6 months preceding the initial interview. His mood was depressed every day with a diurnal variation (worse in the morning). He felt hopeless and helpless about his situation and often cried. He was worried about his finances and lack of a job but was unable to motivate himself to find work. He had to push himself to get out of bed in the morning, and although he planned to look for work, he did not send out resumes or go to job interviews. He had difficulty concentrating and making decisions. He had little socialization as his only contacts, besides family, were people at the gym. He had a decrease in his sexual drive, a sleep disturbance with middle insomnia and, at times, early morning awakening. He had some fleeting thoughts of suicide, but he reported no plans or intent to harm himself.

His past history included a depressive episode at the age of 11 shortly before the divorce of his parents. He was treated with a "medication." There was no history of hypomania.

He was diagnosed as having a major depressive episode (DSM-III-R). His score on the Beck Depression Inventory (Beck et al., 1979) was 24, indicating moderate to severe depression. The therapist gave the patient an option of taking an antidepressant drug (Fluoxetine 20 mg) in combination with 20 sessions of Cognitive/Behavior Therapy as he reported having responded favorably to medication in the past.

The first five sessions of therapy focused on Mr. D.'s inability to find work. The target symptoms associated with this problem were avoidance, indecisiveness, and self-criticism. He felt anxious about job interviews, not knowing what to say about the loss of his last job and his current state of unemployment. As noted previously, he was extremely self-critical and had come to view himself as a failure. Several interventions were chosen to help Mr. D. begin to increase his job-seeking activities. Behavioral interventions (self-monitoring and scheduling of daily activities) were planned. It soon became apparent that Mr. D. was spending much of his time at the gym having almost entirely avoided job-seeking actions. Initially, Mr. D. had difficulty completing his self-help assignments, a manifestation of his avoidance behavior. Once a plan of action for job seeking was determined, the therapist worked on basic assertiveness/interviewing skills that Mr. D. could use in the interviews.

Mr. D. reacted to his previous job-related problems by blaming himself and being critical of his performance. He took excessive responsibility for his actions and concluded that he was not competent enough to achieve in a competitive environment. At this point, the therapeutic emphasis was changed from mainly behavioral approach to one based on cognitive interventions. He responded well to taking "an alternative perspective" to his self-defeating thoughts particularly once the therapist discussed his biased attributions of failure. This intervention was helpful in dealing with his sense of hopelessness about finding a new job. He tended to attribute his current difficulty to his perceived negative characteristics (dishonesty, disloyalty, lack of competence) and at the same time ignored other factors that contributed to his difficulty finding work (the economic recession and his lack of consistent effort). He had trouble asserting himself because his thinking was dominated by these self-criticisms. The therapist helped him with his biased thinking and improved his assertion skills.

Early in therapy, it became evident that one of Mr. D.'s attitudinal vulnerabilities to depression was his view of achievement. He defined his sense of worth by his accomplishments and thus, losing his job had threatened his sense of autonomy.

At session 6 (3 weeks into the treatment), Mr. D.'s symptoms had improved. His mood was brighter, he was crying less often, and he reported having more energy. However, his concentration, sleep, and indecisiveness remained problematic. His score on the BDI was 9, which indicated considerable improvement.

His relationship problems were addressed in the following sessions. Recall that Mr. D. had broken his engagement 2 years previously, and although he had not dated anyone since, a few weeks prior to starting therapy, he had met a woman who had attracted his interest. He was hesitant to contact her but with encouragement he eventually did so. They started dating, and he became extremely anxious about getting close to this woman. When it was time to become more intimate, he would leave.

During the next nine sessions, several interventions were used to decrease the amount of avoidance, anxiety, and indecisiveness Mr. D. experienced in this relationship. Mr. D. "had to be sure" of the outcome of the relationship before taking any chances or making a commitment. He could be intimate only if he was sure they would marry. He had to have a high degree of certainty and control prior to taking that added responsibility. Getting close meant that he would be hurt if the relationship ended. He had too much to lose emotionally and financially. She could find out who he *really* was and reject him. As he said "I am just human."

In most of Mr. D.'s other relationships, his need for "social approval" was notable. For example, at work around people, he tried to please them so they wouldn't hurt him. With time and understanding of his thinking and behavior, Mr. D. became closer to his girlfriend. He responded to several cognitive restructuring interventions and slowly started to understand his underlying dysfunctional attitudes.

One specific problem situation was his intolerance for his girlfriend's smoking. This became a major issue, and he had "to win" in their arguments about smoking. Interestingly, one of the reasons for his previous breakup had been the couple's inability to negotiate issues around religion. He felt that he couldn't give in as it was too threatening to him and his identity. In these situations, he became aggressive and either had to take control or, alternatively, leave.

By session 14, Mr. D. showed a return of several depressive symptoms. He felt angry, depressed, mildly hopeless, and helpless. He was more avoidant than he had been recently. He stopped dating and had avoided seeing his family for their Easter reunion. He wished he had improved more and was anxious about their reaction to him. By this time, he had a part-time job, but he was dissatisfied about his performance and the financial remuneration. These issues were revisited the way they had been in previous sessions with considerable improvement. It was explained to Mr. D. that during the course of recovery from depression, mood fluctuations are to be expected. These times are opportunities to practice his newly acquired skills. The last five sessions focused on his dysfunctional attitudes, a discussion of what to do if symptoms returned, and termination issues. Mr. D.'s attitudes regarding achievement and acceptance by others were challenged as in previous sessions. Although he was becoming increasingly aware, his level of understanding was still fairly superficial. Several events occurred in the last few weeks of therapy that brought more clarity to these concepts. Mr. D. had never mentioned to his ex-fiancée that he suffered from depression. This avoidance was an important issue for him. He wanted to tell her but was afraid she would reject him. He believed that having experienced a depression meant that he was a "weak, inadequate person" and "a failure." He didn't apply these standards to others but strongly believed them. He felt ashamed and embarrassed and concluded that she would reject him.

The homework assignment for Mr. D. was to talk to his ex-fiance and let her know about his depression. Notably, he demonstrated to himself that sharing this information did not result in rejection. On the contrary, he felt closer to her, and she spoke about her own problems. He felt there was more trust in the relationship as she had been caring in response to his disclosure, an important experience to counteract his dysfunctional attitude. In other words, he could utilize an alternative behavior (self-disclosure) that reinforced intimacy and trust.

With respect to other dysfunctional attitudes related to success achievement and perfectionism, at the beginning of therapy his exercising had become extremely competitive. He participated in a marathon and had been very dissatisfied with his performance. The therapist reviewed his performance and asked Mr. D. to get more information about what times would be expected for his level of running. It appeared that Mr. D.'s expectations were extremely unrealistic. He compared his performance to runners with 10 years' experience when he had been running for only 1 year. The goal at that point was for Mr. D. to run for pleasure instead of competition/self-worth. His long-term goal was to balance achievement and social approval. To achieve this goal, he needed to continue to practice alternative actions to these dysfunctional attitudes. He decided to increase his level of self-disclosure to reduce some of his structured exercise time (i.e., run without a watch), and to replace running with other unstructured, potentially pleasurable activities such as reading and crafts.

Another intervention was for Mr. D. to list the advantages and disadvantages of his old attitudes and his new behavior/thinking. This intervention reinforced the need for change. Termination issues were raised during the last few sessions. By the end, Mr. D. expressed some anxiety about terminating. He worried that he might need someone "to talk to," but he did not anticipate any particular problems. By the end of therapy, Mr. D. was self-employed in landscaping. He became reinvolved with his former fiancée, and they were working on their communication. He was still running and involved in training several hours per day, but he expressed the goal of reducing this time.

Challenging Automatic Thoughts versus Exploring Personal Meaning

A common tendency with less experienced therapists and students learning CBT is to adopt a technical or mechanical therapeutic approach. This error is especially evident when applying the CBT framework to the management of the depressed individual. The cognitive distortions (e.g., magnification, selective abstraction for negative information) of the depressed person may appear unrealistic and objectively untrue to the inexperienced therapist. As a result, he/she may resort to challenging or dismissing the patient's statements using counterargument and by offering well-intentioned, but therapeutically misguided, suggestions. While (1) marshaling evidence against distorted, unrealistic thoughts, (2) developing alternative explanations or other conclusions about oneself and the world, and (3) challenging beliefs and assumptions that lead to unrealistic conclusions about the world are important and effective tools of the CBT approach, it is essential to concentrate the therapeutic endeavor on a mutual exploration directed at understanding the meaning and anticipated consequences of these thoughts.

There are several potential hazards that mitigate against a successful outcome when premature or excessive attention is placed on disputing the logic of the patient's ideations, challenging beliefs, and problem-solving strategies. For one, patients, not unrealistically, may believe that the therapist does not understand them, the consequence being a paradoxical enhancement of the very negative thoughts that the therapist is attempting to modify. Therapists may tire of the tenacity with which a patient doggedly adheres to his or her beliefs despite information to the contrary. Therapist frustration, irritability, and anger may ensue (Beck, 1967), thus jeopardizing the patient–therapist bond. Difficulty in solidifying the therapeutic alliance or ruptures in an established alliance may lead to treatment failure or to treatment dropout. Excessive or premature use of these strategies tends to focus the therapeutic process on poorly informed interventions.

In contrast, our experience is that exploration of the meaning and associated consequences of dysfunctional thoughts points the way toward exposing affect-laden beliefs and attitudes. If a significant understanding of the patient's self-referent attitudinal vulnerabilities is to be achieved, it is extremely important to explore the meaning or bases for certain reactions. One useful therapeutic approach is to maintain an understanding of the patient's perceived loss (failure, perceived inadequacy) while intervening.

A question that frequently arises in the course of a CBT supervision is when to intervene with strategies geared toward a reappraisal of certain ideation and when to attempt to access emotions through exploring the meaning-based system of the depressed patient. Choice points present themselves on many occasions during a therapy hour. The therapist must decide when to pursue, change, or alternate between particular lines of inquiry. Factors that guide the therapist in deciding between such process-related strategies include the stage of therapy, level of depression and hopelessness, and the strength of the therapeutic alliance, particularly the patient–therapist bond. With inexperienced CB therapists early in the treatment, too little time is devoted to exploring the meaning-based system compared to the time allocated to the dispute of beliefs and the simple identification of distorted thinking. The aforementioned selection criteria to assess patient suitability for cognitive therapy (Safran, Segal, Shaw, & Vallis, 1990) that bear on the present discussion include rating scales designed to assess the accessibility of automatic thoughts and the patient's awareness and differentiation of various emotional states. These criteria not only help the therapist evaluate patient suitability for cognitive therapy but may also facilitate an exploration of the therapist's understanding of the patient.

EVALUATING AND REASSESSING PATIENT OUTCOME EXPECTATIONS

An essential part of the initial interview involves assessing the problems or issues most troublesome to the patient, obtaining an idea of what are the expectations he/she has for improvement, and deciding with the patient on a circumscribed domain for subsequent CBT intervention. During the initial interview, we routinely evaluate the patient's expectations for change in terms of his/her anticipated behaviors, feelings, and thoughts at the end of therapy. General questions that facilitate patient expression of outcome expectations include the following: "Imagine that you are at the end of an 18- to 20-week course of cognitive therapy. How would you like to have changed? What specific aspects of your self or your behavior would you like to be different, and what aspects would you like to remain as they are?" These are followed up with specific questions directed at elucidating behavioral, cognitive, and affective outcome expectations.

Several times during an 18- to 20-week course of CBT (more frequently as the termination date approaches), periodic reassessments are made of the patient's outcome expectations. Comparisons of these expectations with actual outcome to date are evaluated and discussed. Not only does this procedure foster the patient–therapist collaboration so characteristic of the cognitive approach, but it also provides a forum for refocusing the therapeutic tasks, and in some cases, reappraising the goals of therapy.

This point is exemplified by the following case material from an intelligent, 30-year-old, female patient who initially presented with multiple somatic complaints, severe self-criticism, difficulty relinquishing control in personal relationships, and what she described as "problems with intimacy." The patient had not completed her self-help assignments for weeks 1 and 2, an integral part of CBT that is an important predictor of therapy outcome (Primakoff et al., 1986). After several attempts to make the patient more comfortable with the task and to understand the impediments to this work, the therapist decided to work with the information provided by the patient in the sessions. The therapist began the seventh meeting with the following statements:

"At the very first meeting we had, you outlined a number of problem areas that you wanted help with as well as some of your expectations for how you would like to have changed at the end of therapy. This is our seventh meeting, and I'm wondering what your thoughts and feelings are with respect to these expectations. How well or poorly are we addressing the concerns you had when we first met? What changes have you begun to make, and where do you see room for further change?"

The patient responded that she, too, had been thinking about her progress to date and then wondered out loud whether therapy would really help her since she was aware of a "barrier" to discussing certain issues that she felt were private but believed "should" be discussed in order to improve.

The therapist decided to support the patient's sense of privacy by pointing to the patient's use of the word *should* and suggesting that perhaps she was not ready to discuss such personal matters with the therapist. He added that they could talk *about* the issues without discussing their content. They proceeded to explore the meaning and consequences to the patient of disclosing such information. The patient revealed fears that if other people knew that things in her life were not going well she would be perceived as "weak." With prompting from the therapist, she elaborated on the meaning of weakness and the perceived pity and rejection she anticipated when thinking about disclosing intimate material. She then reported a series of negative thoughts about how such disclosures would be received.

By reviewing the patient's expectations, it became clear that her belief that she could not improve unless she revealed intimate information about herself was impeding therapeutic progress by reinforcing her automatic self-critical judgments. When the therapist and patient attended to the personal meaning and consequences of self-disclosure, the patient concluded that progress could be made with further inquiry and began to discuss her thoughts and feelings.

Combining CBT and Drug Therapy

We have found that attribution theory is helpful in understanding and managing problems arising out of a combined treatment. Therapists treating patients with a combined psychotherapeutic and pharmacological approach may be faced with questions from the patient about how to explain changes or improvement. Some depressed patients attribute improvement to external factors (the medicine), while ignoring psychological aspects of the treatment (internal factors) that may also play a role. Alternatively, the therapist might be faced with the problem of a patient refusing to take medication because of dysfunctional attitudes about the meaning of taking medication (e.g., "If I take drugs I am a weak person. If I take medication I will rely on them to get better and I might become dependent on them to feel good").

Faced with this problem, the therapist can use several interventions. The attribution intervention may help the patient gain a sense of control over his/her disorder. The therapist might explore the patient's previous experience with medications. Of course, CBT and drug therapy may not be given by the same therapist, and the patient's belief that these interventions are independent ways to manage depression may be reinforced. The advantage of one therapist for both interventions is the reinforcement of the integrative approach (i.e., psychological and biological).

As previously mentioned, the management of a depressed patient with a combined CBT/psychopharmacological approach raises some specific issues related to dysfunctional thinking and attributional style. In the case of Mr. D., he readily separated his own action from the actions of the drug. He attributed positive symptom changes to the combination but attributed his attitudinal changes to his own efforts.

Summary

Cognitive/behavior therapy is an evolving system of psychotherapy, but the fundamentals of the CBT formulation and the selection of interventions remain essential. This chapter illustrated issues of patient selection, case formulations, and decisions about treatment intervention. Clinicians interested in using CBT are strongly discouraged from the seemingly simple application of techniques without a clear formulation and systematic consideration of the therapy interventions.

REFERENCES

Beck, A. T. (1967). *Depression: Clinical, experimental and therapeutic aspects.* New York: Harper & Row.

Beck, A. T., Rush, A. J., Shaw, B. F., & Emery, G. (1979). *Cognitive therapy of depression.* New York: Guilford.

Derogatis, L. R. (1977). *SCL-90 administration, scoring and procedures manual.* Baltimore, MD: Johns Hopkins.

Dobson, K. S. (1989). A meta-analysis of the efficacy of cognitive therapy for depression. *Journal of Consulting and Clinical Psychology, 57,* 414–429.

Fennell, M. J., & Teasdale, J. D. (1987). Cognitive therapy for depression: Individual differences and the process of change. *Cognitive Therapy and Research, 11,* 253–272.

Freeman, A., Simon, K. N., Beutler, L. E., & Arkowitz, H. (1989). *Comprehensive handbook of cognitive therapy.* New York: Plenum Press.

Hamilton, M. (1960). A rating scale for depression. *Journal of Neurology, Neurosurgery and Psychiatry, 12,* 56–62.

Persons, J. B. (1989). *Cognitive therapy in practice: A case formulation approach.* New York: Norton.

Persons, J. B., Burns, D. D., & Perloff, J. M. (1988). Predictors of dropout and outcome in cognitive therapy for depression in a private practice setting. *Cognitive Therapy and Research, 12,* 557–576.

Primakoff, L., Epstein, N., & Covi, L. (1986). Homework compliance: An uncontrolled variable in cognitive therapy outcome research. *Behavior Therapy, 17,* 443–446.

Safran, J. D., Segal, Z. V., Shaw, B. F., and Vallis, T. M. (1990). Patient selection for short term cognitive therapy. In J. O. Safran & Z. V. Segal (Eds.), *Interpersonal process in cognitive therapy* (pp. 229–238). New York: Basic Books.

Shaw, B. F., Vallis, T. M., & McCabe, S. (1985). The assessment of severity and symptom patterns in depression. In E. E. Beckham & W. R. Leber (Eds.), *Handbook of depression: Treatment, assessment and research* (pp. 372–407). Homewood, IL: Dorsey.

Stosky, S., Glass, D. R., Shea, T., Pilkonis, P., Collins, J. F., Elkin, I., Watkins, J. T., Imber, S., Leber, W., Moyer, J., & Oliveri, M. E. (1991). Patient predictors of response to psychotherapy and psychopharmacology: Findings in the NIMH Treatment of Depression Collaborative Research Program. *American Journal of Psychiatry, 148,* 997–1008.

Wells, R. A., & Giannetti, V. J. (Eds.). (1990). *Handbook of the brief psychotherapies.* New York: Plenum Press.

7

Brief Social Support Interventions with Adolescents

LAMBERT MAGUIRE

INTRODUCTION

Adolescence is a period of great change and strong emotions. It is also a time when friends are particularly significant and where mutual support, caring, and guidance are all needed. Social networks consisting of fellow adolescents are central in the process of helping teenagers to learn how to respond to difficult situations and crises throughout their lives. Thus the choice of friends becomes particularly important for young teens because these peers are so active in shaping behavior and attitudes. These networks and cliques define one's status and "image" to his or her fellow adolescents (Epstein, 1983).

As youngsters make the transition from family and childhood into peer groups and adolescence, several major decisions are made. They decide to spend less time with their family and more with their peers. In fact, at least half of their time is spent with peers, which is a definite shift for most adolescents (Czikszentmihalyi & Larson, 1984). Such shifts and decisions are rarely conscious, deliberate choices, but they are central life-change transitions that occupy much of the young adolescent's time.

LAMBERT MAGUIRE • School of Social Work, University of Pittsburgh, Pittsburgh, Pennsylvania 15260.

Casebook of the Brief Psychotherapies, edited by Richard A. Wells and Vincent J. Giannetti. Plenum Press, New York, 1993.

For instance, at some level, they need to decide whether their closest friends will be members of the popular clique, the jocks, the brains, the fast crowd, or the "rejects." Such cliques all have varying levels of status, although such perceptions may vary considerably from person to person. But the adolescent must choose a clique or groups of friends who share his or her interests, and that clique also becomes defined or ranked by other adolescents and cliques in terms of their social status or ranks.

The loss of membership in such cliques during early adolescence can be extremely difficult if not traumatic for some youngsters. This is particularly true for girls because girls between the ages of 12 and 16 rely more than boys do on their peers for loyalty, conformity, and intimacy. Young girls spend hours talking to each other, sharing ideas and secrets, and thus further developing their own views of the world as well as their view of themselves (Douvan & Adelson, 1966).

Abrupt and traumatic shifts in the social support system, particularly losses, can be extremely difficult for young adolescents who are so very reliant on these systems. When an especially vulnerable teenager suffers a major rejection or loss, the blow to his/her self-esteem can be devastating, particularly when one's sense of identity is so nebulous to begin with or is already negative.

Fortunately, in the volatile emotional life of adolescents, it is also a truism that self-esteem, behaviors, and emotions can also change dramatically for the better through appropriate intervention, particularly when the clinician is sensitive to the social system of the young client. Brief intervention with adolescents who are suffering from adjustment disorders can and must involve an understanding of how the social system was relevant in the etiology of the presenting problems as well as how to involve the social system in the amelioration of that problem. This social-system orientation to intervention with adolescent adjustment disorders is particularly salient for four reasons: (1) adolescents spend a great deal of time with peers as they move away from the family; (2) clinicians in recent years have come to realize that the 50 minutes that we may spend weekly with clients has significantly less effect than the remaining 167 hours spent away from clinical sessions; (3) the maintenance of positive clinical outcomes can be enhanced by incorporating the ongoing social system into therapy, thus enhancing the likelihood of a continual therapeutic or at least supportive milieu for the client; and (4) social systems can be successfully utilized to become therapeutic aspects of the treatment plan.

From a developmental perspective, clinicians further need to recognize that the social system for adolescents is twofold: family and friends.

In fact, it is not unusual for adolescents to be rather sensitive, if not overreactive, to maintaining this dichotomy, frequently feeling that they need to clearly separate from any identification with the parent.

Research by Offer, Ostrov, and Howard (1981) has somewhat discredited the turmoil theory of adolescence that predominated in traditional psychotherapeutic and particularly psychoanalytic circles, until recent years. Although that long-held view of adolescence has been modified by most researchers and clinicians, it is still generally accepted that young teenagers do need to make the transition from being primarily family oriented to being peer oriented. Furthermore, this transition can be difficult for adolescents who may lack clear identities or who suffer from low self-esteem.

Issues of self-identity are central to early adolescence. Adolescents are still struggling to define their values, goals, and self-concepts. The social support system of the developing youngster is therefore particularly important because these systems serve to provide feedback to the adolescent concerning these issues. They learn from their peers as well as their family whether they are perceived as being worthy of love and support. Adolescents whose family and friends provide the message that they are decent, attractive, good human beings will generally accept that message and base future behavior and attitude upon the assumption that they are both cared for and worthy of care and affection.

Stages of Social Support System Intervention

The five stages of social support intervention are ventilation, assessment, clarification, planning, and restructuring (Maguire, 1991).

In the *ventilation* stage, the adolescent is allowed and encouraged to simply express his/her feelings. In many instances, these involve fears about themselves or what others think of them, or anger or hurt related to feeling abandoned by friends or relatives. Some youngsters easily and quickly begin with this, whereas others may have difficulty in showing such feelings. Boys in particular may have already been acculturated to allowing only emotional expressions of anger as opposed to showing their feelings of hurt, disappointment, or fear.

Assessment may involve a process of diagramming their social networks and then discussing a series of questions in the clarification stage relevant to each network member. The diagram involves using three concentric circles divided into three pie-shaped wedges labeled family, friends, and others (see Figure 1).

Most adolescents enjoy this, or at least will do it as they would a

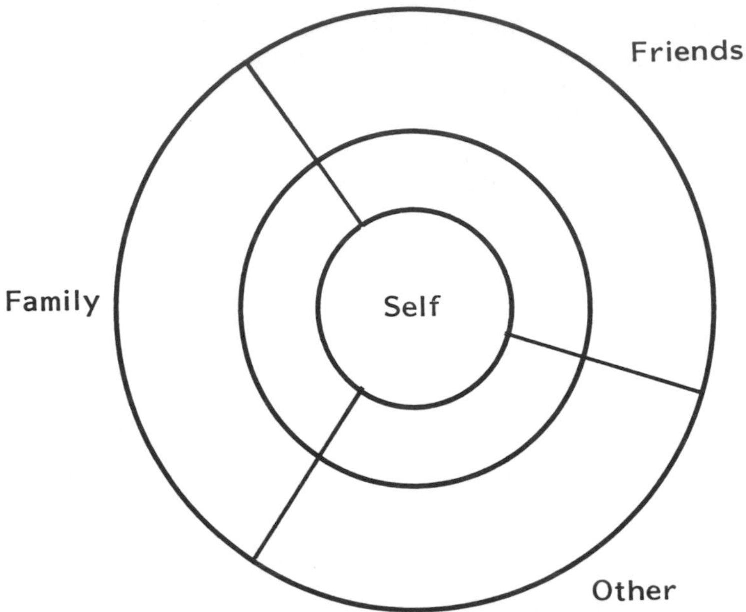

FIGURE 1. Assessing social network membership.

school assignment. They are instructed to fill in the names or initials of their closest friends and put those individuals into the inner circle closest to them. Those who are friends but less close go in the outer circle. The same process is then done for the family space, typically with the teen putting in his or her mother, father, and siblings in the inner circle, and various cousins, grandparents, or aunts and uncles after that.

Clarification is the third stage of social-support system intervention, and it involves more detailed discussions of the previous network and the nature of the relationships. In this stage, the adolescent is then encouraged to discuss and elaborate upon each of the designated people. Specifically, the clinician asks the boy or girl:

What is the relationship (i.e., cousin, neighbor, classmate, etc.)?
How long have you known that person?
What do you "get" from the friendship (i.e., help in school, someone to talk to, a basketball partner, loans, etc.)?
Is the relationship balanced or reciprocal (i.e., do they always have to call the other person, or do they feel used by the other person)?
How often do you see that person—daily, weekly, etc.?

Planning the social system development is the fourth stage. At this point, the clinician is helping the adolescent analyze how past behaviors and attitudes may have hindered the development of caring relationships, and how certain other behaviors may be considered to develop such relationships and social systems.

For instance, typical adolescent clients may have histories of fighting or emotional outbursts that have frightened or alienated peers and teachers. In a supportive and caring way, the clinician needs to get the adolescent to explore how such behavior affects his/her friends. The adolescent also needs to plan his or her approach to friendship development based on his/her experience of who he or she likes or feels attracted to. For instance, discussion needs to ensue concerning past friends and good relationships and how such relationships were initially developed. Examples of peers who are attracted to the client should also be explored in clear, concrete terms, that is, by asking the boy or girl:

What makes you like that person?
What are their positive attributes?
Can *you* display those same attributes?
Do you have other positive traits that you can try to develop to get others to relate to you?
What have you done in the past that alienates others?
Can you stop that behavior, knowing that it alienates others?

Many adolescents in treatment lack the social skills necessary to appropriately initiate relationships. Role playing is often helpful where the clinician takes the role of a peer with whom the client wants to form a relationship. The client can be shown how to meet others and present himself/herself in a way that does not alienate or offend others as he or she may have done in the past.

Restructuring is the last stage and is essentially a monitoring of the linking process. The clinician thus meets regularly with the adolescent and explores their progress and attempts at forming a social-support system. Several failed attempts and discouragement can be anticipated. In fact, adolescents will frequently "forget" or otherwise fail to make the phone calls or go to the sports event or social event or church group or party that they had previously agreed upon. Their fears of hurt or rejection need to be explored and recognized as understandable but as currently barriers in their attempts to develop friendships.

Small, relatively risk-free attempts are strongly encouraged initially. For instance, just going to a school football game to say "hello" to a few classmates might be a good, positive initial task. Again, the use of preexistent groups, teams, clubs, and organizations for adolescents is helpful.

ADJUSTMENT DISORDERS

According to the most recent version of the *Diagnostic and Statistical Manual of Mental Disorders* (American Psychiatric Association, 1987), adjustment disorders are described as inappropriate or maladaptive reactions to some stressful event or occurrence within the client's environment. They occur soon after the stressor, usually within 3 months, and persist for no more than 6 months. Typically there is excessive impairment in the social functioning of the client at home, work, or school. This impairment is not just a brief, single event. It is assumed that the client will return to normal functioning after the source of stress ceases, and in the case of ongoing stress, the client will learn to adapt. The stressors themselves are often significant business setbacks, divorce, psychosocial stress related to illness, discordant family relationships, natural disasters, or persecution. For adolescents, adjustment disorders are often precipitated by divorce or the death of a parent, the undesired move to a new school or neighborhood, rejection by a friend or friends, a traumatic sexual experience or a major fight or disagreement with a close friend or friends that leads to the breaking of a relationship.

CASE EXAMPLE 1

Regina was a 14-year-old girl who came reluctantly into treatment accompanied by her mother. Her mother, Pat, was a 33-year-old, recently divorced woman who was still suffering from the bitter divorce. She described Regina's father as being an immature, irresponsible philanderer who managed his father's grocery store during the day and worked frequently as a disc jockey at night.

In the initial interview, Regina sat as far from her mother as possible as her mother described the last 2 years of behavioral, psychological, and academic disintegration on her daughter's part. Apparently up until seventh grade, Regina had been a reasonably good student at a local Catholic elementary school and had been viewed as a rather quiet but normal, well-behaved girl. However, marital problems became evident at that time, and her father, whom she idealized, left the home to live with a much younger woman. Regina's mother became depressed and angry and took much of her anger out on Regina who both looked and acted very much like her father. Regina in turn began to avoid home and school while occasionally venting her own anger onto her younger sister whom her mother viewed as "the good one."

Regina had already been in treatment for the past 2 months with a psychodynamically oriented clinical psychologist, but all agreed the therapy was not helping. In fact, I began seeing Regina after she was hospitalized with a suicide attempt. Her previous therapist agreed that a more direct approach may have been needed.

As Pat explained in the first session, "I've had it with her. She don't listen to me, she stays out all night with useless bums, she quit school, and her last therapist said she's hopeless. She either straightens out with your help, or she's got to go to some kind of center for kids—like a hospital or detention center. I can't take her."

I asked Pat to leave so that I could get to know Regina better, since Regina would not talk with her mother present. Regina looked at me angrily and said, "Well, I've had it too. My mother is one crazy bitch, and I don't want to live with her anymore either. My dad left her because she's mean and crazy—I don't blame him." As she spoke, her angry affect shifted more toward the hurt and depression that she unsuccessfully tried to cover. However, when I suggested that she must have been very hurt when her father left, she only glared angrily back at me as she attempted to hold back her tears.

The second and third sessions vacillated between tremendous resistance and brief bursts of anger directed at me. Regina was holding back her feelings and clearly did not feel she could or would trust me. Her suicide attempt had been a dangerously concealed call for help, and it eventuated in her being locked up in the adolescent ward of a psychiatric hospital. She did not want to go back to the hospital, and she confided that she currently did not want to kill herself.

In the third session I once again empathically stated that she must have felt terribly alone and hurt to have taken an overdose of pills. I suggested that whatever caused her to do that must have been horribly painful for her. For the first time, Regina looked at me in a way that indicated that I was getting through to her as she said "Yeah, it was rough." At this point there were tears in her eyes, and I said, "If there is anything I can do in any way to help you, I will do it." So the ventilation phase was begun reasonably well by that point.

Session 4 began with an obvious attempt at testing me. She was dressed very seductively and began the session by standing up, walking over to me, and pulling her sweater down partially to show me a new tatoo she had on her chest. Her mother had expressly forbidden her to have this tatoo. Regina was testing to see if I would take her mother's side or hers, while at the same time testing whether I would respond to her seductive behavior.

I gently told Regina to sit down before she finished revealing the tatoo. I also told her that I thought she was a very bright, attractive girl, but what I liked most about her was she seemed so nice and caring in spite of the rough times she had had. Once again Regina stared thoughtfully at me for several seconds as tears began. Then she said, "I don't think I'm so nice and if you really knew me and what I did, you wouldn't think so either."

I said, "Sometimes when rough things happen, like someone you love leaves you and everything seems to fall apart, we feel things or do things, even bad things, we aren't too proud of because we're trying to stop the hurt. That doesn't make you a bad person."

The assessment and clarification stage followed. I explored some of her past interests, abilities, relationships, and social supports. In fact, I asked her to draw her social network for me as it existed about a year ago (Maguire, 1991). I also asked her to describe each person in that diagram.

From the diagram it became evident that she had been very close to her grandmother (her father's mother), and she had a couple of "nice" girlfriends whom she had known for her entire life. We talked about ways of reconnecting with these significant relatives and friends. We also talked about boys and intimate relationships and sexuality. She did not enjoy the sexual relationship with her current boyfriend, Ron, who was very abusive and uncaring. I assured her that relationships with men could be very rewarding and that she was an extremely likeable, caring, and attractive young woman.

Session 5 was unusual in that she continued with some seductive behavior that I rebuffed, again assuring her that I liked her because she was a decent person who was trying to honestly deal with some difficult issues. She vaguely referred to things she had done with Ron who was a drug dealer who was twice her age. She had been involved with him immediately prior to her overdose and hospitalization, and she had avoided all attempts at discussing him up to this point. She was quite defensive about him and her relationship with him.

I suggested to Regina that when we lose someone, like a father, it often makes sense to look for others to help us feel better and to fill that painful void. Sometimes that works and sometimes it doesn't.

Session 6 was a breakthrough. Regina was uncharacteristically tense but controlled when she entered the office. She began by saying, "If my mother or father knew anything about Ron, they'd kill me—or him." I assured her once again that whatever she talked about with me would always be in confidence.

Regina said that she had used cocaine and speed with Ron and that she had been sexually active with him. In fact, Ron had told her to perform a sexual act with a friend of his when they were all using drugs, and she had refused. He beat her, and the suicide attempt followed soon thereafter. She had never told this to anyone before.

I was extremely supportive and told her how proud I was of her that she could talk about this. I also encouraged her to talk about Ron and what he meant to her. She said that I had been right when I suggested before that we sometimes look for others to stop the pain. Ron had initially been very affectionate and supportive, but his behavior became manipulative and abusive toward her rather quickly. She realized that he was using her and that her own use of drugs was dangerous, but she felt she had nowhere else to turn because her mother seemed to really hate her.

In the seventh and eighth sessions, she talked more about Ron, her sexual attraction to him, to drug use and, finally, her feeling of abandonment and feeling unloved and isolated with no way out other than suicide. However, she also confided that she was not trying to kill herself when she took a half bottle of aspirin. She said she did not know what she wanted other than to end her pain.

In sessions 9 and 10, her demeanor and attire began to change noticeably for the better, and she stopped wearing her typical black, seductive clothing and excessive make-up and hairstyle, for a more age-appropriate dress. At this point, we were actively engaged in the planning process. Regina was very open to looking at her past behavior and where it had either helped or hindered her in her attempt to develop friendships with others. She also told me that she had spent the weekend with her grandmother who "still treated her like a little kid," but she loved it. Regina also decided to begin going back to church. In fact, as she began restructuring her social system, she had sought out a fundamentalist preacher/counselor who had been suggested by a girl she knew who had gone through a similar traumatic period. Regina began going to special youth group sessions at this church that she enjoyed because this group and the preacher seemed to be very sure of themselves and assured her that they would help her. They also told her that counseling and therapy were humanistic, liberal, and dangerous because they questioned too much.

My own concerns about this rather dogmatic and authoritarian religious group had to be tempered because unfortunately she was still seeking security and another father figure of sorts. Although I had some discomfort with that particular group, I learned that it had been helpful to a number of other adolescents who had gone through several adjustment-disorder problems. I also learned that while this group was somewhat dogmatic and antagonistic to professional mental health intervention, it was not particularly sinister or antisocial in any other respects. Furthermore, it apparently served as another transitional stage for many young people who had been traumatized by drugs, family upheaval or other severe psychosocial problems. After some period of time with this group, Regina could be expected to leave it when she had sufficient confidence and maturity to deal with life on her own terms.

Clinical Issues

There are several major clinical issues that merit attention in this case:

1. *Brief, directive therapy was the treatment of choice.* This youngster had unsuccessfully been involved in longer-term, insight-oriented therapy prior to her hospitalization. In this instance, such an approach was not advisable. Regina was in a crisis and was not only anxious but frightened as well. She needed clear and immediate direction.

2. *Transference was therapeutically helpful.* Although we rarely give much credence to issues such as transference in brief therapy, this case example demonstrated that the need for an appropriate father figure was a major benefit. Regina needed someone like her father to say he cared for her in an appropriate manner. After her resistance, then seductiveness, then anger, she was able to deal honestly and openly with a father figure in the therapeutic process.

3. *Social system interventions are complimentary to brief interventions with adolescents.* The development of closer relationships to potentially supportive family members and friends can significantly help in the therapeutic process. Therapists have known for many years that the positive gains produced within the traditional 50-minute hour can be easily subverted or nullified by a dysfunctional social system or living arrangement. The therapist who consciously and deliberately utilizes family and friends in the helping process meaningfully enhances his or her impact on the client. The purposeful use of social-system intervention both interacts with, and augments, the intervention that typically occurs on a one-to-one basis between therapist and client.

CASE EXAMPLE 2

Tim was a 17-year-old senior in high school who was referred by his school due to a recent arrest for being drunk and disorderly. His school counselor indicated considerable surprise at Tim because he was considered an ideal student, a class leader, and co-captain of the football team.

However, the counselor said that several teachers had told him that Tim's behavior had become disruptive, and his grades were suddenly uncharacteristically lower.

The therapist's initial superficial impression was that this was an extremely capable, bright, articulate, and attractive young man. He was quietly and politely reserved and appeared to be overly cautious and guarded, but even his guardedness seemed to indicate he wanted to make sure that he was responding positively to the therapist. In short, this was a young man who tried very hard to please.

Tim could not explain his recent arrest except that it was just a party that got out of control. His affect became more noticeably agitated and depressed as he described an incident at the party in which he had beaten up a young man for no obvious reason. In fact, Tim said he hardly knew the boy and felt genuine remorse and embarrassment that he had hurt him. Tim said he had recently began missing school and staying at a friend's house where they would drink beer and smoke marijuana. He said he was able to "coast by" academically because his senior year was easy and teachers were nice to him because he was a football star, a very bright student, and, as he said, "They think I give a damn."

Tim was the youngest of six children in a noveau riche family. The father was a self-made man whose own father was a carpenter who came over from Europe and began working on construction jobs. Tim's rigid and demanding father had turned the business into a very successful company by devoting his life to his work and instilling into his six children a belief that anything less than your best was a failure. As a result, Tim and his siblings were all somewhat similar in being high-achieving, well-liked students with a drive to excel academically, socially, and athletically. Another family trait was a pattern similar to Tim's in which each child would act out or otherwise "fail" the family at some time, usually in late adolescence. The family tried to keep it quiet from other family and neighbors because appearances were extremely important to them.

The therapist had one session initially with the parents alone. Both were well dressed and pleasant, but the father was noticeably uncomfortable in spite of his clear efforts to be involved. The mother did most of the talking, indicating that her four sons had all done well but resented their critical and emotionally absent father. The father angrily glared at his wife but only said, "I don't think that's fair or accurate." The picture that developed of the family was one in which the father criticized his wife and children but also demanded high achievement in all areas. He had grown up rather poor and admitted he still felt unaccepted by his wealthy and better educated neighbors. He was determined that his children would succeed even more than he had even if he had to "force them into it." He did, indeed, care for his children, but their relationship was largely one in which they tried desperately to meet his expectations in order to receive his affection but invariably failed on both counts. Each of his children developed a tendency to work hard but became angry and embittered (and occasionally violent when abusing drugs or alcohol) when they failed to meet their extremely high expectations.

In the ventilation stage, Tim was rather reserved but honestly tried his best to understand his behavior because it had genuinely frightened him that he could mercilessly beat up a peer out of his own fear and frustration related to getting into a good college or keeping his high rank in school. Apparently Tim was waiting to hear from a leading university that two of his brothers had attended, and he found that his anger, frustration, fear of rejection, and failure were all becoming more than he could handle. He knew his violent, drunken outburst was horribly wrong and frightening.

In assessing his problems and his social-support system, he indicated that he felt the problems were related to fears that he really was not good enough to get into the demanding university he wanted. He said that even though people told him he was extremely bright, athletic, good-looking, and popular, he simply did not believe any of it emotionally. He described a dichotomy within himself wherein he intellectually and cognitively knew that he did apparently have all of these positive traits, but he could never feel really good about himself or worthy of any praise he received from others. He adequately assessed his social system as being rather large and active, with him as a leading figure in several cliques at school, but he indicated that he really felt he had only one good friend to whom he was able to confide all of his many doubts and fears.

The therapist had Tim draw his network diagram and explain his relationships with each of his family members and friends. In clarifying these relationships and what they meant to Tim, his relationship with his parents became focal. For the first time in his life, Tim expressed his anger toward his father whom he idealized in spite of his coldness and constant criticism. Tim saw his father as being a good and successful man. He also began to realize that his father had extreme difficulty in expressing his affection in a supportive or caring way. Tim would have been overjoyed if his father would hug him or even say, "I'm proud of you—you've done a great job" or "You're a great kid and I love you no matter how well or poorly you do." However, that sort of caring was simply never shown, and even positive remarks of any sort were all clearly related to achievement.

The therapist helped Tim to plan and reconsider his social relationships and expectations. Tim rigidly maintained that he needed to continue to "force" himself to do his best. The therapist reluctantly but temporary accepted this as the behavior of an anxious and insecure teenager who was overwhelmed with fears of failure. The therapist felt that this was not the time to delve into the issue of deep-seated insecurity and Tim's pattern of denial and covering up poor self-esteem with bravado and a seemingly confident veneer. The plan that Tim developed was to focus more time in dealing with what Tim called his "real" friends. Typically these were long-term friends who did not necessarily share his high social status but were open and genuine in their relationship with Tim.

The majority of the members of his social system as he diagrammed in his network were just acquaintances or classmates or schoolmates who were popular or bright and whom Tim admitted socializing with because they enhanced his prestige and therefore made him feel more secure. In the restructuring phase, the therapist did not discourage him from maintaining these ties, but the focus was shifted toward his two "real" friends. Tim also agreed to talk more with one older brother who had gone through a similar period as a senior in high school when he began acting out, doing poorly, and engaging in fights and alcohol and drug abuse. This brother admitted to Tim that in spite of the high regard teachers, students, and coaches had for him, he was convinced that he was simply deceiving them all with an act. He, too, felt that his father's worst description of him as being lazy, sloppy, and essentially incompetent were all accurate.

Clinical Issues

This case is interesting particularly for what the brief therapist chose not to do. There were three separate and distinct dynamics that could have been explored in depth that the therapist decided would involve long-term psychotherapy and were therefore inappropriate to even open up, given that the patient would soon be leaving for college. The three unexplored therapeutic issues were:

1. *Self-esteem and confidence.* Tim was a young man who compensated for his feelings of inadequacy by maintaining an image of confidence. In fact, a teacher had confided to the therapist that she really disliked Tim because he was so arrogant. The reality was that Tim be-

lieved his father's negative and critical evaluation. However, to open up this central issue without the time to bring it to closure was felt to be inappropriate.

2. *Unresolved anger toward father.* Tim was extremely angry at his cold, rigid, nonsupportive father. Much of Tim's achievements had been accomplished to get the unachievable, that is, love or even positive regard from his father. The therapist did explore with Tim the fact that he was not being realistic in expecting praise and affection from his father and even that required confronting some denial of Tim's. But the deeper issue of a significant anger at what his father had done to him, his brothers and sisters, and Tim's mother in terms of demeaning, insulting criticism, was another area that could not be fully explored at that time for this boy.

3. *Marital tension.* Tim's mother called the therapist at one point and asked for a separate, confidential session. In it she tearfully explained how she had endured this cold and demanding marriage for the sake of her children. Now, as her youngest began to leave home, she was terrified of living with this man whom she had somewhat managed to avoid for 25 years by devoting herself to her children. She wanted sessions with Tim and her husband and herself to look at ways of changing the family. The therapist appropriately suggested that in this instance, the marital issues should be dealt with separately—not as an aspect of the intervention with Tim. Her request was understandable, but the therapist referred her and her husband to a marital therapist and actively followed up the referral. However, the therapist felt that to bring in the issues from 25 years of a poor marriage into the brief intervention with their last child would have opened up a whole new set of concerns that were too significant to be addressed simply as a part of Tim's problems.

Discussion and Conclusions

Brief social support system intervention is ideally suited to adolescents because it helps to develop five resources that are particularly important to them at this life stage (Maguire, 1991):

1. *Sense of self.* By intervening with the social support system of the adolescent, the clinician can help to educate and sensitize family and friends to the crucial concept and identity with which the adolescent struggles. The developing young man or woman needs to know from others whether he or she is smart, attractive, athletic, sensitive, humor-

ous, or in any other way appealing. The family and friends who work in conjunction with the clinician can be helped to realize that by providing genuine and accurate feedback to troubled youngsters that they themselves are lovable and decent people with unique traits and attributes; then the youngster can better develop a clear identity and sense of self, which in turn helps the young person deal with the critical issues of autonomy and separation.

2. *Encouragement and positive feedback.* Clinicians need to work with family and friends to get them to realize that during adjustment-disorder crises, the adolescent needs a positive and caring system around him or her. This is often difficult for the family or peer group who in all likelihood has recently found the target youngster to be obnoxious, rejecting, abusive, angry, or withdrawn and moody. Typically, a family member will not bring the adolescent in until the youngster has already alienated the social-support system and may have even turned it against himself/herself. At such times, it is difficult to get irate parents to be affectionate toward their youngsters. More often, the parent or parents will indicate that they are presently extremely angry, hurt, and disappointed themselves at this youngster, and they do not feel inclined to say or even suggest that the boy or girl has these positive traits.

The clinician therefore needs to instruct and discuss with the parent the fact that the child is currently questioning his/her own self-worth, and much of the behavior that is currently exhibited is the result of feeling that he/she is bad or unworthy of love. This self-identity can only be reversed by being told, by people whom they respect and care for, that they have worth and good qualities.

3. *Protection against stress.* The lives of adolescents are frequently stressful because they are so changeable, busy, and uncertain. Their friends, who they highly value, are all growing and changing and questioning themselves, just as the client is doing. When too much change leads to anxiety, uncertainty, and fear, an adjustment is required.

Youngsters frequently adjust to the stress by looking for stability. It may be in the form of a boyfriend or girlfriend or a parent, teacher, counselor or a member of the clergy. It may also be to negative but frequently powerful influences that make the situation considerably worse. For instance, many frightened adolescents become involved with drugs as a means of escaping stress, or they connect with abusive adults who claim to have answers. This may be in the form of a religious cult or leader or any strong dominant personality. Some alienated adolescents seek protection from life's uncertainties with adults who use them for illegal and/or unhealthy activities. Needless to say, this turns the situation from bad to worse.

Clinicians can instead use networking, case management or referrals to a variety of support groups or treatment groups to counteract the perceived lack of protection from stress. Such groups or helping systems can help to provide the sense of safety and protection needed by helping to provide resources and answers to how to cope and deal with difficulties in their environment.

4. *Knowledge, skills, and resources.* The adolescent who is temporarily depressed and seemingly incapable of appropriate responses frequently needs clear, concrete answers and provisions. The homeless adolescent who cannot be reunited with her abusive parents needs help in getting a job and housing. The depressed school dropout who was recently arrested and waiting in a detention center needs a cognitive framework for comprehending the rationale for his or her depression and the part that his or her own thoughts and behaviors played in maintaining the depression. The drug-abusing boy with limited academic skills or interests but a natural ability with machines needs job training and referral for appropriate work in addition to aggressive treatment for the drug dependency.

In the absence of positive, useful knowledge, skills and resources, negative or incorrect knowledge, skills and resources frequently fill the void. So youngsters are told by opportunistic adults that there is no hope or possibility of change or that the skills to be developed involve selling drugs or hurting people or otherwise breaking the law. In those instances, what began as an adjustment disorder can develop into an illegal lifelong career or a more serious psychological condition leading to severe depression, suicide, alcoholism, or drug abuse.

5. *Socialization opportunities.* Social-support-system intervention complements all types of brief intervention because it inherently involves a "shortcut" in treatment. The basic theory behind social-support-system intervention is that by connecting a client to a network or system of potentially helpful, positive individuals, the clinician can augment his/her own work with the support of others. This socialization opportunity is essentially a linking process wherein the clinician gets the adolescent to identify past or present members of his/her personal networks, and then he or she mutually discusses the practical aspects of how and why it would be advantageous to reconnect to certain past or present friends, relatives, or others.

In many instances, this linkage can provide a relatively quick therapeutic result, particularly when the adolescent is helped to link up to preexistent groups, clubs, organizations, or similarly organized systems. Thus, clinicians encourage youth to discuss and consider joining sports teams, school activities, church organizations such as teen clubs or choirs, or locating self-help or other support groups at school or in agencies where the goal is to get teens to socialize and talk to each other about mutual problems.

References

American Psychiatric Association. (1987). *Diagnostic and statistical manual of mental disorders* (3rd ed.–Revised). Washington, DC: Author.

Czikszentmihalyi, M., & Larson, R. (1984). *Being adolescent.* New York: Basic Books.

Douvan, E., & Edelson, J. B. (1966). *The adolescent experience.* New York: Wiley.

Epstein, J. L. (1983). Selection of friends in differently organized schools and classrooms. In J. L. Epstein & M. L. Karweit (Eds.), *Friends in school* (pp. 73–90). New York: Academic Press.

Maguire, L. (1991). *Social support systems in practice: A generalist approach.* Silver Spring, MD: NASW Press.

Offer, D., Ostrov, E., & Howard, K. I. (1981). *The adolescent: A psychological self-portrait.* New York: Basic Books.

8

Heavy Ideals

Strategic Single-Session Hypnotherapy

Robert Rosenbaum

Introduction

Strategic therapy can be broadly defined as any therapy in which the therapist is willing to take on the responsibility for influencing people and takes an active role in planning a strategy for promoting change (DeShazer, 1985; Fisch, Weakland, & Segal, 1982; Madanes, 1980; Papp, 1980; Rosenbaum, 1990; Weakland, Fisch, Watzlawick, & Bodin, 1974). Strategic therapists tend to work from a systemic epistemology and often see clients' problems as being maintained by their attempted solutions. This being the case, strategic therapists usually work briefly, believing that frequently only a small change is necessary to resolve the presenting problem. To minimize resistance, strategic therapists adopt a nonjudgmental attitude and utilize whatever a client believes or brings to the therapy, in order to help the client make a satisfactory life for him or herself. Thus strategic therapists tend to design an approach custom tailored to each problem and each client they see. Strategic therapists hate boredom and repeating the same old thing over and over. They also prefer to focus their creativity on finding present-time *solutions* rather than on exploring putative past "roots" of a problem.

Although strategic therapy meets clients at their view of the world and pays close attention to the exact language clients use in describing

Robert Rosenbaum • California Institute for Integral Studies, 765 Ashbury Street, San Francisco, California 94117.

Casebook of the Brief Psychotherapies, edited by Richard A. Wells and Vincent J. Giannetti. Plenum Press, New York, 1993.

their complaints in order to stay close to the clients' immediate experience, this does not mean that strategic therapists take all clients' presenting problems at face value. Frequently, resolving the chief complaint involves exploring a complex web of interpersonal relationships and even—dare I say the word in an article on strategic therapy?—the intrapsychic meaning the problem holds for the client.

The following case example is an edited verbatim transcript of just such a case. A woman in her late 20s came in requesting hypnosis for weight control; in the process of resolving her problem, both she and the therapist had some interesting new learnings. The entire case was concluded satisfactorily in a single session lasting approximately 90 minutes. Single-session therapies are not unique nor even especially characteristic of strategic therapy; in fact, research indicates that psychotherapists of all theoretical persuasions see between 30% and 50% of their clients for only a single session (Bloom, 1981; Hoyt, Rosenbaum, & Talmon, 1992; Rosenbaum, Hoyt, & Talmon, 1990; Talmon, 1991); furthermore, a surprising number of these single-session cases—up to 80%—report lasting improvement. This being the case, it behooves the therapist to be aware of the possibility that the first session may be the last. Single-session therapies are not a magical solution or a bromide; many clients need longer treatment, but a surprising number benefit from a single visit to a mental health professional. Recognizing this fact helps to promote a certain set of attitudes in therapists, attitudes that strategic therapists tend to adopt. These include expecting change and recognizing that all stability is maintained through change and that all change is maintained through stability (Keeney, 1983). Secure in this knowledge, the therapist can view each encounter as a whole, complete in itself. Knowing that many clients improve on their own reduces the pressure on the therapist to rush or try to be brilliant. Recognizing that big problems don't always require big solutions, the therapist can help a client break the problem down into small steps that can make a big difference. By taking an attitude that life, not therapy, is the great teacher, and viewing therapy as a way of promoting learning through daily life experience, the therapist emphasizes abilities and strengths rather than pathology and thus promotes change, autonomy, and independence, helping clients to help themselves.

THE CASE OF THE WOMAN WITH HEAVY IDEALS—TRANSCRIPT

In the following transcript, therapist statements are marked by "T:", client statements by "C:", and interpolated comments are in italics.

T: Before we start, I just wanted to mention to you that some colleagues and I have been doing some research, and we found out that a lot of people get better coming in just for a single visit. Now, I don't know if we can solve your problem in just one visit, and certainly if we need to meet more, I'll be glad to schedule as many visits as it takes. But I wanted to let you know that if you want to work on solving your problem today, I'm willing to work hard on this if you are. Would you like that?

By framing the present session as an opportunity for rapid change and indicating that the therapist is willing to work hard if the client is, the therapist rapidly creates an opportunity to strengthen the therapeutic alliance and increase the client's motivation. When doing this, it is important to leave the door open for future visits as necessary; this reduces excessive performance anxiety for the client (and therapist!) and minimizes resistance or feelings the therapist is "efficient but uncaring." Strategic therapy is not an uncaring application of a set of techniques; rather, it is a process where the therapist attempts to rapidly engage the client in the sort of relationship the client will find most helpful. To do this, the therapist must be profoundly respectful of the client. Note how, after making the initial statement, the therapist does not impose the single-session modality on the client; he asks the client for her permission to proceed.

C: Sure, OK.

T: I read the sheet that you filled out [*an intake questionnaire*], and I understand that you want help overcoming your weight problem, and that you'd like hypnosis for that. Tell me a little bit more what you would like to have happen.

C: Basically, I need some kind of, I guess, a mechanism in my brain to tell me that I am not hungry, and that I can do a diet. I've tried to do a diet that is kind of like a fasting-type diet, which I know is probably not the best way, but I think is the right way for me, right now, to get at least half my weight loss off, and I just have difficulty staying on the program, it's like something, if something wrong happens at work, or something, it just triggers me to go back to my bad eating. I eat the wrong foods, sweets, and then plus I don't get enough exercise. . . . It's surprising, I don't eat a lot, but it's the things that I do eat, and then I lay on it, or I just don't exercise at all. That's basically it. I have been overweight the majority of my life. I went down in high school.

T: That's when you were thinner? *[Therapist seeking clues by focusing on past successes or times when the problem didn't exist.]*

C: Yeh, right, or when I was a baby.

T: Were you a thin baby?

C: Well, yes and no. I was a lazy baby, too. I didn't start walking until I was 16 months . . . but hum,

T: A lot of babies who walk late are very intelligent verbally. *[Reframing toward a more positive self-image.]*

C: Oh really! Huh.

T: Did you know that?

C: No, I didn't know that. But, basically my problem is then that I didn't get enough exercise.

T: Even as a baby, you were able to sit back, and watch . . . *[Again, the therapist attempts to offer a positive framing, but the client will reject it and, in fact, give a hint as to the underlying problem that the weight problem serves as a "ticket of admission" for, namely, her relationship with her mother.]*

C: Even as a baby, even as a child, my pediatrician told my mother that she needs to get out and get some exercise. She didn't push me enough, and I guess, I didn't push myself enough either to get out there. I did take a lot of dancing classes, but I did it mostly as an overweight child.

T: Did you enjoy them? *[Finding if she was self-motivated or pushed. The therapist always wants to know sources of pleasure and autonomy.]*

C: I enjoyed them.

T: What kind of dance?

C: Tap dancing, I did ballet, and African.

T: So you can do many different kinds. *[Notice the therapist puts her abilities in the present tense, a subtle suggestion that she can still do these if she wants.]* Have you done any of that recently?

C: No.

T: I hear you telling yourself that you should exercise, and shouldn't do this.

C: I know what I should be doing, but I am not doing it. *[Statement of the problem from the client's point of view.]*

T: Have you ever had a period in your life where you *did* do those things? *[Again, looking for past successes.]*

C: I have never been much of an exerciser. *[Again, the client rejects the therapist's attempt to reinforce positive self-images for the client. This is an indicator that direct reassurance will probably not be helpful for this client. In all strategic therapies, not just in single-session cases, there is no clear boundary between an "assessment" phase and a "treatment" phase. Rather, the therapist constantly makes small interventions, monitors the client's response to the intervention, makes adjustments, and intervenes again.]*

There then follows some routine discussion of background material, including the client's job situation and educational aspirations. The therapist explores sufficiently to rule out any major negative indicators for brief therapy or hypnosis: the client is not suicidal, assaultive, or psychotic, and has no history of drug abuse.

T: What's making you decide that you want to lose weight now? *[Therapists always need to know the current situation for a brief psychotherapy. Why is this a problem* now? *What makes it a problem to the client?]*

C: I feel that I want to get into a profession. I want to become a hospital administrator, and I know that in a lot of professions, overweight is kind of frowned upon, being overweight, no matter how intelligent you are, it is your presentation, the way you look, as well as your educational background. So, I know that I need to get the weight off for that purpose and also for health reasons. I don't want a, as I told my mother, I don't want to die young, which right now I see a lot of people in the hospital that are extremely overweight, and they are dying, and I want to live as long as I can. *[Note the many sources of strength in this statement. Client is obviously attempting to move on with her life. The mention of mother is again a signal that the client sees her mother as somewhat of an obstacle, though she does not say so in as many words here.]*

T: Good reasons.

C: It's just implementing those reasons!

T: How have you tried?

The therapist now inventories past attempts at solution of the problem. Mostly, the client has tried various diets, without much success. The therapist now returns to client's current plans.

C: I'm trying to, I am going through transition right now, will probably start school in the fall, so I would be there for awhile until I can get something else that is more administrative.

T: School in what this fall?

C: MBA, and hospital services administration.

T: Have you had a taste of hospital administration? You must have been on the receiving end of it. *[Therapist knows from the questionnaire the client has filled out that she is currently working in a hospital setting.]*

C: Right, right. No, I haven't. I have been talking to the administrators at my hospital, and they have been helping me, you know, enlightening me.

T: One of the things you put on your sheet is that you like to have a sense of self-control. Tell me about the things in your life that you do have a sense of control over now.

C: I don't have any control. *[Client again rejects the attempt to frame positive self-concept. Note that the client's rejection of therapist efforts may not be "resistance," but rather a tendency to make autonomous judgments. However, she is exercising her autonomy in a way that requires her to denigrate herself. We will see that this is, in effect, the basic pattern of the presenting problem as expressed in her struggles with her weight.]* I am very compulsive in a lot of ways. I'm a chronic shopper; not a chronic shopper, but I do tend to shop a lot. Oh, let's see, what do I have self control of. Hum.

T: When you shop, do you go buy the first thing you see, or do you compare, and . . . *[Seeking to establish whether client does utilize self-control.]*

C: No, I know exactly what I want when I go. I have a real sense for what I am looking for. I love bracelets. I don't really like pendants.

T: And besides shopping, what else do you like to do? *[This kind of information is useful for later interventions, which will seek to build on client's preferences and meet her at her world view.]*

C: I go to the movies by myself a lot. I have friends, but because of my schedule, I go to matinees a lot. I love the theater, the arts, music.

T: There are a lot of things that you like. Do you dabble in any of them yourself in creating them?

C: I used to sing.

T: Ah huh. *[Interested. The therapist also likes music—this may offer an opportunity to meet the client in a genuine empathic encounter. The client is black and the therapist white, so it is important to find common interests that act as bridges between both parties' experiences.]*

C: But, I don't anymore.

T: Uh huh. Why not?

C: I got shy. The older I got, the shyer I got. I didn't want to get up and sing. I used to tap dance. I used to sing for the Junior . . . *[The client then describes how, after an embarrassing incident in which she was singing in public and her voice cracked, she stopped singing. At this point the therapist consults with colleagues behind the one-way mirror,*[1] *then returns and says the following]*:

T: I spoke with my colleagues who are observing us, and it's clear to all of us that you're a young woman who is interested in bettering herself. However, we have a disagreement and can't quite decide: They think the problem isn't that you should lose weight, but that you should learn to accept yourself the way you are . . .

C: I have . . .

T: I think the problem is not so much that you should lose weight, but that once you *do* lose weight you should be able to stay and be the way that you want to be.

Notice that this is an illusion of alternatives. Both sides of the "disagreement" presume that she needs to be more accepting of herself. This intervention results in a major shift in the client's presentation.

C: Okay, they are both right. I think one of my biggest problems right now is my mother. And, I have always been very confident being overweight. I dress nice. I look good. A lot of men did find me attractive, but lately I feel that she is influencing me; she is kind of pulling me down. Not intentionally, she just wants the best for me, and she feels that in society being overweight is a negative thing. And also, you know, being black, it is kind of difficult a lot of time to pursue certain things, that being black, overweight, and a woman, I guess she feels that it's a triple whammy, or whatever, for me. And, I guess she is concerned about my health. She says certain things to me that, I have a complex because of this. My friends notice it, and I have noticed it. I tried to explain it to her, but she says, "Oh no, no, no, I am not doing that to you. You are doing that to yourself."

[1]Moshe Talmon and Michael Hoyt, collaborators on a research project on single-session therapies with the current author. Note that while many strategic therapists (e.g., Papp, 1980) work in teams with one-way mirrors, it is not necessary to do so. Frequently economics and scheduling make cotherapy impossible. It still can be helpful, though, to occasionally step out of a session either to clear one's head, or to consult with a colleague, or simple to punctuate an intervention on your return (which will be attended to better by the client after the break).

T: Does she sort of offer you advice just kind of out of the blue, or does she call you up, or . . .

C: Well, she will say things like—I said one day to her, "Oh my fingers are a lot like daddy's, just the way they are made." "Oh well, they used to be thinner, when you were thinner, they were like mine." Things like that. Just, I was saying something totally general not talking specifically about how big my fingers are, just that they are shaped like my father's like other body parts are, and she will say things like that. I know she means well, but at the same time it doesn't help my self-image.

T: So when she says something like that, you react.

C: I get depressed. And I tend to go, I guess maybe it's a rebellious thing, I'll go out and get something to eat.

T: Do you ever say anything to her?

C: Constantly, but—

T: So, so, let's follow that situation through. You say, "Gee you know my fingers are shaped like Dad's," and she says, "Oh, they used to be thinner like mine." What might you say then?

C: I won't say anything.

T: You won't?

C: I won't. I'm tired of defending myself, a lot of times. So, I tend not to say things because of this.

T: How often do you see her?

C: We live together.

T: You live together?

C: So a lot of times I will stay up in my room if I'm home because I just don't want that kind of interaction. I know that I have been huh, I'd say like, "I'm going on a diet." And the next thing, she turns around and I'm not doing diet things, that type of thing, and she will comment on that. It's the way she looks at me. I think, in a way, I wish I could move out. I can't afford it right now, but I think probably I need to be at a distance because I feel that I am not really being accepted. I'm not meeting up to her potential, I mean, what she expects me to be. And, I think that is some of my problem, too, that I don't feel that I'm successful enough. So, I'm an overachiever. I want to be at the top.

T: Uh huh. You know, I am curious. If you did do just what your mom wanted and lost the weight and did the things she wanted, do you really think she would be happy, or do you think she would find something else to find fault with?

C: I don't know. I have a brother, as you know, and *I have always had the weight of being the ideal child. [This is a crucial statement. It states the problem in one sentence, and also offers an avenue to its solution. It therefore can function as a "pivot chord," a psychological space where a solution can emerge from what appears to be a problem (Rosenbaum, 1990).]* He is a drug addict, and his life has declined in the past 2 or 3 years, and I have always been the one to get the good grades. I have never been a problem child. The only problem that I have had is being overweight, so.

T: Gee, everyone is entitled to some problems, aren't they?

C: Yes, oh yes, yes. And, I figure being overweight is my only problem, and that's not too bad.

T: Uh huh.

C: But, I think to a certain degree, I had more pressure, I think, of trying to be better. Like I said, it is partly me, and then partly not.

T: You say then, does your dad come into this, too?

C: Sometimes. He comments, "You'd be prettier if you were thinner. You're a pretty girl, but if you were thinner, you'd be prettier."

T: And no doubt they do everything correct. *[Stated sarcastically. Siding with client intentionally to establish alliance.]*

C: Oh no. They are overweight. My mother is about 20 lb. overweight. My father is overweight. "But, when I was your age, I was thin."

T: Well, let me ask the question then, if you had a choice between getting your mom off your back or losing weight, which would come first? *[The therapist senses that, while the client has desires to be more autonomous, she is conflicted in this area. To push for more autonomy may meet with resistance. This question, posed as a choice, is a diagnostic probe.]*

C: I don't think your mother can ever be off your back.

T: No, really?

C: No, I don't think mothers will ever be off their daughters' backs. I have friends that their mothers have said certain things to them—"Well, you're not as pretty, you know, as this other girl that she might be competing with." My friends, it is really interesting, some of the mothers are very nice, and they don't bother them about weight, or not having a boyfriend, or whatever, but then I think on the whole, most women do hear from their mothers from time to time.

T: All right. Do you know that if you are carrying your mother on your back and you step onto a scale, the scale is going to be much higher and heavier than it would be otherwise? *[Rather than confront the client directly about "individuating from mother," this speaks in the client's language—i.e., of controlling her weight.]*

C: That's true.

There follows further exploration of client's interactions with her parents.

T: Mm hum. That's interesting that you offer that. You know, my mom would often go on diets, and whenever she would go on diets, she'd lose a lot of weight the first day, a lot of weight the second day, and the third day, my father would start offering her all kinds of sweets. Does your mom ever do something like that? *[Probing to see if mother is subtly sabotaging daughter, in a way which does not force client to feel mother would be portrayed as "bad" if she were doing this.]*

C: No. She usually tries to keep me on the diet as long as possible.

T: She does. Uh. You know, you've sung, and you've tap danced, and you know that when you are singing, for a while when you sing, very often teachers will sing along with you, right?

C: Uh huh.

T: To kind of help you find out what pitch you are singing at.

C: Right.

T: It is easier to sing along. *[Here follows a brief indirect "hypnotic" suggestion.]* It is a good way to teach a kid how to sing. But, you also know that if the teacher never stops singing, it doesn't give you much of a chance how to be on pitch yourself. And you know when the teacher stops, and you are trying to find the pitches yourself, sometimes you will start to get a little sharp and sing a little higher than you should, and then you kind of become aware of it, and so you correct, and you go back and sing right. And then very often you get a little lower than you should, then you correct, until you are able to sing right on key by yourself. But, you can't hear the slight highers and the slight lowers, if your teacher's voice is going along with you. So, how are we going to get your mom . . .

C: It beats me.

T: So, that this is whatever weight you decide to be, it is going to be your weight and not hers.

C: That's right. I don't know. I always see that the only way to get her off my back, about the weight, is to lose weight and let her see that I am trying.

T: I don't know. You sound like such a good daughter. *[Empathizing and adopting client's values.]*

C: Ha, ha. I've got flaws, but yeh, pretty good. *[Client is now able to say positive things about herself, as opposed to earlier in the session.]*

T: And, it sounds like you try hard, but trying hard is different than doing something. Right?

C: Right. Uh huh.

T: And, I don't know whether you want to lose weight or not. *[Purposely challenging client as a way of making sure the decision is her own. It was also said in a way that indicated the therapist didn't care if she loses weight or not.]*

C: I do, I do.

T: You do.

C: I do.

T: I do know that you won't be able to do it and enjoy it unless it is for yourself.

C: That's true. I am trying to get my mind to say that I'm going to do it for myself and for no one else.

T: Okay. Getting back with your mom and this diet, you are living with her, and there are no possibilities of your moving out yet, right? So, one of the ways you have of getting privacy and having your own space is to go up to your room. Right?

C: Uh huh.

T: How about when you are not in your room, do you have ways of having your own space and your own privacy?

C: Not really, because she is retired and she's home a lot.
T: She's around all the time.
C: Unless I tune her out.
T: Can you do that?
C: Sometimes I can.
T: How do you do that?
C: I just ignore her. You know, she is doing her thing, and I just try to tune her out. I try, but that's not always easy when someone else is around.
T: Uh huh. Okay. And, you seem like a very open and honest and truthful person. Those are wonderful traits, but I am wondering with your mom, whether you can ever fudge facts a little bit.
C: Oh, I can. I've done that before.
T: And you can feel okay about this.
C: Sometimes. I think because I went to Catholic school for 12 years that I have that guilt mechanism built into me. Catholic school will do that to you.
T: So you are carrying around a lot of burdens. You are carrying around this guilt inside your head; you carrying this mother on your back; maybe, a little of this shyness.
C: A little.
T: You've gotten over that.
C: Well, I'm not really shy though, I mean, as far as I can get up and do a presentation or something. I just don't get up and sing anymore. That is the basis of my shyness.
T: And what are the things you do now? You talked about going to the movies, and enjoyed the arts. Tell me the thing you enjoy most, which is all your own?
C: All my own, I really don't know. There isn't just one thing that I enjoy the most.
T: Two or three would be fine.
C: I love shopping. I love watching TV, which is kind of a bad thing at times, because I am just sitting there, watching. I watch some soap operas, but I have a tendency, if I'm downstairs, I switch the TV with the remote a lot. I can't stay on one soap opera for very long, because it's just kind of boring at times, that's when I'm at home. Right now, I think I have limited myself in the activities that I used to do. I don't go out dancing. That's another thing I like to do, dancing, but I don't go out.
T: Why is that?
C: For one thing, I am afraid of rejection. You know, going out to these discos, and all the thin women, which is fine for them, and, but, you know, with men, they're not going to ask me to dance usually, so I tend not to set myself up for that type of rejection.
T: Yet, is has always seemed to me that dancers mostly like to dance with good dancers.
C: Uh huh.

T: Is that not true, do you think?

C: No. I mean come on, this is California. Thin is in. I mean, unless you go to a place that maybe is for overweight people, ha, ha. I don't know but a lot of times, I've been there, and know the scene as far as what people are looking for. You can have a beautiful face, but it's the body. I mean, you know, if I weighed 180, maybe they would ask me to dance, maybe. But, on the whole, you are not going to be asked to dance. That's just it. And, there are a lot of heavy women that can dance. I can dance, but, and I probably dance better than a lot of my friends do, but—

T: I bet you are light on your feet.

C: Ha, ha, but they would be asked to dance before I would, so a lot of times, when they call me up and ask me to go out I don't. Because, I just don't want to deal with that type of rejection.

T: But, you are used to that. You see, I am a little worried. I am a little worried that when you lose weight, you are going to have to battle the shyness again. I mean what are you going to do when all these people are asking you out to dance? *[Restraint from change as a way of estimating and avoiding resistance; by pointing out the negatives of getting better and indirectly suggesting she might be better off to keep her symptom, it makes it easier for her to decide if she really wants to change and, if she does, give up the symptom.]*

C: I'd go. (laughs)

T: You mean, you're not going to feel shy? *[Notice this is all in the context of* when, *not* if *change will occur.]*

C: No. When I am with my friends, well, I'd go out with my male friends because I know I have a dance partner, so that's fine. But going out with a group of females, I don't do that. But, I don't think that if I lost the weight, I would be shy, and not go out.

T: Uh huh. But, it would be nice to find out, wouldn't it?

C: It would be.

T: Okay. I think that there are a few things we can work on together that would be helpful for you, and hypnosis is one of them, and we can do that today, but I think for the hypnosis to work, there are going to be a few other things that you are going to have to do in terms of the dieting. Just as you know that hypnosis won't work without dieting, right. Well, dieting won't work without doing a few other things. Okay. I don't want to treat you with hypnosis now unless we can get an agreement to do these other things. *[This is an "anticipation" technique in which the "cure" precedes the treatment technique. It is rather like syncopation in music. Getting the client to agree to this technique will essentially solve the problem before any "treatment" (i.e., hypnosis) is administered since it will indicate the client has already made a fundamental change in attitude.]* Now, I want to run them by you.

C: Okay.

T: This isn't going to be a blank slate. *[Encouraging autonomy, implying the client will have to make her own decisions about the therapeutic program.]* The first thing is, in terms of the progress of any kind of weight loss you have, okay. Have you thought about how you are going to set this up with your mom, and what you are going to tell her, and what part she is going to play in all this?

C: No.

T: What have you done in the past?

C: I usually, sometimes, I will tell her to try to help me along, and then at times I don't ask her because if I go off, and go on a binge, or whatever, I don't really need that force coming at me saying, "You know, you are supposed to be on a diet, or you should be on the diet," that type of thing. So, I have decided that I would not involve her when I made up my mind to diet. I'd just start it, do it, and not worry about telling her.

T: Think she'll notice?

C: Oh, yeh.

T: Do you think she will say something when you start doing this.

C: She probably will.

T: You see, I think that's a problem with the strategy that you have. The idea behind this strategy, I think, is wonderful, and to do it on your own for yourself. But in practice, when you're in the house with another person whose got her eyes on you, like glue, it is going to be hard to do it.

C: Yes.

T: Hiding it doesn't work.

C: No.

T: Because it's going to be visible as you lose weight. Enlisting her isn't going to work because that's going to make her be part of it. But, I will tell you what idea I have on this, which is, I think you should announce to your mom that you're going, when you are ready but not before, but when you are really ready to lose weight *and keep it off [interposing an indirect suggestion]*, then I think you should announce to your mom that you are going on a diet, and I think that you should tell her that you are going to post a schedule of the number of calories that you have eaten each day and your weight each day on the refrigerator, okay—Let me finish. And, I want you to fill that chart in each day, and ask her to check it, *but when you fill in the chart, I want you to lie. [Alleviating the weight of being the ideal child by keeping her true progress secret.]* I want you to give her the information, but give her wrong information.[2]

[2]A colleague told me she thought telling a patient to lie is immoral. I was surprised, on rereading the transcript, to find I had said such a thing, since I value truth highly. Yet I also found that, while I felt embarrassed at having this chicanery exposed to public view, I could not find it in me to feel guilty about this intervention.

I think the intervention feels justified because, on a deeper level, in effect I was urging the patient to tell the truth; it just so happens that the truth, in this case, involved

C: Okay . . . (smiles)

T: So that she doesn't know what's happening, but she thinks she does. Now that's true of parents anyway. Now your brother knows how to do this already.

C: Oh yeh, he's good at it.

T: He's good at it. That's right. You might even learn a little something about him because I will tell you a secret. To be a good hospital administrator, you are going to have to learn how to do this. Okay. So this is good practice. Now, I have a prediction that when you do that you are going to get flustered and guilty. *[It is always useful to anticipate any difficulties so that, should they come up, the client will feel prepared.]*

C: You are probably right.

T: Am I right?

C: Uh huh.

T: So, it is better practice yet, then. But, I want to form this way of your doing this, so that you will have your mom off your back, and whatever she says you know it's not going to affect you as much because you know it is based on false information.

C: Oh, okay. So lie. (smiling broadly)

T: What do you think about that?

C: That sounds pretty good, actually.

T: But let me say something that I kind of notice, as I am saying this, your face, your eyes look a little teary. *[Monitoring affect, looking for resistance and subsidiary issues which could interfere with the intervention.]*

C: Yeh but, I don't know what they're teary about.

T: What's that about?

C: I know I'm not crying or anything, . . . I guess.

admitting she had been lying. Each time she had gone on a diet because of external pressures from her mother, to some extent she did so insincerely. Some part of her held back, because she and her mother were colluding in a lie: that the patient could be an ideal child. She had been overtly compliant while covertly fighting her mother.

This lack of wholeheartedness in her effort in itself prevents her from being an ideal person or an ideal child; it also accounts for her previous failures in dieting. At the same time, as long as her mother was her partner in her efforts, she could blame her mother for her difficulties (though she could not acknowledge this explicitly to herself or others). When the patient writes down her calorie intake on a list, posts it on the refrigerator for her mother to see, but makes up the figures, she no longer has mother as a partner in her diet or, by extension, in her life. At that point, the patient must face the fact that she alone is responsible for her own actions.

All prevarication and misleading of others has its root in self-deceit. Of course, we are all imperfect; we must struggle to engage in wholehearted action. Telling the patient to lie is really telling her to be truthful to herself, to accept her imperfections and acknowledge her humanness. Once she acknowledges this truth to herself—that she, like all of us, has a capacity to be less than ideal—then, and only then, she gains the ability to be truly honest.

T: Hum, hum, you know what?

C: What?

T: I think that it is going to be a little sad to grow up and leave your mom behind, which is what this is.

C: Oh yeh, oh yeh. It was hard for me to come back and live with them.

T: Was it? When did that start?

C: In '84 . . .

T: Do you think they'll feel sad when you finally do move out and they'll be off on their own.

C: Back again. Well, yeh. They were on their own for about 5 years.

T: Now, I don't want you to do this unless it makes sense.

C: It makes sense, because I would be in control. Yeh.

T: Okay. That's number one, and number two, and you are not going to like this one, I don't think it would be useful to start the hypnosis unless I have an agreement from you that you are going to start practicing your singing again and your tap dancing. *[Prescribing two things in the hope that she'll be willing to do one.]*

C: Oh, ha, ha. How about the singing? Let's make a deal. Come on. How about just singing? Tap dancing, no, not right now.

T: Tap dancing later.

C: Yeh.

T: Now you can start by singing in your shower.

C: I do that all the time.

T: You do that all the time. Then, we have to make it a little harder.

C: How about voice lessons?

T: Voice lessons. I like that idea. Would you be willing to start those? I think that is an excellent idea. And you know, you said that you need some exercise, well, that's the exercise I prescribe to start. *[Going with her idea to encourage autonomy but channeling it in the direction of recognizing already existing strengths.]*

C: Okay.

T: Because, you know, it takes a lot of exercise to really train your voice. But, I want you to have the experience of going high and going low, and then finding the middle range, where you feel most comfortable. *[A metaphor for the weight control issue and her finding what's right for her.]* Okay. And, it takes a certain amount of energy to sing well.

C: Uh hum, it does.

T: Okay. And so, it will be good to channel some of that energy into that activity. Okay?

C: Okay.

T: We have an agreement.

C: We have an agreement.

T: Let's shake on it then. (C and T shake hands.) Okay, I have the feeling that you are the kind of a person that really keeps her word. Am I right?

C: Except about the dieting.

T: Oh, but that's to yourself.

C: Yeh.

T: That's a different matter. *[Again, an indirect suggestion that the client's task is to find a way to be true to herself—i.e., be more autonomous.]* Okay. Now, you wanted to have hypnosis. Have you had any experience with hypnosis before?

C: No.

T: Have you any idea what it's like or what it involves?

C: I know kind of what it involves . . .

T: Okay. What's your idea of what it involves?

Here the hypnotherapy is initiated with eliciting the client's preconceptions about hypnosis. With this client, encouraging autonomy is crucial, so a more direct trance induction is used in which her consent is solicited at each stage, together with frequent suggestions to enter trance in her own way, at her own pace. Finding the right depth of trance becomes a metaphor for finding the weight at which she will feel most comfortable, her own person. The induction utilizes her interest in music, since this is an area with many helpful metaphors; it is also an area the therapist can genuinely "connect" with the client as a shared interest.

T: So you know how you can become absorbed in a piece of music and just follow a jazz theme . . . and sometimes there is a very big sound, and the *big* sound *is beautiful*. And sometimes, the music is real *light*, and that *can be pleasant*, too . . . you know how music sounds like it's all around you, and outside of you, but inside of you as well. 'Cause you know when you sing, you bring beautiful sounds from inside of you and you let them out. And, when you listen, you take beautiful sounds from outside of you, and you let them in . . . *[Then an arm levitation is induced, after which the following simple suggestions are given]* . . . arm starts to feel heavy, and the arm which starts to feel heavy, is going to get heavier and heavier. . . . You can allow to be pulled down, little by little, down towards your lap. That's good. Little by little that arm gets heavier and heavier. And you might notice that it is hard to tell exactly where it is, but when it touches the fabric, at its own time, and in its own pace, you will be able to *let all the heaviness flow out, and let go of the heaviness,* and let that arm relax completely. Very good. And that *heaviness will go away* and become relaxed, and *the heaviness won't return. [Simple indirect suggestions for weight loss]* I would like you to notice that this other arm has been floating in air . . . and I would like you just to *enjoy some of the sensation of lightness,* that arm levitation. And, really enjoy it, as it is pulled up towards the face. And when it touches the face, but not before, you will go into a very deep trance. . . . And while that's happening, I'd like you to do something about your arms that you know, but you haven't remembered for a long time, which is that your arms help you keep your balance. And as you walk forward, they swing back and forth to help you stand up straight, and to help *you stand on your own two feet [Suggestions for autonomy]*. . . . And then when

> you sit down, you can *relax and feel good about yourself.* And, it's a funny thing about the swinging of the arms, when you notice it you can feel self-conscious *[dealing with shyness],* and you don't know what to do with your arms. But, when you just go ahead and *walk on your own,* your arms will automatically *find the proper balance* which is *just right for you,* and nobody can tell you the proper rhythm or number of times to swing your arms for each step that you take. But, your inner mind lets you adjust that, until you find what is just right for you. And, when your hand, that hand, touches your face, you will be able to get very relaxed. And, the hand will drop down after it touches the face, and you enter a very deep sleep. . . .

An embedded metaphor follows in which a person stores up fuel to be burned at need, and is criticized by neighbors for having too much wood stockpiled on their porch. The story is interrupted and the client is enjoined to imagine herself going into a department store with her mother (utilizing her fondness for shopping as a familiar experience). She selects a number of clothes herself, and then goes into a "changing room" and draws the curtain, so that she is by herself, away from her mother. Within the changing room, she is asked to imagine herself dressed warmly, wearing several layers of clothing.

> And you're looking kind of flushed and warm, and when you feel that and see that I'd like you to just nod your head. Now going *at your own pace, in your own time,* I'd like you to take off one layer of the clothing. And, you know how it feels to take off a jacket, or a skirt, or a pair of stockings. And the feel it has on your skin as it just slips off, and the sound it has as it comes off. And you know the relief you have, as you slide it off, and you feel lighter, and more comfortable, and less enclosed. And when you have taken off a layer of clothing, nod your head. And I'd like you, when you're ready, to take off another layer of clothing, and keep on taking layers off, little by little. And I'd like you to stop taking layers off when you are down to your underwear. And then, when you are ready to really appreciate, and find the most beautiful spot on your body, I'd like you to take off those last layers of clothing. And enjoy the relief that's there, in feeling lighter, and really appreciate the beauty, that is your body's alone, and the uniqueness that is there. Because you know, everyone has a unique set of fingerprints, and everyone has a unique set of facial features, and even our footprints are unique, as we travel onto where we want to go. And, I'd like you to be aware of how these are yours, and really enjoy them. And of course within your body, you have a unique system.
>
> I have a friend who says that kids are born with two ears for listening. The left ear is for the father, and the right ear is for the mother. But, they are born with one brain, and that is so they can have thoughts for themselves. *[Another autonomy suggestion]*
>
> And when you are ready, I'd like you to imagine putting the clothes back on now, layer, by layer. And it doesn't feel bad to have just

a layer of underclothes, but then you put on the next layer after that, and the next after that, and I want you to keep on putting on layers, until you are all the way back to where you started from—to that uncomfortable, overdressed warmness. And you know, there is a reluctance to do that, empty feels good, free. And, I like you to put them back on, and when you've got all those layers back on again, I'd like you to nod your head. That's good. And, now this time when you're ready, I want you to *take off just as much as you want to until you feel really comfortable, at your own pace, at your own time*. And, when you reach that comfortable place, nod your head. Okay, and you have taken those clothes off now, and *having found what's comfortable to take off, from now on you can keep them off*, while I tell you what happens in the other story.

All through the fall, and through the early winter, that neighbor would nag her about having too much wood on her front porch. But, she used that wood all winter, and all winter, the porch got emptier and emptier, and she used that wood to warm himself. And in fact, that winter happened to be a particularly cold one, and a difficult one, and she needed all of that wood for that time, and she was happy that she could burn it off. *[Long pause]*

And, you know she had the joy of watching a nice warm fire. And, you know one of the things that joy makes us do is it makes us feel like singing. And, when you start your singing lessons, and you will sometimes sing a little too high, and you will sometimes sing a little too low, and after a little bit of practice, you are going to sing just right for your own pleasure. Now, your inner mind is going to be able to absorb and remember whatever is useful here for you. And, I'd like you to take the time now to absorb whatever is useful, and let go of whatever you want to let go of. And, whatever you let go of, won't have to come back. And, there is one more thing that I want you to do tonight, which is when you go home, I want you to sit down or lie down and take a load off your feet. And, you can do that best by taking your shoes off. And once you take them off tonight, I want you to keep them off, and enjoy the sensation of walking around barefoot. And, take the time now to absorb whatever is useful, and let go of anything which isn't necessary. And, you can come back up out of this trance simply by taking one, two, or three deep breaths and opening your eyes.

C: (Long pause, then opens eyes.)

T: Is there anything you'd like to share with me before we stop? You did very, very well then. Here's what I think would be useful. Uhm. I think after a hypnosis session, it is useful to kind of let things filter down and absorb them for awhile. Usually, for at least 3 or 4 weeks. Of course, if you'd like to, we can make an appointment now before then. But if you feel you have enough to go on for now (she nods), then at the end of 3 or 4 weeks, or at least before 2 or 3 months, I'd like you to give me a call, and let me know how things are going. If you don't call me, I am going to try and remember to call you, okay. Because I want to know how things are going. I would especially like you to call me after you have had your first voice lesson because I am curious how it will go. And, I will tell you, I know that it is not so easy to get these things arranged, because I have been trying to get myself piano lessons for a while. *[Notice how in the preceding the therapist gives the client a wide range of choices, again to respect her autonomy. Also, the therapist attempts to maintain a sense of connectedness even while letting go and separating.]*

C: I play the piano.

T: Do you really?

C: Yeh.

T: Aw, you have some things to teach me then. But, I've been trying for a few months. So, if you will pursue yours . . . okay. And you can quiz me when you call (about the therapist taking lessons). *[The idea here is to let the client feel she can be "one-up" on the "parental" therapist.]*

C: Uh hum. Okay.

T: So, I'll be hearing from you in a little bit then?

C: Okay, in about a month.

T: Sounds good.

C: Thank you, and goodbye.

Follow-Up

The client never called back for a follow-up appointment. Six months later, as part of a research project, the client was contacted by telephone by an independent research associate ("R" below).

R: How are you doing now?

C: The problem is much improved. I lost weight again, and I've kept it off. I feel more focused and busy. I am going to graduate school, and plan to move to a better place which will give me more interesting job opportunities.

R: What do you think made the changes possible?

C: Making a firm decision, which is mine, and trusting my will power.

R: What do you remember from the session?

C: I remember the whole session. I went only once. The talking and the relaxation helped a lot.

R: Do you recall anything that was particularly helpful?

C: The insight. Realizing that my attempts to please my mother and her expectations of me put a heavy weight on me. After the session, I realized that the only time in my life when I did not feel this need was when I went away from home to college. So I decided to go back to school again and in this way to become myself again. The rest fell into place relatively easily, because I was able to stand up behind my own decisions.

R: Did you find the single session sufficient?
C: Oh, yes.
T: Thank you very much for taking the time to speak with me.

Comment

The follow-up indicates a successful resolution to this case. The follow-up also indicates the client ascribes the success to herself, not to the therapy. This, of course, is precisely what we would wish. The goal of a strategic therapist is to become unneeded by the client as soon as possible and to help the client recognize his or her own strength and power.

When asked what was most helpful, the client mentioned "relaxation" but attributed her changes not to the hypnosis she originally requested, but rather to the insight she gained. Clients usually remember sessions very differently than do therapists, and frequently the most important part of their therapy experience may have little to do with technique or even anything the therapist did intentionally.

A therapist friend of mine, a psychoanalyst, once told me about a case she saw for several years without success. Then, rather abruptly, the client started making rapid progress and within a relatively brief period of time resolved many major issues and successfully terminated the analysis. My friend was somewhat puzzled as to the cause of the change, but assumed some previous interpretation had finally "sunk in." A few years later, she followed up on the case, and asked the client what had made the difference. The client responded: "Oh, I remember very well. There was this one session you came in and you had a cast on your leg. You'd apparently had some sort of accident. I figured then, that if you could come in and be willing to work hard with me even though you'd been hurt, I'd better start working hard myself."

Strategic therapies give us many useful techniques, but we must not forget that the technique is not the therapy (Minuchin & Fishman, 1981). Virtually all schools of psychotherapies achieve roughly equal outcome. This clearly indicates that specific techniques, while important, are not the critical issue. Common factors across all schools of therapy account for much of the variance in outcome. The simple act of talking with another human being who is interested and is trying to be helpful, of getting a different perspective on a problem, and of feeling supported and reminded of one's strengths, can do wonders.

As therapists, we carry around our own sets of "heavy ideals"; ideas and concepts about how therapy "should" proceed, about what we "ought" to do as therapists. We may need to recognize that the techniques we use are helpful mainly because they give us, the therapists, something to do, a way of controlling our own anxiety, so that we don't get in the way of the therapeutic process, which basically relies mostly on the client's inner resources. When we can accept this, we will be less likely to label ourselves or label our clients; letting go of the heavy weight of mutual manipulation, we can become more able to engage our clients in an authentic fashion. The basic "strategy" of strategic therapy, finally, is to find a way to be one human being connecting with another: In meeting the client's autonomy, we rediscover our own freedom.

Acknowledgment

Support for this project was partially provided by the Sidney Garfield Memorial Fund administered by the Kaiser Foundation Research Institute. The opinions reported here are those of the author and do not necessarily reflect any policies of Kaiser-Permanente.

References

Bloom, B. L. (1981). Focused single-session therapy: Initial development and evaluation. In S. H. Budman (Ed.), *Forms of brief therapy* (pp. 167–218). New York: Guilford Press.

DeShazer, S. (1985). *Keys to solution in brief therapy.* New York: W. W. Norton.

Fisch, R., Weakland, J. H., & Segal, L. (1982). *The tactics of change.* San Francisco: Jossey-Bass.

Hoyt, M., Rosenbaum, R., & Talmon, M. (1992). Planned single session therapy. In S. Budman, M. Hoyt, & S. Friedman (Eds.), *The first session in brief therapy: A book of cases* (pp. 59–86), New York: Guilford Press.

Keeney, B. P. (1983). *Aesthetics of change.* New York: Guilford Press.

Madanes, C. (1980). *Strategic family therapy.* San Francisco: Jossey-Bass.

Minuchin, S., & Fishman, H. C. (1981). *Family therapy techniques.* Cambridge: Harvard University Press.

Papp, P. (1980). The Greek chorus and other techniques of paradoxical therapy. *Family Process, 19,* 45–57.

Rosenbaum, R. (1990). Strategic psychotherapy. In R. Wells & V. Giannetti (Eds.), *Handbook of the brief psychotherapies* (pp. 351–404). New York: Plenum Press.

Rosenbaum, R., Hoyt, M., & Talmon, M. (1990). The challenge of single-session psychotherapies: Creating pivotal moments. In R. Wells & V. Giannetti (Eds.), *Handbook of the brief psychotherapies* (pp. 165–192). New York: Plenum Press.

Talmon, M. (1991). *Single session therapy: Maximizing the effect of the first (and often only) therapeutic encounter.* San Francisco: Jossey-Bass.

Weakland, J., Fisch, R., Watzlawick, P., & Bodin, A. M. (1974). Brief therapy: Focused problem resolution. *Family Process, 13,* 141–168.

9

Brief Treatment of Anxiety Disorders

LARRY V. PACOE AND MICHAEL A. GREENWALD

INTRODUCTION

This chapter describes a brief cognitive/behavioral therapy for a young man experiencing panic disorder with agoraphobia and dependent personality. Although some may quarrel with the appellation *brief* when applied to a case seen for approximately 37 visits, we believe, together with Budman and Gurman (1988), that brief therapy is best defined by its planned character, attitudes of the therapist about therapy objectives, maintenance of clear and specific foci, high level of therapist activity, and flexible use of interventions and time. Wells (1982) takes a similar view in what he has characterized as "goal-oriented extended treatment."

Brief therapy with complex cases, then, is a matter of efficiency and focus, and involves interventions targeted at specific points of intervention that are present, have the potential ability to change, and that are maximally likely to have a positive effect on the problem or problems (see Levine & Sandeen, 1985). Cases in which a client's interpersonal style, social history, or other characteristics exist that make it difficult to

---

LARRY V. PACOE • Departments of Psychiatry and Psychology, University of Pittsburgh, Pittsburgh, Pennsylvania 15213. MICHAEL A. GREENWALD • Program in Counseling Psychology, Department of Psychology in Education, University of Pittsburgh, Pittsburgh, Pennsylvania 15213.

Casebook of the Brief Psychotherapies, edited by Richard A. Wells and Vincent J. Giannetti. Plenum Press, New York, 1993.

change in a very brief interval may nonetheless be excellent candidates for a brief treatment approach. The remaining portion of this section will describe historical and empirical bases of the approach employed with this client.

Brief cognitive and behavioral treatments for panic disorder, together with conceptual models and treatment outcome studies, have evolved in the past two decades. Barlow (1988) and Michelson (1987) offer excellent reviews of cognitive and behavioral treatments, together with descriptions of treatment strategies and their empirical standing. Early behavioral treatments involved intensive and prolonged in-vivo exposure to phobic situations, assisted by a therapist who would accompany clients into a graduated hierarchy of phobic situations, helping them stay until high levels of phobic anxiety abated. Variations on this approach included the addition of various coping skills (e.g., relaxation, paradoxical intention, etc.) in order that clients could be helped to more readily remain in phobic situations and contend with their anxiety symptoms.

As time progressed, the therapist role focused more on instructing clients in self-directed practice (e.g., Matthews, Gelder, & Johnston, 1981), also called programmed practice (Greenwald, 1987), as an addition and ultimately as an alternative to therapist-led exposure. An example of such an exposure plus coping skills approach can be seen in Michelson et al. (1986). Guidano and Liotti (1983) proposed an integrated cognitive and behavioral approach to agoraphobia, based on a constructivist congnitive/developmental conceptualization, which involves a stepwise treatment, addressing individual behavioral difficulties (the need to acquire anxiety management skills), and the cognitive organization of the disorder, or the defensive cognitive stance. Beck and Emery (1985) provided additional conceptual and therapeutic suggestions for the cognitive/behavioral treatment of agoraphobia. Empirical support for the value of cognitive therapy in the treatment of panic was provided by Michelson et al. (1990). The work of Clark (1988) and colleagues (Clark & Salkovskis, 1987) was quite important in highlighting the role of cognition and misinterpretation of bodily sensations in panic, including those associated with hyperventilation, which resulted in a cognitive model of panic that takes into account physical and cognitive features. Clark and Salkovskis also contributed to the technique of panic evocation (in which clients are directed to expose themselves to panic symptoms directly) as a means to decondition fear of panic and reattribute the significance or specific physical symptoms of panic. (For a full description of an integrated group cognitive/behavioral intervention, with details concerning these procedures, see Greenwald [1990].)

Thus, effective combination treatments for agoraphobia developed that were initially behavioral in nature and evolved to combination treatments addressing cognitive and somatic aspects of the disorder. Recent treatments emphasize the activity of the client in systematically approaching and mastering panic symptoms in phobic situations and developing the capacity to test and reformulate ideas about the dangerousness, predictability, and controllability of panic sensations, as well as dysfunctional beliefs about the self.

Specific clinical problems that occur among these clients include a strong prohibition against experiencing affect and arousal, relative difficulty recognizing the connection between their psychological distress and the contexts in which it occurs (Guidano & Liotti, 1983), a fear of loss of personal control interwoven with fear of social disapproval (Beck, 1976), the illusion that it is possible and necessary to exert direct control over emotions, and a view of their environment as constraining and intolerable. Often, significant assertion deficits and strong feelings of personal weakness or incapacity are present as well. These characteristics were certainly apparent in the client to be described below, and his wishes for control and symptomatic relief of panic prompted his appearance for treatment.

Case Identification and Presenting Complaints

Marc is a 28-year-old college professor, who presented with the chief complaints of nocturnal panic, severe phobic anxiety, and phobic avoidance of 4 years duration. He had developed a 10-mile safety radius beyond which he would not drive, and a several block walking radius beyond which he would not venture out alone unaccompanied. He avoided isolated areas where he feared he could not immediately obtain help if he should require it. Panic attacks at the time of referral were rare, due to his severe avoidance of phobic situations. He feared that his anxiety might precipitate a heart attack and thus actively sought out situations in which he could not be "stressed." He had read that "strong emotions can kill you," believed this, and therefore avoided not only situations in which he might experience panic, but also those in which interpersonal conflict could lead to "strong emotions." His fear of "stress" also extended to all levels of physical arousal, and so he avoided any physical exertion. He lived with a profound sense of vulnerability, self-criticism, and constant fear. Precipitating events at the time of onset included family conflict, death of a grandparent, and near death of one of his children.

At the time seen, he was working an extensive schedule with significant research and academic demands contributing to a moderate amount of work stress. He is married and has three children. He referred himself to treatment after reading a newspaper article detailing the results of one of the authors' research projects involving successful behavioral treatments for panic. His expressed aims of treatment: to reduce phobic ideas and behavior, decrease his worries about heart attack, to increase his capacity to travel, and to decrease his strong level of fear associated with feelings of anger.

RELEVANT BACKGROUND INFORMATION

Marc had made several attempts to deal with his anxiety problems by means of psychotherapy, and all failed. The first was a group behavior therapy program designed for agoraphobic individuals, and it focused on graduated exposure to phobic situations via group outings and individualized assignments. He did achieve some mild improvement in symptoms of avoidance and panic. When this treatment was reviewed in detail, however, it became evident that he may have misinterpreted instructions (or may have been given poor instructions) for exposure: He understood that he was to approach phobic situations until he experienced high levels of anxiety and then immediately retreat if his anxiety were to become too great for him to handle. This interpretation of the instructions for practice threw him into the teeth of his fear of "strong emotion" and the belief that he would have a heart attack should he experience "strong enough emotion." Complying with these instructions required him to "risk his life" in terms of his beliefs, and this introduced a complicating element into the therapy that interfered with its effectiveness. These concerns were not addressed in the previous therapy. In other words, not attending to his beliefs that his panic could not be controlled (save through escape) and that intense anxiety was dangerous to his life, left these key aspects of his problem unchanged. This we believe to be a central factor in the failure of this treatment.

His second attempt to deal with his anxiety by working in psychotherapy was to see a psychiatrist who specialized in treating adults who had been abused as children. He found this treatment to be rather threatening and discontinued when he learned that a symptomatic treatment was available. We believe that his fear of "strong emotion" made this perhaps very appropriate choice of a therapy that could conceivably address core issues inaccessible to him at the time. In addition, he made two brief counseling trials during his university years that yielded mixed benefits: an unstructured 1-year trial of supportive therapy had no effect on symptoms, and a 6-month trial in which he received specific instructions, goal setting, and homework reduced his panic attacks to zero. Even so, considerable phobic avoidance remained at the end of these treatments. Thus, the challenge in providing care to this client was to provide a brief treatment that would not be superficial and that would address the foci of symptomatic control, the wish for control, strong emotions, fear of interpersonal conflict, and his anxiety-related behavioral avoidance that were not fully addressed in the earlier work, and at a pace and in a sequence that could be tolerated.

Relevant social history: Marc's father was a problem drinker, who was verbally abusive to him, his younger sister (by 3 years), and his mother. The couple divorced when Marc was 4. Marc's father reportedly sexually abused his daughter during visitation periods following the divorce, when the child was 7 to 9 years of age. Marc described himself as feeling "as though there was a war going on with Dad." He found himself in the role of peacemaker and was extremely deferential to his father as a way of trying to protect himself, his mother, and his sister from father's abuse. This took a great toll on Marc, who experienced chronically high levels of tension and fear. At age 6, his hair reportedly fell out "due to stress," and he suffered from asthma. From age 12 to 18, he experienced a quiet period in life as there was no contact with father during this time. His sister has had an extensive history of psychiatric and physical problems throughout her life and currently lives with his mother. College provided a welcome respite for Marc, and he was successful academically and socially. He met his wife on campus, and his life was relatively free of panic symptoms. Nonetheless, significant anxiety concerning conflict, self-confidence, and autonomy was present, and he had developed a lifestyle in which he was highly dependent upon his partner for support and accompaniment. Episodic symptoms of panic were addressed during brief counseling trials described above.

Diagnostic and Assessment Interview

In addition to a standard intake interview, ADIS-R (DiNardo et al., 1985) questions were administered that helped to confirm the diagnosis of panic disorder with agoraphobia. A detailed behavioral assessment of panic symptoms and phobic situations was conducted, together with detailed inquiry concerning phobic precautions and rituals (see Barlow, 1987). The Millon Multiaxial Clinical Inventory MCMI-II (Millon, 1976) and Burns Anxiety and Depression measures (Burns, 1989) were administered. The client qualified for diagnoses of agoraphobia and dependent personality. Additional clinical impressions suggested a sincere, somewhat obsequious and fearful interpersonal style, significant motivation for a systematic "control-oriented" treatment aimed at dealing with phobic symptoms (this was, after all, why he sought out this treatment). Strengths included intelligence, excellent organizational ability, and values consistent with a cognitive/behavioral intervention (e.g., he values reason, problem solving, stepwise approach, is willing to collaborate, and to assume responsibility for effort involved with change). We initially agreed upon a 12- to 15-visit treatment trial, renegotiable as needed, with the aim of helping him achieve the aforementioned goals.

First Phase of Treatment

The previous attempts at therapy highlighted the need for Marc to be able to develop a sense of control early in therapy so that he could approach the more central issues with sufficient comfort to continue to successfully work on the core issues in his problems. His beliefs about panic being uncontrollable and the dangerousness of both the panic and "strong feelings" in general were keys to the current maintenance and to the eventual mastery of his panic and feelings. The theoretical underpinning for this approach is laid out in Guidano and Liotti (1983). An outline of their strategy for treating agoraphobic clients begins with the essential need to provide for the client's need to feel some level of control as the first step in treatment. Helping this patient establish and maintain some level of perceived control was the key strategy for the initial approach to this therapy.

A two-stage treatment model was conceptualized. The first stage was directed toward his need for control over his symptoms, and it focused on his belief that he could not control his panic. The first step was to give him detailed information about anxiety, panic attacks, arousal, and to offer a cognitive model for understanding his anxiety. Emphasis was placed on the "feed-forward" cycle of panic described by Beck and others (e.g., Beck & Emery, 1985) in which symptoms of arousal are misattributed as signs of imminent death or dyscontrol, leading to increased arousal and further panic. He was taught about the process of misattribution, as well as its links to the alarm response and how it operates (Barlow, 1988). In general, the treatment rationale included a discussion of the cognitive model of panic (Clark, 1988), and he was taught about the misinterpretation of sensations and the role of overbreathing in panic (Clark & Salkovskis, 1987; Michelson et al., 1990).

One of the first behavioral techniques employed was training in diaphragmatic breathing, as a means for helping him learn to control feelings of anxiety and panic. Once mastered over the course of several sessions, Marc was helped to evoke panic via hyperventilation (see Clark & Salkovskis, 1987) and to reduce it with the diagphragmatic breathing procedure. Thus, he learned to repeatedly practice evoking first low, and later moderate to high levels of anxiety triggered by hyperventilation, and then decrease it with a self-control skill. This was a direct means of helping him to experience control and to provide him with experimental evidence to begin to challenge his belief that he could not control his anxiety. Additional anxiety-eliciting sensations were discovered, evoked, and "controlled" in session (e.g., jumping rope to accelerate heart rate), and homework was assigned so that he would gradually employ panic evocation at home and in other settings (see Greenwald, 1987, regarding generalization).

Panic evocation related directly to his training in cognitive therapy, as a means for eliciting his beliefs about the dangerousness, predictability, and controllability of panic sensations, and for conducting behavioral experiments to test the validity of these beliefs (see Beck & Emery, 1985; Burns, 1989; Clark & Salkovskis, 1987; Michelson et al., 1986). He could elicit the sensations he usually associated with panic and experience the fact that his predicted death, or even panic, did not necessarily follow. His belief about heart attacks was deliberately and persistently challenged in the same manner, first in the office in small steps in which arousal was elicited and damped with coping skills, and later, at home and during programmed assignments in which exercise was prescribed. Initially he was led to test his beliefs about his capacity to control; later, he was led to test the necessity for control, by eliciting arousal and simply waiting until his system calmed itself. A program of regular physical exercise was initiated at the outset of treatment, after he had been successful in the office, and then extended to supervised exercise at home with his family and later to running and biking in his safety zone.

A direct attack on the concept of safety zone and other related phobic avoidance was initiated during this first phase of treatment as well. The behavioral approach of in-vivo graduated exposure was described anew, and a detailed discussion of self-directed practice helped to prepare him for between-session programmed practice (see Greenwald, 1985). In particular, he was coached to seek out situations in which he could expect moderate levels of phobic arousal and remain in those situations until his anxiety abated, employing anxiety management skills as needed (see Greenwald, 1990; Michelson et al., 1986, 1990, for descriptions of the clinical procedures and treatment rationale). Because his previous therapy instructions had "failed him," he was accompanied during two visits and coached in vivo, to be sure he could implement the anxiety management skill (breathing) when and where needed. Therapist accompaniment was always an option to him during the therapy, but it proved to be a rare occurrence after his initial successes with panic evocation in session and two successful therapist-assisted exposure visits. During the first and well into the second phase of treatment, programmed practice assignments, for example, specific assignments for entering and remaining in phobic situations, were made, and these were discussed during the first 15 minutes of each session. The discussion emphasized collaboration in problem solving, goal setting, and implications of these experiences for testing his beliefs about anxiety. Over time, he was led to assume more and more responsibility for goal setting and troubleshooting of assigned tasks.

The first phase of treatment, then, emphasized acquisition of cognitive therapy and behavioral skills (anxiety management and self-directed exposure) that addressed his wish for control and for symptomatic relief of panic and avoidance.

SECOND PHASE OF TREATMENT

This phase of treatment focused on the client's sense of constraint and vulnerability as a more general characteristic of his life. In particular, his ideas about control, its role in his life and its necessity for his sense of security, and his expectations and beliefs about himself and others were targeted. This material was elicited in two ways. First, it was uncovered in his thought records and in sessions via Socratic questioning. Second, it was elicited interpersonally, early in treatment, when the client revealed his fear that he would be berated by the therapist for not doing his homework. This afforded an opportunity to begin to identify a pattern of the client's expectations of others being critical, being punitive, and humiliating him. A fear of losing important relationships was also identified.

During the earlier sessions, the phase 2 focus of treatment was secondary to the primary goal of helping him to successfully challenge his beliefs about lack of control over anxiety and his beliefs about his vulnerability to the devastating effects of strong feelings. As his control over anxiety improved and he began to feel more confident in his ability to initiate and maintain control over important aspects of his experience and his behavior, he was more available to deal with situations that evoked panic or threat, and with his ideas about controls, himself, and others. Thus, an agreement to direct our attention to underlying ideas and beliefs, and other circumstances that elicit strong feelings of threat, could be reached and collaboratively approached.

The issue of a critical stance toward self became more apparent, after 10 or 12 sessions, when he discussed how critical he was of himself for not making more progress to date, and how he saw each setback as a major failure. The pattern of self-criticism was made more apparent, together with questioning to help him to consider a more sympathetic stance. In subsequent sessions, this theme was highlighted when it appeared in many of his thought records; the pervasive quality of his self-criticism (and imagined criticism from others) became more evident to him. At this point, he had improved symptomatically to the point where it was possible to evaluate therapeutic progress and determine together whether new goals were indicated.

Marc had learned that he could still function though anxious and no longer defined himself as an anxious person. He had discovered that his progress owed much to his decision to do things regardless of how he felt, and his daily programmed practice (setting out to deal with anxiety every day) decreased his feelings of incapacity. With these accomplishments recognized, it was possible to formally initiate Phase 2 and address the issues uncovered and noted earlier as a main focus of attention. In this way, we could approach threatening emotional material gradually, and upon a foundation of mastery of anxious feelings, without the specter of a heart attack as a likely outcome of exploration.

The goals of Phase 2 were oriented to schema related to self-criticism, the need to please people, to avoid conflict, and feelings of vulnerability. In the early sessions of Phase 2 (sessions 17–18), the focus was on his need to control criticism and to control others by being extremely critical of himself and by being compliant. This led to a historical examination of the relationship between his own self-criticism and his early experience with his abusive, alcoholic father who set extreme standards of conduct and administered abusive punishment when his standards were not met. To help Marc more fully understand the role that his father played in his contemporary behavior, he was assigned homework in which he wrote an autobiographical review of his father's history and of his relationship with his father. There was a particular emphasis on his dad's world view and his rules of behavior. He also was asked to write a letter to his father, to practice expressing difference of opinion and his own feelings. These exercises were intended to provide him with the experience of understanding the historical origins of his beliefs about his self-criticism and his understandable fear of retaliation in the face of assertion. At about this time in treatment, Marc began to introduce examples of current interpersonal difficulties, for discussion and problem solving, in which these themes played out. These were addressed via modeling, role playing, and coaching of assertion skills and testing anxiety-related cognitions.

The developmental review of his childhood experiences was intended to help him form a compassionate understanding of the roots of his behavior with the aim of weakening the contemporary credibility of these beliefs. Thus, a fresh framework could be provided for his own behavior. He was able to see his excessive compliance as adaptive behavior for a child who needed to relate to a more powerful and aggressive adult. His peacemaking decreased the possibility of family violence and protected him, his mother, and his sister. This reframing led to considerable relief, as the behavior that so shamed him as an adult served some comprehensible and useful purpose as a child who was trapped in an impossible situation.

This realization quickly led to the client discovering that he talked to himself as if he were a child. He had long been aware (it had been pointed out to him early in therapy) that he spoke to himself in thought records in the second person ("you . . ."), but it became more clear to him that he was inadvertently referring to himself as a sternly and harshly judged child. He began to see the relationship between this harsh judgment and the self-torture and worthlessness that he felt. He was instructed to actively refer to himself in thought records using the pronoun *I* and to experience himself as an adult who could make active choices and independent evaluation. During practice in a phobic situation, he observed a sequence in his thinking that amounted to a major turning point in his therapy: He realized that he was punishing himself for being anxious and that this was not necessary—in fact, it made things more difficult. "Once I realized this, it was liberating! I was punishing myself because I was not perfect. I didn't need to be. Once I could forgive myself for not being perfect, my anxiety symptoms decreased. When I could forgive more, I could do more."

More assignments relating to an alternative self-view were initiated, including the practice of making trivial mistakes and attempting activities in which perfection could not be readily attained. In addition, assertion training was employed to help him learn alternative ways of dealing with others, rather than automatic compliance, and to help counter his prediction of attack or harm by others, should he express his preferences, differences, or his own feelings. This was undertaken in connection with a number of challenging interpersonal situations at home and at work.

This work led to the client being able to take an even more active role in his therapy, helping him to "declare war" on his residual fears.

The belief that he had no control over his fear was yielding to the alternative belief that as he moved toward his fears, they lost their hold on him. He set out to approach more distant practice objectives as a way to further strengthen his new beliefs about himself. Residual fears of weakness, incapacity, and expectation of being overwhelmed were dramatically reduced. Mutually defined homework included assignments in which he experimented with experiencing strong emotions such as rollercoaster rides, watching sad or frightening movies, or recounting painful experiences from the past, and these challenged his belief that if he experienced "strong emotions" he would have a heart attack or be otherwise overcome. Repeated experiences like these further weakened his initial thoughts about the harm of strong emotions to his health, and he came to develop the contrasting belief that *avoiding* the experience or strong emotion could be unnecessarily stressful. This latter discovery permitted him to confront those at work whom he had had some discontent with, and finally, to discuss painful and unresolved issues with family members and hold his ground.

In the final portion of the treatment, his goals, our interventions and methods were reviewed in detail, together with what he learned, and plans were made for extending and consolidating his gains (see Greenwald, 1987). Specifically, his responsibility was increased, future problems and solutions were practiced, and plans for follow-up defined. A detailed review of reactions to sessions was conducted, and sessions were faded to monthly contacts.

Clinical Issues

Clinical details have been sufficiently addressed above and do not bear repeating here. Instead, we will summarize what we feel to be key points of the therapy:

1. Teaching the client specific skills for achieving what *he* wanted at the outset of treatment, with detailed coaching that solved the technical problems (escape vs. habituation) of earlier treatment.
2. Helping him to first control, reframe, and ultimately accept physical sensations of arousal and anxiety.
3. Providing treatment at a pace and sequence he could tolerate.
4. Addressing underlying beliefs about the self that contributed to his avoidant, fearful, and self-deprecating stance.
5. Helping establish new schemata and new behaviors that permit a contrasting style of interaction with others and compassionate self-evaluation.

REFERENCES

Barlow, D. (1987). The classification of anxiety disorders. In G. L. Tischler (Ed.), *Diagnosis and classification in psychiatry: A critical appraisal of DSM-III* (pp. 223–242). Cambridge, England: Cambridge University Press.

Barlow, D. (1988). *Anxiety and its disorders: The nature and treatment of anxiety and panic*. New York: Guilford Press.

Beck, A. T. (1976). *Cognitive therapy and the emotional disorders*. New York: Meridian Press.

Beck, A. T., & Emery, G. (1985). *Anxiety disorders and phobias: A cognitive perspective*. New York: Basic Books.

Budman, S. H., & Gurman, A. S. (1988). *The theory and practice of brief therapy*. New York: Guilford Press.

Burns, D. (1989). *Feeling good workbook: Using the new mood therapy in everyday life*. New York: Morrow.

Clark, D. M. (1988). A cognitive model for panic attacks. In S. Rachman & J. D. Maser (Eds.), *Panic: Psychological perspectives* (pp. 71–89). Hillsdale, NJ: Erlbaum.

Clark, D. M., & Salkovskis, P. M. (1987). *Cognitive treatment for panic attacks: Therapist's manual*. Unpublished treatment manual. Oxford, England: University of Oxford, Warneford Hospital.

DiNardo, P. A., Barlow, D. H., Cerny, J., Vermilyea, B. B., Vermilyea, J. A., Himadi, W., & Waddell, M. (1985). *Anxiety Disorders Interview Schedule—Revised* (ADIS–R). Albany, NY: Phobia and Anxiety Disorders Clinic, State University of New York at Albany.

Guidano, V., & Liotti, G. (1983). *Cognitive processes and emotional disorders: A structural approach to psychotherapy*. New York: Guilford Press.

Greenwald, M. (1985). Programmed practice. In A. Bellack & M. Hersen (Eds.), *Dictionary of behavior therapy techniques* (pp. 170–173). New York: Pergamon Press.

Greenwald, M. (1987). Programming treatment generalization. In L. Michelson & M. Ascher (Eds.), *Anxiety and stress disorders: Cognitive-behavioral assessment and treatment* (pp. 583–616). New York: Guilford Press.

Greenwald, M. (1990). Group cognitive and behavioral treatment of agoraphobia. In M. Seligman & L. Marshak (Eds.), *Group psychotherapy: Interventions with special populations* (pp. 263–292). New York: Grune & Stratton.

Levine, F. M., & Sandeen, E. (1985). *Conceptualization in psychotherapy: The models approach*. Hillsdale, NJ: Lawrence Erlbaum Associates.

Mathews, A. M., Gelder, M. G., & Johnson, D. W. (1981). *Agoraphobia: Nature and treatment*. New York: Guilford Press.

Michelson, L. (1987). Cognitive-behavioral assessment and treatment of agoraphobia. In L. Michelson & M. Ascher (Eds.), *Anxiety and stress disorders: Cognitive-behavioral assessment and treatment* (pp. 213–279). New York: Guilford Press.

Michelson, L., Marchione, K., Dancu, C., Mavissakalian, M., & Greenwald, M. (1986). The role of self-directed in vivo exposure practice in cognitive, behavioral and psychological treatments of agoraphobia. *Behavior Therapy, 17*, 91–108.

Michelson, L., Marchione, K., Greenwald, M., & Dancu, C. (1987). Cognitive-behavioral treatments of agoraphobia: Tripartite outcome of cognitive therapy plus exposure vs. relaxation training plus exposure vs. exposure alone. *Behavior Research Therapy, 25*(5), 319–328.

Michelson, L., Marchione, K., Greenwald, M., Glanz, L., Testa, S., & Marchione, N.

(1990). Panic disorder: Cognitive-behavioral treatment. *Behavior Research and Therapy, 28*(2), 141–151.
Millon, T. (1976). *Millon Multiaxial Clinical Inventory.* Available from National Computer Systems. Minneapolis, MN.
Wells, R. A. (1982). *Planned short-term treatment.* New York: Free Press.

10

Treatment of Anger with a Developmentally Handicapped Man

Laura Black and Raymond W. Novaco

Introduction

Therapeutic interventions for anger and aggression have progressed significantly in the past decade, yet the treatment of this very problematic emotion/action complex remains neglected among seriously disordered populations. Recent work by Howells and his colleagues (Howells, 1989; Howells & Hollin, 1989; Levey & Howells, 1991) has certainly provided an impetus to addressing problems of anger, aggression, and violence among institutionalized patients.[1] Most assuredly, the management of patients' aggressive behavior presents formidable challenges to clinical staff who must be concerned with risks to themselves and to the welfare of other patients. Moreover, a patient's inability to control aggressive behavior will certainly forestall discharge and perpetually remain a liability for social adaptation. Because assaultive behavior is often mediated

[1]In addition to an insightful discussion of anger treatment for seriously violent psychiatric patients, Howells (1989) provided an informative case study that might interest the readers of this volume.

Laura Black • State Hospital, Lanark, Scotland ML11 8RP. Raymond W. Novaco • School of Social Ecology, University of California at Irvine, Irvine, California 92717.

Casebook of the Brief Psychotherapies, edited by Richard A. Wells and Vincent J. Giannetti. Plenum Press, New York, 1993.

by anger, treatment procedures that aim to provide clients with anger-control capabilities are important therapeutic resources, especially because they seek to promote anger regulatory competency through the development of coping skills that have larger implications for psychosocial adjustment.

Among the clinical populations for whom treatment of anger and aggression has been neglected are the mentally handicapped. A review by Schloss and Schloss (1987) of social skills research in the field of mental retardation indicates that aggression and "negativistic attitudes toward authority" are "major factors leading to poor occupational adjustment of the mentally retarded" (p. 109). Their conclusions in this regard dovetail with the observations of Blunden and Allen (1987) about the repercussions of "challenging" or "offending" behavior among people who are mentally retarded, emphasizing the importance of their learning coping strategies for dealing with feelings of anger and frustration. Indeed, it is frequently the lack of anger-control coping skills that prevent people who are mildly retarded from being accepted for community placement or that results in their rapid exclusion from placement facilities. This case study aims to show how an individualized cognitive/behavioral treatment approach to anger management was implemented with a man who had long-standing difficulties with anger and aggressive behavior.

The treatment approach was a modification of the Novaco (1983) procedures, which have been shown to be effective in a number of clinical intervention studies, involving a wide range of patient types.[2] One intervention study, conducted by Benson, Rice, and Miranti (1986), experimentally evaluated the treatment approach with mentally retarded adults. The Benson et al. study was a comparative group analysis of the Novaco anger treatment components, although the full treatment procedure was not used, and a problem-solving component was added. Thus, they conducted a component analysis with four conditions: relaxation training, self-instruction, problem solving, and a combined treatment. The results were significant reductions on anger and aggression measures across groups, but there were no significant differences between groups. The absence of a control group makes interpretation

[2]These studies have included psychological clinic outpatients (Novaco, 1975, 1976), child and adult psychiatric inpatients (Bistline & Frieden, 1984; Dangel, Deschner, & Rasp, 1989; Lira, Carne, & Masri, 1983; Novaco, 1977; Spirito, Finch, Smith, & Cooley, 1981), forensic patients (Atrops, 1979; Howells, 1989; Stermac, 1986), institutionalized and non-institutionalized delinquents (Feindler, Marriott, & Iwata, 1984; Schlichter & Horan, 1981), and college students (Deffenbacher, 1988; Deffenbacher, Story, Brandon, Hogg, & Hazeleus, 1988; Hazeleus & Deffenbacher, 1986; Moon & Eisler, 1983).

difficult, but the combined treatment condition should have produced differentially stronger effects. In an earlier report of this study, Benson, Miranti, and Johnson (1984) speculated that the combined treatment condition "probably suffered from too many skills trained in too little time" (p. 7). Their treatment procedure was conducted in groups of 5 to 9 persons over 12 weekly 90-minute sessions.

Considering the importance of anger management for mentally handicapped patients, the present case study seeks to extend the anger control treatment, improving upon several procedural limitations of the Benson et al. study, especially the neglect of the self-monitoring, cognitive restructuring, and behavioral coping skills components of the Novaco procedure. On the other hand, the particular attention given to problem-solving by Benson et al. was noteworthy and is convergent with Castles and Glass (1986), who found that training in interpersonal problem-solving skills was highly beneficial for mentally handicapped adults. Hence, we gave explicit attention to this element.

Because this case study seeks to apply a cognitive/behavioral treatment to a mentally handicapped person, thereby examining whether treatment efficacy extends to this population, some modifications were required regarding treatment procedure and length. Although the Novaco (1983) treatment is designed as a 12-session procedure (the various experimental evaluations have involved 5 to 12 sessions), here the main treatment phase was 28 sessions of 40 minutes, so as to accommodate the client's cognitive capacity. Four sessions were devoted to self-monitoring, 4 to cognitive preparation, 10 to arousal reduction, and 10 to cognitive/behavior skills, including problem solving. The total treatment session time, however, was only 40 minutes longer than that involved in the Benson et al. study (1,120 minutes vs. 1,080 minutes).

Case Identification

Peter is a 47-year-old man with a mild degree of retardation. He has many functional skills but has been in a residential facility for over 30 years. He was referred to the Department of Clinical Psychology by his consulting psychiatrist because of intense anger, often expressed in socially inappropriate ways. Hospital staff had observed repeated occurrences of both verbal and physical aggression. Improvement in anger control was necessary for him to be successfully relocated to community living facilities. To ascertain the verbal level at which treatment would be conducted, the British Picture Vocabulary Test was administered, resulting in an age equivalence of 10 years, 1 month. At the time of the referral, he was working in a sheltered workshop outside the hospital. When he considered life outside the hospital, he was ambivalent, being unsure about his ability to cope.

BACKGROUND INFORMATION

Although the early case notes are sparse, Peter's childhood was chaotic. He disliked his stepfather, whom he describes as often drunk and abusive to his mother—"I felt horrible; because of what he was doing; I felt like killing him." Family difficulties resulted in admission to a children's home at the age of 6.

That placement was unsuccessful, as he became "difficult to manage, violent, and antisocial," according to the case notes. He described his foster parents as "bad people" from whom he ran away. He was admitted to a large mental retardation facility at the age of 13. There, his life continued to be unstable, as he was relocated from one ward to another on 12 occasions.

Peter found it upsetting to "rake over" his past. He said that he very much missed his family, and he was frustrated by unsuccessful efforts to trace and contact them. However, he felt that things were improving lately. He had attained 1 year of work experience outside of the hospital and had developed a friendship with a hospital employee, whom he often visited at that person's home. He was also awaiting admission to a local technical college that had literacy and numeracy classes.

DIAGNOSTIC AND ASSESSMENT INTERVIEW

Given Peter's verbal ability, his unfamiliarity with interviews, and his initial defensiveness, a multimodal assessment was done, similar to the illustrative case example provided by Howells (1989) that was guided by the Novaco (1979) model of anger components. The anger-assessment information is thus categorized in terms of situational triggers, cognitive influences, somatic arousal, and behavioral manifestations. The methods of assessment included self-report scales, interview, staff ratings, and archival records. The self-report measures consisted of modified forms of the Novaco Provocation Inventory (Novaco, 1975, 1988), the Castles and Glass (1986) Problem-Solving Assessment, and the O'Malley and Bachman (1979) Self-Esteem Inventory. A semistructured interview was adapted from Novaco (1983). Clinical staff provided daily ward behavior ratings of anger pertaining to 10 observable anger responses and their severity, and they also provided weekly ratings of social behavior on four dimensions pertaining to appropriate coping styles. Data were also obtained from the ward incident book and discussions with staff.

Situational Triggers

Peter's anger was predominantly activated during interpersonal exchanges, especially when any limits were placed on his behavior ("People are always on my back"). He strongly disliked being asked to comply with many aspects of the ward routine, and a weight-reduction diet produced particular havoc. When asked who annoyed him, he stated, "anyone at all, if they get on to me." He was rather intolerant of other residents on the ward, being dismayed about their personal hygiene and table manners. He became incensed if there was any noise when he was watching television. He would report the misdeeds of others immediately to nursing staff, and if there were no immediate consequences, he would feel aggrieved. The staff described him as impatient and as easily becoming cross. Although they were sympathetic to his frustrations with institutional life, they felt that he lacked flexibility and compromise.

Cognitive Determinants

The problem-solving assessment provided the richest information about cognitive factors. In response to a number of provocation vignettes, Peter asserted that the annoying behavior of others was deliberate and targeted toward him ("for spite against me," "just to get me annoyed," "just to get me going," "to see me lose my head"). Regarding attributions, Howells (1989) highlighted the importance of appraisals of the intentions and motivations of others, calling attention to clients' automatic assumptions of malevolence, especially deliberate harmdoing. Indeed, blame was an important dimension for Peter, not only with regard to his blaming of others but also with regard to the prospects of him being blamed by staff. He would automatically assume that he was being blamed, and he held a generalized construction of this ("I get the blame for all sorts"; "I get the heavy end of it, and others get off with it"). Staff indicated that if they asked to speak to him, he would become visibly anxious, believe that he was being reprimanded, and not listen to what was being said. He would take things personally and take offense when none was meant. He would focus on being singled out for correction and ignore positive interactions. He had a distinct tendency to ruminate, stating, "If I've been angry, I keep saying things to myself, keep it going." He had a "black-and-white view" of the world, reflected in his characterizations of fellow residents, who either "couldn't help it" or "knew better."

Somatic Arousal

Peter said that once he became angry, it took quite a while for him to cool down. He was worried that if he "lost the head" that he would "really make a mess of someone." He described himself as a "worrier" and as "nervous." When he became angry, he was aware of a sharp pain in his chest, shakes in his legs, and generalized bad feelings. Physiological arousal measures (blood pressure and heart rate) were not taken in this case, which had a strong behavioral focus.

Behavioral Manifestations

Initially, Peter was quite defensive, asserting that he was able to "walk away" from provocation and "count to 10," adding that "I want to hit them, but I don't." He later admitted that he had physically assaulted staff and other residents and that he feared being transferred from the hospital to somewhere more secure or to being discharged to "walk the streets, because my family don't want me." He was annoyed that he had been referred for anger management by the clinical team and suspicious about where information would be sent. However, once reassured, he was able to admit that he was worried about his anger, fearing that he might do some "real damage" to someone.

During the 16-week baseline period, 31 anger-related behaviors were recorded on the staff rating scales, which included 1 act of physical aggression, 20 occasions of verbal abuse, 4 instances of slamming doors, and 6 angry protests of unfairness. The staff also stated that he was intimidating, having flicked a lighter in a resident's face and also threatened violence and otherwise acted belligerently.

The most serious incident during the baseline phase involved noise from others while he was watching a television program. Peter told everyone there to "shut it, or else," and when a staff member came to investigate the argument, Peter escalated the conflict, shouting that the nurse was "picking on him because he was easy to upset." Then, he insulted the nurse, tried to hit him, and threatened to report him to a superior.

Summary

Having spent all but 6 years of his life in institutional care, it is hardly surprising that Peter has failed to develop socially appropriate ways of dealing with stressful events and interpersonal conflict. Although he actively seeks social contact, enjoys the company of people whom he trusts, and has an affable manner, he nevertheless suspects people's motives, assumes the worst in ambiguous situations, and rarely gives people the benefit of doubt. He often believes that he is being blamed unfairly, is very easily hurt, and is quickly defensive. Aware of having a reputation within the hospital, he will deliberately provoke arguments and fights to assert his position. Anger arousal has been functional in achieving this goal.

Treatment Approach

The cognitive/behavioral therapy for anger problems specified in the Novaco (1983) treatment manual was modified to fit the special needs of a mentally handicapped client. In line with the original approach, the general aims of treatment were to prevent anger arousal when inappropriate or dysfunctional, to regulate anger and anger-engendering cognitions when activated, and to promote the execution of behavioral coping skills for dealing with provoking events. The complexity of the treatment approach, however, required modification. The cognitive-preparation phase was subdivided into a self-monitoring and an information phase, each of which had four sessions. The skill-acquisition phase was subdivided into arousal reduction and coping strategy subphases, each having 10 sessions. The application training phase was incorporated throughout treatment and during the 16-week follow-up, during which Peter was monitored to evaluate his acquisition of coping skills.

Session Format

Treatment was begun following the baseline behavior ratings by staff. Treatment sessions were approximately 40 minutes in length. Each began with a general review of the week, whereby Peter was encouraged to discuss anything that he considered to be of significance. His anger diary recordings were then reviewed, at which time he would describe any incidents of provocation and how he coped with them.

Then, there was a brief discussion of the session objectives and a review of the previous session. Approximately 20 minutes were then devoted to the session's treatment agenda. At the end, the session's work was reviewed and homework was set.

Self-Monitoring Phase

The first four sessions focused on gathering daily diary ratings of anger intensity. Because Peter only had rudimentary literacy and numeracy skills, the first session concentrated on the concept of gradation (more than/less than), using a simple visual analog scale. On a line marked "not" at one end and "very" at the other, he was presented with sets of three pictures that depicted the concepts of size, age, and number. Peter successfully ordered the pictures on the line in their order of magnitude. Following a discussion of various emotions, he was able to repeat this procedure with depictions of happiness, sadness, and anger. He was then instructed to complete an anger diary, twice daily, place a cross on the line to indicate how he was feeling.

Overall, the self-monitoring phase went smoothly except for an explosive outburst prior to session 3 when Peter ripped up the diaries and told staff that he did not wish to continue treatment. However, he did come to the session as scheduled. He first stated that he considered treatment to be a waste of time but worried that he would get into trouble for tearing up the diaries. After listening to his feelings, he was given reassurance that treatment was voluntary, as was completing the diaries. He then disclosed that he had heard that he might be transferred to another ward because of hospital construction work. This precipitating event and his reaction thus provided a useful opportunity for both assessment and client education, which are objectives of the cognitive-preparation phase. As discussed in Novaco (1985), the emotion/action complex that the client's anger problem entails can often materialize during treatment and constitutes one of several special challenges for therapists doing anger treatment. It is essential that the therapist sees such occasions as opportunities to implement treatment, rather than being derailed by viewing the client's expressions of annoyance, frustration, or impatience as negative judgments of the therapist's competence.

Information Phase

Four sessions were devoted to ensuring Peter's comprehension of the treatment rationale and its key concepts; it was a period of further assessment of Peter's personal anger patterns. Anger was put in the context of other emotions, was differentiated from harm-doing behavior, and was explained as having both positive and negative functions. Peter was defensive about his inability to manage his temper, and so his view of himself as "being bad" was changed to "feeling bad." He was helped to see that someone has a right to be angry but not to act aggressively. He seemed genuinely surprised to learn from the therapist that she at times had to struggle with controlling angry feelings and that some situations were more difficult than others. As she described the likely consequences of losing one's temper at work, he was able to follow the scenario and began to realize that this was a skill that had to be learned by everyone. A crucial concept was that our behavior can make any given situation better or worse. He had some difficulty in understanding that although stress can lead to irritability and a lowering of one's provocation threshold, one still had a personal responsibility to behave in a socially appropriate manner in stressful circumstances.

A simplified version of the Novaco (1979) anger model was discussed, emphasizing the point that thinking, feeling, and acting are interlinked. Particular attention was given to the idea that anger can be a signal to constructive problem solving. Peter came to understand the escalatory nature of provocation, ruefully commenting that his need to "get the last word" had often prolonged incidents. Semistructured interviews, keyed from his responses to the provocation inventory, assisted in the analysis of his anger patterns. The future course of the treatment process was outlined, emphasizing the learning of stress coping skills and the self-regulation of anger.

Overall, Peter did well through this phase, although he said that he sometimes got bored with "all the talk". He began attending some occupational therapy sessions at the hospital and a special education class at a local technical college. He also went for an interview at the local housing association. However, there was another anger episode when he was transferred to another ward. Again, he ripped up his diaries and failed to attend the next two sessions. Nursing staff provided him with reassurance, as he eventually settled on the new ward and then resumed treatment.

Arousal Reduction Phase

Progressive relaxation training and self-instruction were the foci of the next 10 sessions. The previous informational phase material on stress was reviewed, and he was urged to attend to somatic cues as traffic signals (especially red and amber). He was aware of feeling tense much of the time, and he agreed that it was important to learn ways of being more calm generally, of regulating the degree of anger arousal, and of being able to STOP AND THINK before "losing the head."

In approximately five sessions, he learned an abbreviated progressive relaxation program (Lindsay & Baty, 1986). Having grasped the influence of private speech on the genesis and maintenance of anger, he learned to generate self-instructions for use in conjunction with a simplified relaxation induction (Ost, 1987). Behavioral strategies for remaining calm were also rehearsed, such as going for a walk to cool off, talking to others directly about problems at appropriate times rather than ruminating and becoming more angry, and taking a hot bath for general relaxation. A relaxation-induction tape was made for practice back on the ward, but he preferred to use it in the hospital garden, where it was more private.

The later sessions were spent in role play, using rapid relaxation in vivo. This involved several steps in coping with a provocation: (1) instructing himself to STOP; (2) taking slow, regular breaths and instructing himself to BE CALM; (3) walking away from the situation (as a short-term strategy, until more proficient ones were acquired); and (4) self-reward for coping. The self-instruction that Peter found to be most useful was, "Be calm, be good." He generated this himself, which is an important aspect of efficacious self-instruction. Regarding the arousal reduction component, he remarked that: "Relaxation gets everything out of your mind," and also "Your mind tells you to be calm."

During this phase of treatment, he did have a fight with a fellow resident, which resulted in his loss of a pass for a few days. However, the following week, he was slapped by a female resident (an event having high provocation potency), yet he did not retaliate physically.

Cognitive/Behavioral Coping Skills Phase

The general treatment strategy is to teach the client to view anger situations as problems needing to be solved, rather than as threats calling for attack. When faced with provocation, the core coping skills are self-monitoring and being task oriented. Task orientation involves both cognitive and behavioral proficiencies. Because the pretreatment assessments revealed cognitive distortions and impulsive behavior, special attention was given to cognitive reappraisal, problem-solving skills, and self-instructional controls.

Two sessions were devoted to the likely effects of cognitive distortions on his behavior and constructive ways that he might view the behavior of others in more benign terms. Several sessions were concerned with problem solving, involving the generation of alternative solutions, the anticipation and evaluation of consequences to himself and others, and the responsibilities of decision making. The latter step involved making a choice between alternative solutions generated with consideration of consequences for himself and others.

Peter learned to use the fingers of one hand to prompt himself for these problem-solving steps, with the arousal of anger serving as a cue for coping. These skills were integrated with his newly acquired arousal reduction abilities. Self-instruction facilitated his coping efforts. When faced with provocation, prompting himself by enumerating sequentially with his fingers, he instructed himself: (1) "STOP," (2) "Stay Calm," (3) ask "What can I do?" (4) ask "What will make things better?", (5) direct himself to do it, and (6) reward himself for successful coping.

Communication skills and appropriate assertive behavior were also taught. These and the other coping skills were modeled and rehearsed in role play and through role reversal. He was reminded of the escalatory nature of provocation and to remain task-oriented, focusing on thinking and acting in a constructive manner aimed at problem resolution. Overall, this phase was difficult for Peter, and he did need some reassurance to continue. A cartoon representation of the problem-solving steps was provided as a reminder.

In view of Peter's intellectual handicap, the 10 sessions devoted to this phase were not fully adequate. More time was needed to deal with cognitive distortions, problem solving, and behavioral coping strategies, and he was ready to develop further skills in these areas.

TERMINATION AND FOLLOW-UP RESULTS

Over the course of treatment and follow-up, there was a progressive decrease in clinical staff ratings of socially inappropriate responses to anger arousal. These results are presented in Figure 1, where it can also be seen that Peter's diary self-reports of anger, in contrast, show increases in anger occasions. However, there was a considerable decrease in his report of anger during the arousal reduction phase, suggesting that this component was particularly useful for him. Our interpretation of this general increase in anger self-report is that Peter grew accustomed to and more comfortable with recording anger incidents as treatment progressed. We discuss this further below with regard to issues of institutionalization and empowerment.

During the 21-week follow-up phase, Peter came for weekly discussions of his diary and his experiences in using the anger control coping skills in vivo. During this time, he became increasingly impatient about

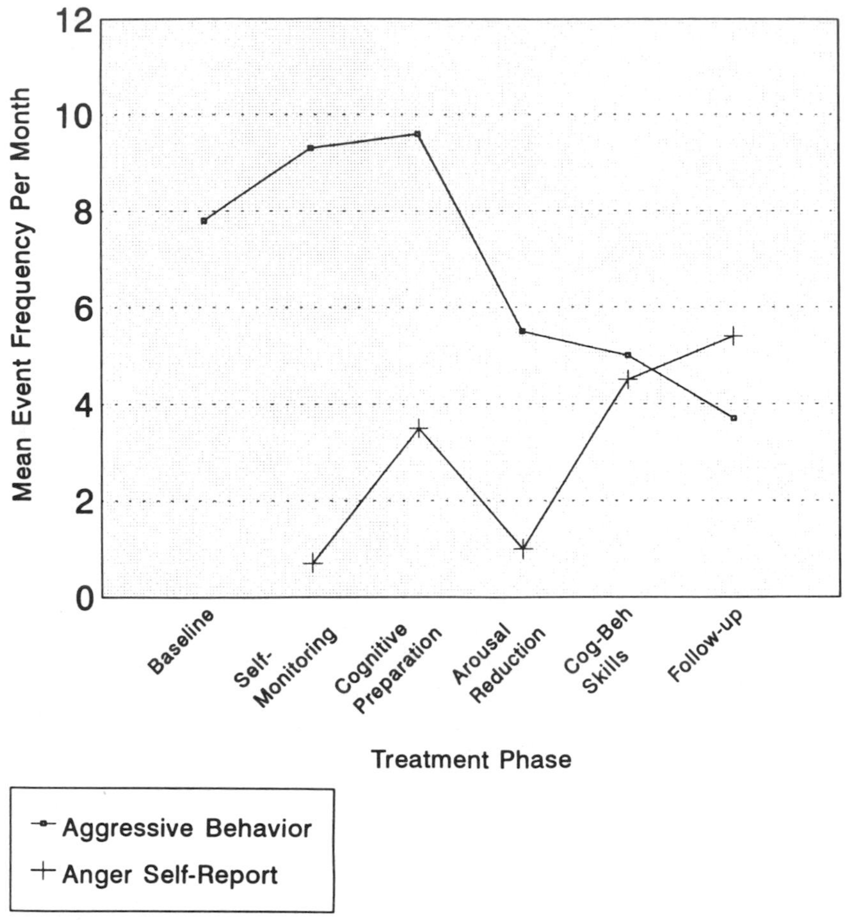

FIGURE 1. Occasions of anger (self-report) and aggressive behavior (staff ratings) across treatment phases: average monthly frequencies.

obtaining a community placement, and he began to doubt whether he would ever be able to leave the hospital. In this period, he recorded 28 anger incidents, but the staff recorded only 5 occasions of inappropriate anger, which suggests that he had achieved greater control over his behavior when angry. This interpretation (as opposed to an anger suppression interpretation) is reinforced by comparing clinical staff ratings of his social behavior at baseline and follow-up. Weekly ratings were done on four behavioral attributes, and favorable results occurred on each of them. The ratings were performed on 6-point scales ("not at all"

= 0 to "very" = 5) and were obtained for 8 weeks during the baseline phase and 21 weeks during the follow-up. Comparing the rating means for the respective phases, Peter improved in being "tolerant and able to compromise" (*M* = 2.5 vs. 3.8), "considerate of others' needs and views" (*M* = 3.0 vs. 3.5), "sociable" (*M* = 2.3 vs. 3.8), and "irritable or easily upset" (*M* = 3.7 vs. 1.7). In addition to the strong decrease in rated irritability, the rated improvements in prosocial behaviors support our inference above that he had achieved increased self-control of anger and aggressive behavior.

Indeed, he was subsequently able to move to a shared tenancy in a housing association and is receiving coordinated services through the social work department. Peter has asked to maintain contact with his friends and therapist on the ward, and this has been arranged for him. He said that it felt strange to be leaving the hospital, which had been his home for 30 years.

Clinical Issues

The success of cognitive/behavioral interventions, which emphasize self-regulatory capacity, can hinge on the adequacy of the self-monitoring component. The stress inoculation approach to anger control has strongly emphasized this treatment element as a fundamental skill, yet it is often neglected by both researchers and practitioners. We have shown here that, even with a mentally handicapped client, self-monitoring should be an integral part of the treatment and assessment process. In the field of mental retardation, more generally, there is a dearth of the use of self-report materials. Our use of a visual analog behavioral diary and other such scales (which helped him to master the concept of gradation) was effectively implemented for assessment purposes and facilitated Peter's sense of increased self-control. Indeed, various occasions of his rejection of the diary keeping provided important information about his anger experiences and the ways in which he coped with them. Moreover, we again emphasize that therapists who treat angry people must be able to view occasions of client frustration, annoyance, or rejection as opportunities to address the very problem for which the person is in treatment rather than become demoralized by the disappointment of noncompliance with the treatment regimen.

Another issue is that some clients referred for anger management without acknowledged personal motivation can resent be labeled as being deficient in this area. Peter initially denied having anger difficulties, intently demonstrating this by ripping up the diaries on two occasions during the self-monitoring phase, in which he recorded only two incidents of anger arousal in the 12-week period (yet he was far more forthcoming in completing the anger inventory, perhaps because of receiving more personal contact from the therapist).

Although the aims of treatment were generally achieved, the cognitive/behavioral skill component needed additional time, especially with regard to the modification of cognitive distortions, fostering problem solving, and developing assertive behavior. Verbally presented vignettes facilitated the identification of cognitive distortion subtleties, especially with regard to the intentions that he ascribed to other people. His inclination to perceive malevolence was significantly lessened over the course of treatment, but many years of overlearned cognitive appraisal habits are not so rapidly undone.

Overall Evaluation

Peter gained considerable benefit from treatment, as evidenced by the outcome assessment results and by his success in obtaining a shared tenancy. About 1 year later, at this point, he continues to cope successfully with the demands of living in the community. Although mentally handicapped, Peter was relatively skilled and verbal; hence it remains to be determined whether clients with greater mental handicaps could also benefit from this cognitive/behavioral intervention approach. However, we have demonstrated the effectiveness of this treatment for someone whose mental status may have been thought to preclude its successful application.

In addition, we have addressed a nagging question about whether an "anger control" treatment, when applied to clients who are disenfranchised (such as low-social-status institutionalized patients), would merely lead to the suppression or removal of an important human emotion. To the contrary, our results show that at posttreatment Peter was more able to acknowledge anger and felt reassured about his entitlement to these feelings. We consider it important to empower people to recognize this potentially problematic emotion but also to enable them to express it in socially acceptable, dignified, and useful ways.

Acknowledgments

Preparation of this chapter was partially supported by a grant to the second author by the John D. and Catherine T. MacArthur Foundation Research Network on Mental Health and the Law. We also thank Paul

Dickens at Royal Scottish Hospital and Chris Cullen at the University of St. Andrews for their assistance.

REFERENCES

Atrops, M. (1979). Behavioral plus cognitive skills for coping with provocation in male offenders. *Dissertation Abstracts International, 39*, 5053-B.

Benson, B. A., Miranti, S. V., & Johnson, C. (1984). *Self-control techniques for anger management with mentally retarded adults.* Paper presented at annual meeting of the Association for the Advancement of Behavior Therapy, Philadelphia.

Benson, B. A., Rice, C. J., & Miranti, S. V. (1986). Effects of anger management training with mentally retarded adults in group treatment. *Journal of Consulting and Clinical Psychology, 54*, 728–729.

Bistline, J. L., & Frieden, F. P. (1984). Anger control: A case study of a stress inoculation for a chronic aggressive patient. *Cognitive Therapy and Research, 8*, 551–556.

Blunden, R., & Allen, D. (1987). *Facing the challenge.* London: Kings Fund.

Castles, E. E., & Glass, C. R. (1986). Training in social and interpersonal problem-solving skills for mildly and moderately mentally retarded adults. *American Journal of Mental Deficiency, 91*, 35–42.

Dangel, R. F., Deschner, J. P., & Rasp, R.R. (1989). Anger control training for adolescents in residential treatment. *Behavior Modification, 13*, 447–458.

Deffenbacher, J. (1988). Cognitive-relaxation and social skills treatment of anger: A year later. *Journal of Counseling Psychology, 35*, 234–236.

Deffenbacher, J., Story, D., Brandon, A., Hogg, J., & Hazaleus, S. L. (1988). Cognitive and cognitive-relaxation treatments of anger. *Cognitive Therapy and Research, 12*, 167–184.

Feindler, E. L., Marriott, S. A., & Iwata, M. (1984). Group anger control training for junior high school delinquents. *Cognitive Therapy and Research, 8*, 299–311.

Hazaleus, S. L., & Deffenbacher, J. (1986). Relaxation and cognitive treatments of anger. *Journal of Consulting and Clinical Psychology, 54*, 222–226.

Howells, K. (1989). Anger-management methods in relation to the prevention of violent behaviour. In J. Archer & K. Browne (Eds.), *Human aggression: Naturalistic approaches* (pp. 153–181). London: Routledge.

Howells, K., & Hollin, C. (1989). *Clinical approaches to violence.* Chichester: John Wiley & Sons.

Levey, S., & Howells, K. (1991). Anger and its management. *Journal of Forensic Psychiatry, 1*, 305–327.

Lindsay, W. H., & Baty, F. (1986). Abbreviated progressive relaxation: Its use with adults who are mentally handicapped. *Mental Handicap, 14*, 123–126.

Lira, F. T., Carne, W., & Masri, A. M. (1983). Treatment of anger and impulsivity in a brain damaged patient: A case study applying stress inoculation. *Clinical Neuropsychiatry, 4*, 159–160.

Moon, J. R., & Eisler, R. M. (1983). Anger control: An experimental comparison of three behavioral treatments. *Behavior Therapy, 14*, 493–505.

Novaco, R. W. (1975). *Anger control: The development and evaluation of an experimental treatment.* Lexington, MA: D. C. Heath.

Novaco, R. W. (1976). The treatment of chronic anger through cognitive and relaxation controls. *Journal of Consulting and Clinical Psychology, 44*, 681.

Novaco, R. W. (1977). Stress inoculation: A cognitive therapy for anger and its application to a case of depression. *Journal of Consulting and Clinical Psychology, 45*, 600–608.

Novaco, R. W. (1979). The cognitive regulation of anger and stress. In P. C. Kendall & S. D. Hollon (Eds.), *Cognitive-behavioral interventions.* New York: Academic Press.

Novaco, R. W. (1980). Training of probation counselors for anger problems. *Journal of Counseling Psychology, 27,* 385–390.

Novaco, R. W. (1983). *Stress inoculation therapy for anger control: A manual for therapists.* University of California, Irvine.

Novaco, R. W. (1985). Anger and its therapeutic regulation. In M. Chesney & R. Rosenman (Eds.), *Anger and hostility in cardiovascular and behavioral disorders* (pp. 203–226). Washington, DC: Hemisphere Publishing Corporation.

Novaco, R. W. (1988). Novaco Provocation Inventory. In M. Hersen & A. S. Bellack (Eds.), *Dictionary of Behavioral Assessment Techniques* (pp. 315–317). New York: Pergamon Press.

O'Malley, P. M., & Bachman, J. G. (1979). Self-esteem and education: Sex and cohort comparisons among high school seniors. *Journal of Personality and Social Psychology, 37,* 1153–1159.

Ost, L. G. (1987). Applied relaxation: Description of a coping technique and review of controlled studies. *Behaviour Research and Therapy, 25,* 397–410.

Schlichter, K. J., & Horan, J. J. (1981). Effects of stress inoculation on the anger and aggression management skills of institutionalized delinquents. *Cognitive Therapy and Research, 5,* 359–365.

Schloss, P. J., & Schloss, C. N. (1987). A critical review of social skills research in mental retardation. In R. P. Barrett & J. L. Matson (Eds.), *Advances in developmental disorders.* Vol. I. (pp. 107–152). Greenwich, CT: JAI Press, Inc.

Spirito, A., Finch, A. J., Smith, T. L., & Cooley, W. H. (1981). Stress inoculation for anger and anxiety control: A case study with an emotionally disturbed boy. *Journal of Clinical and Child Psychology, 10,* 67–70.

Stermac, L. E. (1986). Anger control treatment for forensic patients. *Journal of Interpersonal Violence, 1,* 446–457.

11

Brief Relapse Prevention with Substance Abusers

VINCENT J. GIANNETTI

INTRODUCTION

This chapter presents a brief, structured model for preventing relapse among drug and alcohol abusers. Relapse prevention is a form of substance abuse counseling which is usually delivered after an intensive inpatient or outpatient program and oriented toward the development of adequate coping skills that facilitate long-term abstinence and sobriety. The model of relapse prevention described in this chapter is based largely upon cognitive/behavioral psychotherapy and social learning theory. Although substance abuse disorders represent a complex of genetic, physiological, social–cultural, and psychological components, relapse prevention can be conceptualized as essentially a problem-solving process and a reorientation of life attitudes and values. This involves developing the client's repertoire of skills in coping with stress, conflict, and frustration (remedial coping) as well as reorienting the client's attitudes and values so as to create a world view that is inconsistent with the abuse of substances (transformational coping).

The treatment consists of 16 sessions with 4 booster sessions encompassing self-observation and monitoring, homework assignments, bibliotherapy, and the use of guided imagery and role play. The model is

VINCENT J. GIANNETTI • School of Pharmacy, Duquesne University, Pittsburgh, Pennsylvania 15282.

Casebook of the Brief Psychotherapies, edited by Richard A. Wells and Vincent J. Giannetti. Plenum Press, New York, 1993.

eclectic, drawing mainly on therapeutic concepts from cognitive and behavioral approaches. The philosophy of the approach recognizes that the treatment of addiction involves remediation of cognitive/behavioral deficits in coping with stress and the usefulness of a philosophical reorientation for long-term abstinence.

ASSUMPTIONS IN TREATMENT

There are three basic assumptions to this approach:

1. *Substance abuse is learned behavior.* Principles of conditioned learning operate throughout the natural history of substance abuse. This includes the initiation of use, the development of tolerance and dependence, and relapse after treatment and abstinence. The initial stage of use begins with stress-induced negative affect in a context where comforting chemicals are available and use is encouraged. Both negative and positive reinforcement maintain, strengthen, and increase the use. The use of the chemical removes the aversive stimuli of stress and provides the reward of pleasurable experiences in its place. As tolerance and dependence increase, the original reasons for use become obscured and negative reinforcement becomes a primary factor. The substance abuser is now using to prevent the onset of painful physical and/or psychological consequences of abstinence due to tolerance and dependence (McAuliffe & Gordan, 1974; Wikler, 1973). This is the critical shift that Alcoholics Anonymous speaks of "when the drink takes you." In addition, secondary positive and negative reinforcement develops. Cues in the form of rituals, places, people, feelings, and thoughts can all become associated with the primary reinforcer's (addictive substance) ability to provide pleasure and alleviate pain. The exposure to these cues can precipitate relapse and reinstitute the cycle of addiction (Childress et al., 1986; Schuster & Johanson, 1981; Stewart et al., 1984).

2. *Cognitive processing mediates stress related emotions* (Beck, 1976; Ellis, 1962). Emotional distress is a result of regressive and primitive automatic thoughts and self-talk engaged in during periods of coping with the inevitable stresses of life. These automatic thoughts are the immediate intervening cause of emotional upset rather than the external events that precipitate them. They precede affect, are outside immediate awareness, are taken for granted as accurate, and are habitual and stereotypical. These automatic thoughts and self-talk represent a cumulative, learned, familiar cognitive map with which the person negotiates life. Coping with and transcending stressful life events is possible through substitut-

ing rational attitudes, beliefs, and processes for irrational thoughts that are the cause of emotional disorders. Irrational thinking refers to both the content of thinking as well as the process of arriving at conclusions about life events. Rational thinking is objective, factual, oriented toward problem solving, and seeks the maximum amount of fulfillment while respecting the limitations of the situation and responsibility to others. Rational thinking results in acceptance of responsibility for self, competency in dealing with stress and conflict, and the development of an internal frame of reference for self-acceptance and esteem. Irrational thinking is egocentric, absolutistic, dichotomous, global, one sided, and idiosyncratic. In addition, certain global assumptions concerning the world, self, and others form the core of a cognitive schema that ensures that the interpretation of reality will be distorted resulting in self-defeating behavior, low self-esteem, emotional distress, and lack of self-efficacy (Beck, 1987; Ellis & Harper, 1975).

3. *Substance abuse represents a dysfunctional means for coping with negative emotions and difficult life tasks through self-medication (Brown, 1985; Franklin, 1987; Kandel & Raveis, 1989; Khantzian, 1985).* Westermyer (1976) refers to the substance abuser as a "folk pharmacologist," self-medicating with available drugs in order to receive relief from symptoms of emotional or physical distress. Although the motives for engaging in substance abuse reported in the literature have been diverse, a common underlying theme for all of the diverse motivations is the desire to provide a painless and effortless route to accomplishing common life tasks. These tasks include establishing an autonomous identity, achievement, intimacy, balance, relaxation, and meaning and purpose in life (Dohner, 1972). In addition, substance abuse as a form of self-medication is culturally conditioned in a medication-oriented society that has evolved a technological bias toward solving complex social and psychological problems through chemical intervention (Illich, 1976; Koumjian, 1981; Ray, 1978).

COGNITIVE/BEHAVIOR TREATMENT OF SUBSTANCE ABUSE

The approach described in this chapter utilizes cognitive/behavior theory and techniques applied specifically to relapse prevention with substance abusers. Cognitive/behavioral therapy has as its central assumptions the following: (1) people respond to their mental representations of their environment, not their environment per se; (2) thinking, doing, and feeling are interrelated; (3) learning is active and reflective involving the acquisition of rules and skills that may be either adaptive or maladaptive, and (4) skill acquisition and the modification of maladaptive cognitive representations is the basis for constructive change (Heide & Mahoney, 1980).

There has been an emerging literature in the treatment of substance abuse disorders from the cognitive/behavioral perspective. The following discussion of basic relapse dynamics and prevention is a selective summary and distillation of Ellis et al. (1988), Marlatt and Gordon (1985), and Brownell et al. (1986). Relapse involves the return to the use of comforting chemicals to cope with stress and negative emotions as the result of the inability to tolerate frustration long enough to develop functional coping and problem-solving skills (discomfort, anxiety) and difficulty in accepting the mundane and routine in life manifested as the need for continuous sensation seeking. Once the relapse occurs, the belief that an initial relapse itself means that the addict is worthless and doomed to continued failure (abstinence violation effect), and a reinforcement of the addict's lack of self-efficacy in meeting the demands and challenges of life maintain the pattern of abuse. High-risk situations for relapse include indulging negative emotions, interpersonal conflicts, and social pressure. The typical relapse event involves a high-risk situation where coping skills are inadequate leading to a decreased sense of self-efficacy with positive expectancies for use to provide relief and gratification. A series of rationalizations for use and minidecisions are made that provide the platform for relapse that results in guilt, depression, and decreased sense of self-efficacy (hopelessness), with a return to addiction. Cognitive behaviorally oriented relapse prevention consists of the following interventions designed to prevent this relapse cycle:

Decuing behavior. This technique involves the identification of people, places, situations, and emotions (secondary reinforcers) that act as a cue for craving and subsequent relapse. The client is asked to keep a diary of emotional states and situations that precede craving and to briefly discuss them in the session. The therapist then takes the role of the client, and the client is given the task of identifying, labeling, and disputing the irrational thought processes responsible for the emotional distress. Prior to this exercise, a brief explanation and demonstration of how irrational thinking causes emotional upset is presented in the session with an assignment to read and outline a popular book on cognitive therapy (Ellis & Harper, 1975).

Stimulus control. This technique consists of an avoidance/substitution exercise. Because people, places, and situations associated with substance abuse have reinforcing properties, clients are asked to develop a plan that will allow them to substitute alternate rewarding behavior (positive addiction) while avoiding prior behavior associated with substance abuse (Glasser, 1985). The development of alternate, nondestructive sources of satisfaction is especially critical in mitigating against the experience of deprivation and discomfort anxiety associated with "giving up" gratifying drug-related experiences.

In-vivo desensitization. Because substance abuse represents a pattern of escape/avoidance behavior when confronted with stressful situations, the abuser loses the ability to tolerate frustration while engaging in problem solving. The abuser then becomes less competent and more anxious in stressful situations that reinforce the exclusive dependence upon chemicals to cope. The client is asked to identify what is being avoided or escaped through abuse. The client is then first exposed to the situation in the session rehearsing positive self-talk, disputing negative self-talk, and developing a concrete set of situation-specific skills to manage the problem. An assignment is then given to seek out formerly stressful situations and test the newly developed skills. Modifications and elaborations in skills can then be made based upon the results from the "real-world" testing of the new skills. The most critical attitude in this exercise is the suspension of judgment regarding outcome until the data are present (scientific attitude) and the perception of mistakes and problems in performance as "opportunities to learn, grow, and hone skills" rather than evidence of personal inadequacy (relabeling).

Anticipated relapse (fire drill). This exercise is designed to prevent the abstinence violation effect by having the client imagine in the session a relapse and to describe *in detail* the thoughts, feelings, and behaviors associated with the relapse (Hypnosis, guided imagery, and posthypnotic suggestions can enhance this exercise.) The client is then responsible for developing a comprehensive plan to recover from the relapse using all of the concepts and skills learned up to that point in therapy. The plan should be written up outside the session in terms of a contract detailing the steps the client is committed to when and if a specific relapse occurs.

Long-term goals and transformational coping. The client is asked to generate a list of personal situations that are problematic and difficult. The concept of economy of emotional energy is introduced by having the client rate which problems are "realistically changeable" and which ones are not. The client is then assisted in accepting, letting go, and reinvesting energies in solving problems that are amenable to change. This involves helping the client to dispute the irrational belief that life *must* be the way I want it to be, to understand that chemicals give the illusion of control over life when total control over the contingencies of life is impossible, and to develop a healthy detachment (life as journey versus destination) regarding the vicissitudes of fortune and failures. Acceptance and detachment from the unchangeable limitations of life can be facilitated by having the client repeat the limitation, for example, chronic disease, divorce, death of a loved one, and so forth, with the subsequent suffix "I don't like/want it, and I accept it." When the client can fully own the statement with all the implied feelings and implications, acceptance is usually accomplished.

What the client assesses as realistically changeable can form the basis for long-term changes the client would like to make. The client should be encouraged to set goals that are specific, challenging, attainable, and lead to increased competency and satisfaction. Goals should be broken down into subgoals with specific times and dates for accomplishment, and the client should be encouraged to continue to develop new goals with specific plans for attainment. Investing energy in goal-directed behavior that enhances competency, provides gratification, creates order and structure in life, and focuses energy is part of the psychology of optimal experience.

Transformational coping in dealing with the vagaries and crises of life involves the development of the "autotelic self." The autotelic self has self-contained, personally chosen rather than socially conditioned goals for life. The pursuit and continuous development of these goals form a lifelong project of continued growth and involve the transformation of stress into opportunities for the development of a greater complexity in consciousness and an increase in the repertoire of skills to both enjoy and continually master life challenges. The development of the autotelic self involves setting self-generated goals, total immersion and focus upon activities necessary to accomplish attainment of the goal, the ability to sustain attention and focus in order to anticipate problems, and the ability to enjoy the immediate here-and-now experience of the challenge and activity.

The development of a set of unified goals that give meaning, purpose, and structure to life is the basis of a change in orientation that leads to optimal psychological experience (Csikszentmihalyi, 1990). If the client comes from a religious tradition that is meaningful for him/her, spiritual principles such as expressed in the "serenity prayer" and other spiritual concepts can be used to support the ideas of acceptance, detachment, coming to terms with limitations in life as well as an understanding of life as process rather than winning and accumulation (May, 1988). However, spirituality should not be foisted upon the client who has had a negative religious formation history or no spiritual formation or interest.

Case Study

The following case illustrates a selective application of the previously discussed techniques to relapse prevention.

The client, John, is a health professional who has developed a sedative–hypnotic addiction over the course of a 5-year period. He was detoxified in a hospital, sent to an intensive day program, and referred for aftercare. He is 56 years of age, has a history of migraine headaches, and was recently diagnosed with hypertension for which he is receiving medical care. John continues to smoke a pack of cigarettes a day, has recently suffered the abrupt loss of a long-term relationship, and is currently living alone. He was married once (22 years) and divorced and has three adult children who all live out of state. His children visit and call him regularly.

John is gainfully employed and has adequate financial resources to support himself. The effects of his addiction upon his employment have been minimized because the client was self-employed with a reliable staff to conduct business. He was referred because of the author's involvement in working with impaired professionals. The physician who referred became aware of the problem in the course of his medical treatment of the patient.

The early sessions begin with an explanation of the philosophy of the approach with an emphasis upon the structured and time-limited nature of the therapy. The client is told that the sessions are limited because an individualized, finite set of skills can be developed and applied to provide adequate coping and living skills sufficient for sobriety. The client is responsible for developing an individualized risk profile and set of solutions using structured exercises, self-observation, and monitoring. The first sessions focus upon remedial coping skills, whereas the remaining sessions upon transformational coping. Background information regarding drug and treatment history as well as other information is collected toward the end of the session and is kept to a minimum. It is extremely important, from the moment of first contact with the client, to establish the intensity, urgency, and immediacy of the sessions. Therapist qualities that work best with this approach are an intensely caring yet confrontive, nonjudgmental attitude that holds the client responsible, but not blameworthy; a pragmatic and scientific approach toward solving problems; and the ability to see the humor with the pathos while having an appreciation for the enjoyment of life in spite of the inevitable limitations and pain. Excerpts from the first interview illustrate two critical issues in this session.

T: John, I understand from Dr. Smith that you've been referred after you were evaluated at a local program and you requested a private practitioner.

C: Yes.

T: What was it about the program that you decided not to continue with therapy?

C: The therapist spent a lot of time talking about spirituality and focused upon my drinking. I never had a drinking problem, but I am an addict. The therapist kept insisting we talk about drinking. After the appointment, I called Dr. Smith and asked if he could recommend someone else and that's how I got your name.

T: I'm glad we have the opportunity to work together. Before we start, I would like to restate what Dr. Smith told you concerning continuance in treatment. Because of state licensing laws, I am obligated to keep Dr. Smith informed of your progress and inform him if you decide not to continue in treatment. I would like your agreement to these conditions.

C: I have no problems with the conditions.

T: Good. Our therapy will be approximately 16 sessions or less. The number is not as important as the fact that we will focus upon a new set of skills that you will develop to assist you in managing your life without the need for chemicals. I would like to check out if we are operating on the same assumptions. There are all kind of theories about addiction that people have. I have found that the original reasons and theories about why people become addicted may be interesting but not useful if not connected to what's happening now. In other words, the question I would like you to continue to ask both in and outside the sessions is what is it about my thinking, acting, and feelings that sets me up to use chemicals. Once you can actually observe and experience what you are doing "that sets you up," you can then make new decisions about how you want to change so that chemicals are no longer necessary in your life.

C: Most of the theories I learned were in pharmacology. It was my favorite subject. I always enjoyed studying all the theories and did well in pharmacology. In fact I wanted to pursue research in pharmacology at one time.

T: (Smiling) I think you may have just proved my point about theories, John. I appreciate you helping me out so early in therapy.

C: (Smiling back) Yea. I guess it didn't help me.

T: Before we end the first session and assign some out of session work, I would like to pursue the conflict over drinking you apparently had with the other therapist.

C: Yea. He just kept focusing on my drinking. I have a drink occasionally. I am not a regular drinker. Maybe once a week if I go out to eat. And then I usually only have two drinks. I know I had a drug problem, but I can honestly say drinking was not a problem.

T: I would prefer not to focus upon whether you have a drinking problem or not. You recognize that you have a problem with chemicals by your presence here. It seems to me at the minimum, we would both agree that alcohol lowers inhibitions, and you already understand the concept of cross-addiction. I would like you to reflect back upon the benefits you have derived from alcohol and the current risks it may pose to your abstinence. If you are willing to take risks, and as you are well aware they are considerable for you, for your intermittent drink, then you may have a problem. In any case, I would like you to carefully evaluate the risks and benefits and let's discuss it in the next session.

C: OK, but it's no big problem for me.

T: Good, then we won't spend a lot of time and energy on it. I would just like you to spend some time listing all of the benefits and risks of continued intermittent drinking for both your short-term and long-term sobriety. Let's not forget including your general health.

T: For next week, I would also like you to reflect back upon the times you used chemicals or had a strong urge to use. Simply describe the situation and then recall as accurately as possible what you were feeling, thinking, and doing. We can use the material for discussion in the next session.

C: OK. Do you want any format?

T: No. Just describe your feelings, thinking, and doing as specifically as possible. We are interested in what specific feelings, thinking, and actions lead to taking a chemical. Situations such as the people you are with or the places you are in may be included.

Commentary and Continuation of Early Sessions

The liberal use of "we" is intentional in that it encourages the client to see therapy as a cooperative endeavor. Also, humor can be especially effective technique for redirecting clients as well as testing for ego strength. The essential beginning point is that clients "set themselves up" for relapse by what they think, do, and feel or through the situations they place themselves in. In subsequent sessions, the relationship between thinking, doing, and feeling will be explored and related to how clients make a series of "minidecisions" that lead to relapse. It is essential for the client to see that a series of decisions usually outside of awareness sets the stage for relapse long before the first drink or drug. Finally archaeology, theorizing, and talking about addiction are discouraged. The client has established in the first session his belief that he may be able to drink despite his drug problem. The next session begins with a discussion of the assignment and continued work on decuing behavior and stimulus control.

T: Let's take a look at what was associated with your urges to use. Describe for me a situation in which you felt like using that stands out in your mind.

C: I sit around the apartment after reading, and I feel bored. I'd really like to go out, but the woman I date I really don't like. I've been out of the dating scene now for a while. I'm tired of the singles functions. When I do go out Joan really irritates me. She's always complaining. But I really go out with her because it's something to do. Sometimes it's OK, but more often than not I get irritated.

T: Bored, irritated, and sounds like you're feeling hopeless. In other words, I can't do anything to meet anyone that I can really enjoy being with and I'm upset because I "have to be" with Joan.

C: That's about it. You may be exaggerating the hopeless part a little.

T: OK. What would the drug taking do for you in this situation?

C: Probably nothing. Only make things worse.

T: That's the "just-out-of-rehab-John" talking and obviously that's a healthy attitude. You know that the drug can easily take away those negative feelings and help you feel good for a while. But, how about dealing with the negative feelings that seem to get you thinking about taking a drug. How can you take care of the boredom, irritation, and discouragement? My point here is that emotional distress, if not taken care of, leads to drug taking that very effectively relieves the distress, but as you are *more* aware than I am, at a big price.

C: I don't know. There isn't much I can do now. I can't stand the singles functions. Even the professional singles functions. Whenever I go it seems to me that everybody there is a loser. I was even an officer in one of the singles club. I just met some real winners (sarcastically).

T: I still hear you saying two things to yourself. I can't/won't meet anyone, and I'm angry with myself because I have to associate with "losers." I keep hearing anger and some hopelessness. I'm forced to be with people I don't want to be with, and I'll never really be with people I want to be with. Let me hazard a good guess here. Underneath it all it sounds to me that you may be beginning to believe that you're a loser for not being able to get your relationships together with people you want to be with.

C: Yea. I'm feeling some of that. Wouldn't you? It's hard out there. It's especially hard when you're older, and I don't exercise as much anymore because of my knees and hypertension. I'm carrying more weight.

T: You're not feeling as good about yourself and the way you look.

C: That's right. Thirty pounds, 15 years, and heart disease, and you could be sitting in my seat.

T: OK, there are a number of feelings. Let's focus upon the three basic ones. This may be a slight exaggeration but see if you can agree if we can work with these three feelings. Things seem to be hopeless for me now. I'm angry because I have to settle for less than I want from relationships, and I am losing my attractiveness and abilities to do things.

C: That's about it.

T: OK. I want to suggest to you that hopeless, angry, and unattractive feelings are more a function of your thinking than the situation you find yourself in. If you can suspend judgment for a minute, I want to suggest that you can rarely change emotions by willing them away. However, you can change emotions by directly changing how you think and talk to yourself about the situation you find yourself in. You'll also find that a change in how you feel will provide a platform for acting differently and taking more responsibility for actively changing what you don't like about your life. Let's try and demonstrate this idea of changing your thinking and see what results we get. If it works I hope you can adapt it to other situations. Can we give it a try?

C: OK. Why not?

T: Let's take that feeling of hopelessness. What are you saying to yourself when you're feeling hopeless? What thoughts come to mind?

C: Well, things just aren't going to change. I'm going to continue to work, see my kids from time to time, and do a lot of reading—which by the way, I enjoy. The work is OK, and I do well financially, but it is routine. I just don't see myself meeting anyone I can really have a good time with. I'll continue to live by myself and go out with women I'm not crazy about.

T: I have a simple question. How do you know for sure, I mean now with *absolute* certainty, that the scenario you just painted will happen? Is it at all possible that either by chance or some action you take, even a stab in the dark, that the scenario could change? Is there any possibility that it may not happen as you predict?

C: Well, there's always a possibility that things will work out differently.

T: Yes. For the better or worse, but they may be different. So to be accurate, we would have to say that we can't predict how the future will be for you.

C: Yes, but I mean probability. I think it probable that things will stay the same since I have just not had a lot of success lately—at least over the past 10 years.

T: That's fine with me. As long as we both know that we both recognize that we are dealing with probabilities not certainties. Now, just to be clear, I hear you saying that because I have not met anyone in the past, I won't meet anyone in the future. Whatever happens in the past is destined to and must be repeated in the future. Can you convince me of the accuracy of that statement.

C: Well, no. I just think it probable.

T: OK. What controls the probability?

C: Part of it is the situation I found myself in.

T: Try saying, "the situation I placed myself in," and tell me which is probably closer to the truth.

C: Well, there are some things I did control and some I didn't.

T: OK, good. Now let's get off the philosophical level and relate all of this to what's happening in your life now. You agree that your future is not certain. You can't with absolute certainty make predictions either positive or negative, and the past does not have to determine the future. You also have some, even if limited, control over your situation by making new decisions. For example, while it may sound absurd, you could decide to leave the area, sign up for duty with an international health organization, and travel the world assisting other countries with medical problems. You would certainly break out of the routine of your present job and certainly meet new and decidedly different people. This is not a suggestion, and it may not suit you at all. But, we would both agree that this decision could radically change your life. I use a somewhat radical decision to point to the richness of possibilities for more than just superficial changes. The decisions you make may be more modest, but they will certainly lead to change. For the next session, I would like you to brainstorm a list of all the possible changes you could make in your life so as to increase the probability that you could connect with a person you could build the kind of relationship you want.

Commentary

Demoralization is a common attribute of psychotherapy clients and in particular clients with drug and alcohol problems (Frank & Frank, 1991). While the client in this case can verbalize the fact that drug taking will only exacerbate problems, long-term abstinence will not be maintained by this attitude alone. While there are potentially many issues that could have been addressed, including the client's view that he can drink occasionally, I find it especially critical to "prime the therapeutic pump" by assisting the client in challenging and changing his belief that he is destined to live a routine life bereft of any significant relationship and the best he can hope for is a financially comfortable life reading in his apartment with occasional convenience dates. Each client and therapeutic situation is unique, and the issues may differ. However, it is essential that clients begin to adopt the attitude that the future cannot be predicted with any certainty, and the past does not determine the future.

This frees the client to experiment with change. Toward the end of the session the issue of occasional drinking was dealt with by discussing both the positives and negatives. The client begrudgingly admitted that the negatives outweigh the positives. This led to a contract in which the client agreed not to drink for 3 months. After the 3 months the contract would be reviewed with the client reporting all of the positive and negative changes in the client's life as a result of not drinking. The next sessions focused upon brainstorming, problem solving, and commitment to making small changes.

T: Let's take a look at some of the suggestions for change you came up with.

C: I came up with a lot, but I don't know how effective any of these will be.

T: Well, I'm really pleased you put some time into the assignment. The effectiveness of the solutions would not be known until we "test them out" and "see the results." At this stage, we want as many as possible so we can increase the probability of finding one that works.

C: I could go the obvious route and take out a personal or sign up with a dating service. I'm not sure I like these.

T: Let's talk about them first without evaluating them. That can come later.

C: OK. I could try to join different singles groups or organizations. I could ask my sister-in-law for some introductions of people she might know, and I could ask the people at work. I know I'm not supposed to evaluate these, but I would feel too needy if I asked people at work.

T: I know it's difficult for you to suspend evaluation. Any other solutions?

C: I could become active in a local synagogue, and I could volunteer with any number of organizations and meet people that way.

T: Great. You've come up with a number of solutions. Rather than try one or two and then evaluate them, let's try as many as possible. I'd like a 3-month commitment. Just try as many things as possible and feasible for you, and after 3 months we can see if your relationships are more satisfying.

C: OK, but I'm really not sure if anything is really going to work or if it's worth the effort. I have my work, I go out occasionally, and enjoy my reading—maybe not exciting but no hassles.

T: Not bad for the short term, but it really hasn't worked for you in the long term. You're telling me that you experience a certain amount of boredom and may I add meaninglessness—you're not happy with the quality of your relationships and at times, in the past and even now, you want to escape it all with a drug. Let's build in some change and novelty and see if your relationships might not change so much that you begin to find them more rewarding—obviating the need for taking a drug to dull the pain.

Commentary

This session focused upon developing an action plan that had as its major goal increasing the client's contact with new people and activities. The development of an action plan involves generating as many solutions as possible without evaluating them and choosing as many solutions as would be feasible that could increase the probability of success. The final step is taking an experimental attitude by making a contract to try the solutions for 3 months and then evaluate the changes and outcomes. The critical psychological attitude is to assist the client in suspending all assumptions and predictions about the outcome of the interventions until "the data are in." This is quite complex because it involves learning to act in spite of negative feelings and nagging doubts based upon past experiences and failings. Also, with addicted clients an immediate-gratification orientation and an inability to tolerate frustration are the result (some would say precursor) of drug-taking behavior.

For the newly recovering addict, the fear of social interaction and relationships without help from a chemical can be intense. The essential toxic attitude here is the erroneous and widespread belief that I "must" feel good in order to and while taking action. Much of the psychological and spirituality literature argues otherwise. The Zen of "right action and right attitude" and "act without concern toward outcome" as well as the existential position of "truth exists in action" are examples. Of course, there is also support in the psychological literature for attitudinal and affective changes occurring as a consequence rather than a prerequisite for behavioral change. However, clients are not Zen monks, existential philosophers, or behavioral scientists. The interventions and solutions should be designed as much as possible to be intrinsically rewarding while assisting the client in tolerating frustration. In other words, while a change in the client's philosophy and assumptions about life is a necessary step in therapy, it is not usually sufficient if the experience of change is bereft of even the most rudimentary rewards.

Getting the client to recognize a preference for feeling good but to cease demanding that good feelings must accompany change is part of the change in the erroneous assumption that "things must be as I want them to be," or what Ellis calls "musturbation." This philosophical change involves changing an absolutist and certain attitude about how present and future reality must and will be. Once the demand for feeling good is given up, then clients can make changes building in as much reward as possible from doing the activity without concern for outcome.

Another problem at this point is fear operating as a aversive condition that reinforces avoidance of change. Worst-case scenario is an excellent way of desensitizing clients to fears involved with change. By having the client express their worst fears, imagine in the session having their worst fears unfold and then practice strategies in coping with the feared event, the groundwork can be set for the risk taking involved in change. In this case, the client's main resistances to trying new ways of meeting people were his concern about appearing "needy" and his perception of people who use dating services, personal ads, and singles clubs for meeting people as "losers." The themes of appearing "needy" and his generalized perception of other people who are seeking relationships as "losers" were explored in detail. Although the temptation might be to see these labels as projection, exploring the nature of the attribution process and the cognitive processing involved in these attributions can facilitate learning discrimination skills, rational thinking, and reducing overgeneralizations.

T: I find your fear of appearing "needy" interesting, and I'd like to explore it a little further. I'm not exactly clear about what you mean when you say "appearing needy."

C: What I mean is, I guess, being too intense and depending too much on other people in relationships. I like to depend on myself for things.

T: What things?

C: I'm really not sure what things, but I just like to stand on my own two feet.

T: OK. Let's discuss briefly what you could reasonably be expected to do for yourself and what is it impossible or not desirable to do by yourself. The point here is a certain amount of independence is healthy. But don't forget, even the Lone Ranger had Tonto. It is sometimes not possible or even desirable to be totally independent. Let's talk about some examples, and then I want you to think of specific examples of when more happiness, fulfillment, and success are produced by "interdependence." Let me begin, and you can follow. I saw Paris as a student alone, and I saw Paris with somebody else. It was nice alone but better with someone else. Now can you give me some examples.

C: (Smiling) Well, sex is better with someone rather than by yourself.

T: Good example. Certainly in an intimate relationship there is an honest recognition on both sides of a desire to be connected to someone, but is that being "needy," as you put it?

C: I'm not sure. Maybe. I guess not.

T: We need to distinguish between I prefer, I want, and I need. Obviously we can do without sex or relationships or most anything which is not absolutely necessary for survival such as food, water, and oxygen. However, to pursue preferences and wants without making them an *absolute prerequisite* for happiness and not becoming bitter and discouraged when we are disappointed in the pursuits of wants means that you never have "to be needy," as you put it. However, you can have wants which you can pursue with the full understanding that you'll win some and lose some and that's OK. It's OK to be vulnerable and have strong wants as long as you don't make their attainment an absolute prerequisite for fulfillment. Can you give me more examples of situations where it is more fulfilling to be interdependent rather than independent?

Commentary

The client gave examples such as eating out, discussing books, and some work situations. An assignment was given to practice discovering the wants and preferences of people with which he interacted and making an attempt to be responsive. Also, the client was given the assignment of matter of factly expressing wants and preferences in a nondemanding manner to colleagues and friends and to report back how this exercise changed his relationships. Along with this exercise, the client was asked to attempt to meet as many new people as possible in the next month by using a combination of methods that he mentioned such as asking for introductions, joining new organizations, and trying a professional dating service. The emphasis was upon meeting and learning as much as possible about new persons using whatever means the client felt comfortable with. This exercise assisted the client in taking the focus away from himself because the emphasis is upon "learning to appreciate the qualities and stories" of others without expectations or preconceptions regarding a relationship. Although dependence and substitution of dependent relationships for an addiction can be common problems of recovering persons, it is more critical to assist recovering persons in developing relationship skills and an understanding of healthy interdependence rather than encouraging isolation or overinvolvement in relationships while recovering.

In order to consolidate some of the gains in cognitive restructuring and problem solving learned and discussed in the prior sessions a relapse rehearsal (fire drill) was done in the next session.

T: I'm going to give you some relaxation skills, and I want you then to close your eyes and imagine a movie screen in front of you. (A brief trance induction follows.) Can you see the movie screen?

C: Yes.

T: I want you to take a moment and flesh out a scene where you feel would be the "most likely scenario" for you to relapse. Where are you, what are you doing, and what are you thinking and feeling.

C: I'm home alone in my apartment. I've got things to do, but they are the same old stuff. I'm not interested, and I feel that there is nothing for me to do that's interesting besides reading.

T: What are you feeling?

C: Bored and feeling that I should call someone to get together? But I don't want to because no one really interests me. So I feel I should get together with people I ultimately know I won't enjoy being with.

T: What else are you feeling?

C: Frustrated and angry because I'm in a situation where I'm going to lose either way.

T: What do you feel like doing?

C: Well, I could pop a few pills, have a drink, and put on some music and just relax. Maybe I'll go out then for supper with someone, and it really won't matter as much whether I really enjoy their company.

T: Now, if you could, what would your irrational self be telling you about this situation. What are you thinking in the situation and then how are you talking to yourself about those thoughts.

C: How did I find myself in the same old situation. I should have planned for having interesting activities and people I could have enjoyed myself with. It takes too much energy to find people I enjoy and I can be just as relaxed here reading and getting mellow.

T: Ok, now what are you really saying to yourself about yourself and the world in which you are living in.

C: I screwed up again. If I do take some chances and try new things they won't work anyway. Besides I work too hard during the week. I shouldn't have to work to enjoy myself on the weekends.

T: Ok, what do you need to change about your thinking so that you're thinking more constructively? Let me play the old, addiction-prone irrational you in the apartment, and you play the new, healthy you using the constructive and rational thinking skills that you've learned. We are talking now in your apartment. Let me start and you refute what I'm saying. But please try and be a little gentle with this poor soul who would rather pity himself, sulk, and nod off rather than taking some constructive action.

Commentary

A conversation between the client and therapist ensues with the client now systematically challenging assumptions of helplessness, incompetency, and the belief that life should and can be "passively enjoyed." The client was able to bring up independently the issue of unnecessarily working so hard and intensely. An extended dialogue concerning "values," that is, the value of having more time with less money, how much money is "enough," and freeing up more energy to pursue interests and relationships took place. The therapist (playing the client) pursued the argument that acquisition of money and things brings satisfaction. As a result of the refutation of this, the client made a commitment to cut back on work and came up with an action plan that included pursing activities including a volunteer organization, a local political advocacy organization, and a organization that sponsors a variety of events such as biking, sailing, skiing on weekends, thus reducing time alone in the apartment. Also, the therapist (client) made a number specific suggestions for avoiding the drug taking in the apartment such as calling a friend or sponsor, visiting his children on the spur of the moment, and leaving the apartment for a movie, hockey game, or play. The suggestion of giving himself permission to ask for assistance and honestly discuss feelings and thoughts with people without feeling "needy" was volunteered by the client. In addition, writing on a piece of paper all of the irrational thoughts preceding the urge to use and then reading them out loud while refuting them was suggested. Finally, the client developed a plan specifying the steps to take if a relapse happened. After the role play and "fire drill" were completed, the client had a new set of attitudes and an action plan which was a real alternative to drug taking. The client now felt that he had a choice and both the short-term and long-term consequences of choices were processed before the session ended.

The next sessions focused upon practicing in actual situations the skills and concepts learned (in-vivo desensitization). The exercises were oriented toward desensitizing the client toward fears of losing independence, appearing needy and dependent in relationships, and not asking for what he wanted from others. The client was given an assignment to initiate a dialogue with his children concerning his desire to be more involved and connected with them. This involved rehearsing the scene of speaking with his children while refuting the thoughts of being rejected, feeling weak for honestly sharing his loneliness with his children, and actively challenging his "Lone Ranger" script. The client was given the assignment to not only share his feelings but to attempt to find out in as much detail as possible the desires and feelings of his children. This type of dialogue was labeled as "you–me talk," and specific skills such as risking self-revelation, nondefensive listening, learning to solicit the other's perspective, and respecting and enjoying differentness were discussed. The client was then encouraged to engage in you–me talk with as many people as possible when appropriate familiarity is established. Taking responsibility for structuring relationships, risk taking, and anticipating and comfortably dealing with rejection were discussed.

The client reported in a subsequent session that he had a positive and emotional discussion relating his need for more intimacy and support with his children. His distancing, pseudoindependent style, and caretaking without allowing himself to be "taken care of" were all identified by his children. The client was now better able to take responsibility for how he set up relationships so he could remain "in control," by not appearing "needy," and how he "shot himself in the foot" in relationships. Finally, the client was asked to create a description of life goals that he would still like to accomplish. The assignment was given from the perspective of writing the last chapters of his life, that is, what was still missing, or what did he still want to accomplish? The strategy for the attainment of these goals would then form the discussion in the future follow-up sessions along with any problems that surfaced since the last session.

Summary

As a result of discussions in follow-up sessions with the client, the following changes were noted. The client reported a greater ease in establishing relationships and less aversion to taking risks. The client was more able to recognize and articulate wants and desires without castigating himself. Although the client had not met "anyone special," he did report that he enjoyed the new people he met as a result of some of the organizations he joined. In addition, the client had plans to sell his business and retire in Florida near his sister and work part-time. Finally, the client decided to study history in college, a subject he had a intense love of, but never pursued formally. He was contemplating a part-time teaching position after he completes his study. Although he did report urges to use "occasionally," the client felt he now had "more to lose" by using, and he had "tools to deal with setbacks."

This case illustrates how small and subtle changes in thinking, acting, values, and goals can generalize to significant change. This approach allows clients to take basic skills and changes learned and developed in therapy and continue to elaborate on them in their lives, thus increasing their sense of self-efficacy in directing their lives and avoiding addictive behavior.

References

Beck, A. T. (1976). *Cognitive therapy and the emotional disorders.* New York: International Universities Press.

Beck, A. T. (1987). Cognitive therapy. In J. Zeig (Ed.), *The evolution of psychotherapy* (pp. 149–163). New York: Brunner/Mazel.

Brown, S. (1985). *Treating the alcoholic: A developmental model of recovery.* New York: Wiley.

Brownell, R. D., Marlatt, G. A., Lichenstein, E., & Wilson, G. T. (1986). Understanding and preventing relapse. *American Psychologist, 41,* 765–781.

Childress, A. R., McLellan, T., & O'Brien, C. P. (1986). Abstinent opiate users exhibit conditioned craving, conditioned withdrawal and reductions in both through extinction. *British Journal of Addictions, 81,* 655–660.

Csikszentmihalyi, M. (1990). *Flow: The psychology of optimal experience.* New York: Harper & Row.

Dohner, V. A. (1972). Motives for drug use: Adult and adolescent. *Psychosomatics, 13,* 317–324.

Ellis, A. (1962). *Reason and emotion in psychotherapy.* New York: Kyle Stuart.

Ellis, A., & Harper, R. A. (1975). *A new guide to rational living.* Englewood Cliffs, NJ: Prentice-Hall.

Ellis, A., McInerney, T. F., DiGuiseppe, R., & Yeager, R. J. (1988). *Rational-emotive therapy with alcoholics and substance abusers.* New York: Pergamon.

Frank, J., & Frank, J. (1991). *Persuasion and healing* (3rd ed.). Baltimore, MD: Johns Hopkins University Press.

Franklin, J. (1981). *Molecules of the mind.* New York: Touchstone Books.

Glasser, W. (1985). *Positive addiction.* New York: Harper & Row.

Heide, R. J., & Mahoney, M. J. (1980). Cognitive strategies for medical disorders. In J. M. Ferguson & C. B. Taylor, (Eds.), *The comprehensive handbook of behavioral medicine,* Vol. 3 (pp. 99–111). New York: S P Medical and Scientific Books.

Illich, I. (1976). *Medical nemesis.* New York: Pantheon.

Kandel, D. B., & Raveis, V. H. (1989). Cessation of illegal drug use in young adulthood. *Archives of General Psyschiatry, 46,* 109–16.

Khantzian, E. J. (1985). The self-medication hypothesis of addictive disorders: Focus on heroin and cocaine dependence. *American Journal of Psychiatry, 142,* 1259–1264.

Koumjian, K. (1981). The use of Valium as a form of social control. *Social Science and Medicine, 15,* 245–249.

McAuliffe, W. E., & Gordon, R. A. (1974). A test of Lindesmith's theory of addiction: The frequency of euphoria among long-term addicts. *The American Journal of Sociology, 79,* 795–840.

Marlatt, G. A., & Gordon, J. R. (Eds.). (1985). *Relapse prevention.* New York: Guilford.

May, G. (1988). *Addiction and grace.* New York: Harper & Row.

Ray, O. (1978). *Drugs, society and human behavior* (2nd ed.). St. Louis: Mosby.

Schuster, C. R., & Johanson, C. E. (1981). An analysis of drug seeking behavior in animals. *Neuroscience and Bio-Behavioral Reviews, 5,* 315–324.

Stewart, J., DeWit, H., & Eikelboom, R. (1984). The role of unconditioned and conditioned drug effects in the self-administration of opiates and stimulants. *Psychological Review, 91,* 251–268.

Westmeyer, T. (1976). *A primer on chemical dependency: A clinical guide to alcohol and drug problems.* Baltimore, MD: Williams and Williams.

Wikler, A. (1973). Dynamics of drug dependence: Implications of a conditioning theory for research and treatment. *Archives of General Psychiatry, 28,* 611–616.

12

Single-Session Experiential Therapy with Any Person Whatsoever

Alvin R. Mahrer and Martine Roberge

Introduction

Experiential psychotherapy (Mahrer, 1989a) is a way for any person to undergo transformation into a substantially new person. In each session, the person is shown how to move toward optimal "integration" and "actualization" by following a four-step sequence: (a) being in a moment of strong, full feeling and accessing or opening up an inner, deeper experiencing; (b) appreciating and welcoming this inner, deeper experiencing; (c) undergoing a radical, transformative shift into being this inner, deeper experiencing in the context of earlier life scenes; and (d) being and behaving as this integrated, actualized new person in this new person's extratherapy world. Regardless of who the person is and what the opening concerns are, each session is an invitation to undergo a profound process of becoming and being as profoundly new, happy, problem-free, and optimally integrated and actualized as the person is ready and willing to achieve.

Alvin R. Mahrer and Martine Roberge • School of Psychology, University of Ottawa, Ottawa, Ontario, Canada K1N 6N5.

Casebook of the Brief Psychotherapies, edited by Richard A. Wells and Vincent J. Giannetti. Plenum Press, New York, 1993.

A Friendly Invitation to Try an Alternative Set of Cherished Truths about Psychotherapy

Almost every therapist has a personal package of cherished truths about psychotherapy. You have firmly entrenched beliefs about how to make sense of your patients, how change occurs, what is to change, and the directions of change that are worthwhile for each patient. Other approaches are seen through the perspective of your own cherished truths. If other approaches do not conform to or even violate your cherished truths, these other approaches are seen as alien, lesser, incomplete, and inadequate. As you read this chapter, we offer you a friendly invitation to set aside your own cherished truths and to allow yourself to get inside another set of cherished truths. When you are done, you will go back to your own set of cherished truths, but of course we hope your ways of seeing how and what therapy can achieve will be enlarged a little.

Every Session Proceeds through Four Steps

The core of this therapy is a four-step sequence. It is the same four steps for every person and for every session.

1. *Being in a moment of strong, full feeling and accessing the inner, deeper experiencing.* The purpose of the first step is for the person to be in a moment in which the level of feeling is strong, intense, full, saturating. The feeling may be pleasant and joyful, or it may be unpleasant and painful. The feeling may be strong and loud, as when the person is yelling, laughing hard, sobbing. Or the feeling may be strong and quiet, as when the feeling is one of awe, wonder, bliss, absolute peacefulness, shock, frozenness, numbness. The feeling is full, saturating when the bodily sensations fill the whole body. This state of strong, full feeling may last but a moment, or it may be a plateau that persists over a few minutes or more.

The reason why this state of strong, full feeling is useful is that something inside the person is activated, is raised up a bit, is made alive and present. The state of strong, full feeling is like a crucible that accesses some inner quality or process or way of being. What is deeper inside is the underside of the strong, full feeling, a connected accompaniment of the strong, full feeling. We call this the person's inner experiencing (Mahrer, 1989b). It is an inner, possible, available way of being or experiencing. It is one of many "deeper potentials for experiencing" inside this person, but it is the particular one that is activated and raised up by the strong, full feeling. We describe it by describing the nature of this particular experiencing as it is right now in this person. It is the experiencing of letting go, setting free, opening up; it is being prized, loved, cared about; it is the experiencing of being better than, competing with, outdoing; it is the experiencing of being soft, passive, yielding. Whatever it is, the accessing of this person's inner experiencing is the precious jewel, the goal of the first step.

2. *Welcoming and appreciating this inner experiencing.* The purpose of the second step is to welcome and appreciate the accessed inner experiencing. The person is to keep it here, let it be, give it a home. The person is to enjoy it, treasure it, feel good with it. The person is to know it, identify it, describe it. The person is to receive and accept it.

3. *Being the inner experiencing in the context of earlier life scenes.* The third step enables the person to disengage and get out of the ordinary, continuing, everyday person that he or she is and to thoroughly and completely be the person who is the inner experiencing. This is a radical shift, a wholesale transformation into being a whole new person who literally is the inner experiencing. This is accomplished within the context of an earlier life scene, some incident or moment that you identify from any earlier time in the person's life.

4. *Being and behaving as the new person in the context of the prospective extratherapy world.* The purpose of the final step is for the person to gain a taste, a sample of what it is like to be and to behave as this new person in the extratherapy world. The person is to be and to behave as this inner experiencing in life scenes of tomorrow and beyond. The person undergoes what it is like to be this new person in prospective life scenes. When the person leaves the session, it may be as this substantially new person, or it may be as someone who has gained a live taste and sample of what life can be like as this new person. In any case, there is to be some commitment to some new way of being and behaving that comes from and provides for the new experiencing, even in a small, safe way.

EXPERIENTIAL THERAPY IS FOR ANY PERSON WHATSOEVER

This therapy is for any person who is ready and willing to have a single session that proceeds through the four steps. This means that some persons may not be ready and willing today, but perhaps they will be ready and willing in a few days or next week or so. That is fine.

What is the most sensible way of seeing if this person is ready and willing to have a session? Try it out. The contract is for this single session, not an extended series of sessions. This means there is no presession evaluation, assessment, or screening. It means that readiness and willingness to proceed through the four steps have nothing to do with what, in other approaches, is referred to as the "presenting problem," or the nature and degree of "pathological condition" or "psychodiagnosis." This therapy is for males and females, old and young, sophisticated, and those not especially so. Readiness and willingness to achieve the four steps of a session are for any person whatsoever.

PRACTICAL LOGISTICS OF THE SESSION

Arrangements for the session are made with the person, rather than with a referral source or relative. You work with this person and not with a couple, a family, or a group. You and the person sit or lean back in chairs that are large and comfortable, with large footstools. The chairs are right alongside one another, facing in the same direction. The person's eyes are closed from the very beginning and throughout the entire session. Your eyes are closed, too. The room is soundproofed. The session ends when you and the person finish the four steps and when both of you are ready to end the session. Typically this takes about 1½ to 2 hours or so. If you want to have another session, and the person is agreeable, you schedule one.

All by itself, each session is a complete minitherapy (Mahrer, 1988). A person may have only this one session, although most everyone wants to have more sessions. Most persons have sessions for a year or so and return later for sets of three to five sessions or so. Some have only 1 or 2 or 10 to 20 sessions. In any case, each session is its own complete minitherapy.

THE PERSON'S STANCE AND ROLE

In the opening of the session, you show the person (client, patient) how to put virtually all his or her attention on some feeling-connected attentional center, issue, image, or scene. This is the person's stance throughout the entire session. He is always focused on something connected with feeling. He is always living in some scene, whether it is real or fanciful, in the present or future or past. Even when he says something to the therapist, it is while he is engrossed in this scene, attending to this or that. Rarely does the person focus most of his attention on the therapist. Never does the person sit face to face, eyeball to eyeball, in back-and-forth conversation with the therapist.

The person's role is to be the one who carries out the four steps. It is the person who carries out the actual work, who is the active doer. This is why the person's immediate readiness and willingness are paramount.

The Therapist's Stance and Role

Throughout the whole session, all your attention is on the immediate scene before you. You are always seeing something, always living and being in some scene, always attending to whatever is there in front of you. Every time the person says and does something, you are postured so that these words, said in this way, are as if they are coming in and through you. This is why it is absolutely essential that your opening instructions enable the person to put all his attention on whatever is central and feeling connected, and to have this feeling as fully as possible. From then on, throughout the session, you are so close into the person, so closely blended into and intertwined into the person, that his immediate words are as if they are coming in and through you. And then his words, said in the immediate way, will evoke scenes and images. You see what his words put here for you to see. Indeed, each time the person says something, you may be furnished with new images and scenes.

Your role is to proceed through the four steps of the session. In the first step, everything you do is aimed toward enabling the person to move toward a level of strong and full feeling and to be ready to receive the inner experiencing that is accessed. In the second step, your role is to welcome and appreciate this accessed inner experiencing, whatever it is. In the third step, your role is to show the person how to locate the earlier life scene, and to wholly be this inner experiencing in this scene. Finally, you are programmed to show the person how to undergo the wonderful possibility of being and behaving as this new, inner experiencing in the prospective extratherapy world.

In proceeding through the four steps, your role is coach, guide, the one who shows the person what to do and how to do it. You are the competent one, the one who is skilled in undergoing the four steps. Your role is also the one who accompanies the person throughout the four steps. You go through what the person goes through right along with the person. You undergo these changes at least as much as the person does, in each session.

This stance and this role mean that you have virtually no private thoughts, no inferences. You are not a separate therapist who attends mainly to the patient, who focuses on the patient while formulating impressions about the patient. You do not relate or interact mainly with the patient. You are neither empathic nor accepting, building rapport, nor establishing a working alliance. What you do and say are not interventions. You are not treating a problem or pathological condition.

The Effectiveness of the Session Is a Function of the Therapist, Not the Person

Experiential therapy is suitable and useful for any person, providing the person is ready and willing for each step in this session. However, this therapy is not for every therapist. It is the therapist who almost singlehandedly determines whether or not this session with this person is successful and effective.

The therapist must have an adequate level of competence and skill in carrying out the methods. The more you can develop and expand your skills, the more likely you are to achieve the four steps. Therapists who lack the requisite skills will probably not have sessions that are successful or effective.

It is relatively easy, quick, and objective to tell if you have achieved each of the four steps. It is much easier than to wait for some way of assessing the consequences of an extended series of sessions. If you do not achieve a step, you have work to do in learning the proper skills or in developing greater competence. The problem lies minimally in the person or the goodness of fit between this person and this therapy; the answer lies in your own competencies.

Your opening instructions are critical. From the very beginning, all of the person's attention must be on a feeling-connected scene or center, and feeling is to be as strong and full as possible. From then on, you must receive the scenes and images that are evoked when you allow the person's words to be as if they are coming in and through you, and to have the feelings that occur with these words in this immediate scene. The effectiveness of the session requires that all of your attention is on those evoked images and scenes. You must totally live in these alive, real, wholly engrossing scenes. Accomplishing this is a risky leap, but a truly effective session requires wholesale live engagement in the immediately evoked scene. Furthermore, you must be fully open to receiving and welcoming any feeling or experiencing whatsoever. In the culmination of the first step, you especially must be ready, willing, and competent to receive the activated inner experiencing. This is critical because the subsequent three steps revolve on the received nature of this inner experiencing.

The degree of success depends on your own readiness and ability to go through the four steps along with the person. In other words, you are to open yourself to as much change as you are inviting the person to go through. Indeed, your own readiness and willingness should match or exceed that of the person in each step.

This therapy offers you the roles of coach and accompanier. This means you are asked to decline all the gratifications of fulfilling all the roles that go with your attending mainly to the patient, and having the patient attend mainly to you. You are to decline the common stance of therapist and patient attending exclusively to one another as the two of you relate and interact and co-construct mutual role relationships (Mahrer, 1978, 1986, 1989c; Mahrer & Gervaize, 1983).

The degree of success depends on the degree to which you understand persons in terms of varying potentials for experiencing that can be integrated with one another, and that the person can be and behave on the basis of. If your conceptualization is cordial, you can achieve the four steps. If your conceptualization is not cordial, success is limited.

The Useful Resources

This experiential psychotherapy has evolved and changed over about three decades. However, the best book on how to do this therapy is given in a manual explicitly written for practitioners (Mahrer, 1989a). The four steps in each session, and the methods of reaching these four steps (Mahrer, 1989a,d, 1990b), are now different from, and better than, those given in earlier publications (e.g., Mahrer, 1986, 1989c). Because a fair proportion of sessions include work with dreams, the theory and methods of dreamwork with persons and with oneself are given in another book (Mahrer, 1990a). The underlying comprehensive theory of human beings is contained in another resource (Mahrer, 1989b). These three books should be sufficient to enable you to do this therapy, although you might be interested in listening to tapes of sessions. To do that, please contact the first author of this chapter. He and his colleagues have written 10 books and approximately 135 chapters and articles dealing mainly with the theory, practice, and research of psychotherapy, including this therapy, but the above four resources are probably the most useful.

CASE IDENTIFICATION, BACKGROUND INFORMATION, AND PRESENTING COMPLAINTS

Nicole left a message that she would like an appointment with you. When you return her call, you and Nicole agree to have a session next Thursday at 4:00, and you let her know the session may go on for 1½ to 2 hours or so. Let her know the fee and that she is to pay when the session is over. Tell her where your office is located. If a professional colleague had called and wanted to refer Nicole, tell her to ask Nicole to call you directly. If the professional colleague or Nicole are inclined to tell you things about Nicole, you can say thank you, but you do not need that information.

The important information that you and Nicole need is the inner, deeper experiencing that is accessed when you both attain the first step of the session. This means that virtually everything that is ordinarily included as case identification, background information, and presenting complaints is not relevant, helpful, or useful for your work. None of that kind of information would lead you to proceed differently in this session with Nicole. Indeed, placing yourself and Nicole in the roles and in the role relationships necessary to gather such information would mean that you could not carry out the session, and would seriously interfere with carrying out the four steps. Accordingly, you do not gather such information, either in a phone conversation, in presession informational questionnaires or inventories, or in the initial session.

DIAGNOSTIC AND ASSESSMENT INTERVIEW

The same considerations apply to what is ordinarily described as a diagnostic and assessment interview. Your work involves you as the one who shows Nicole how to proceed through the four steps, and to undergo the four steps along with Nicole. Your role is not that of diagnoser or assessor or interviewer. Your work requires that you and Nicole access the inner, deeper experiencing in her in this session. None of the information that diagnostic and assessment interviews provide can access Nicole's inner, deeper experiencing in this session. Indeed, placing yourself and Nicole in the roles of diagnoser and diagnosee, assessor and assessee, interviewer and interviewee will seriously interfere with your work and prevent you and Nicole from undergoing the four steps of the session.

Treatment Process

The purpose of this section is to walk with you through the single, initial session with Nicole. It might have been the only session. If we are successful, you may be inclined to see what it can be like to use this approach in your own work. If you would like a transcript of this session, contact us.

Step 1. Being in a moment of strong, full feeling, and accessing the inner experiencing. You greet Nicole at the waiting room. She appears to be in her 30s or 40s, and she is about average height. The two of you enter the office. You tell her to sit in that chair, to remove her glasses. You sit back, close your eyes, tell her to close her eyes, and keep them closed the whole time. You will do the same. Ask if she is ready to begin. She is. Your opening instructions are critical:

"Think of anything that makes you have strong feeling. Put all your attention on whatever makes you have really strong feeling. When you think of it, when you see it, you feel like falling apart or laughing like hell, or being really mad or scared stiff or worried, really worried, or really proud of yourself or like crying. Put all your attention on it. See it. Maybe it's a scene or just something you see. It may be an incident, something you did, something about you, something that happened. . . . You're probably seeing something already. All right, let yourself have the feeling, the strong feeling. There's something that's guaranteed to make you have a strong feeling. Have it as much as you can. Make the feeling happen as much as you can. When you are ready, show all the feeling that is connected to whatever you are thinking of, seeing, putting all your attention on. You are the only one who can see it and who can show the strong and full feeling. You have to be ready. When you are ready, then you go ahead. You are seeing something. Have the feeling, and show it. All the way."

As you say all this, all your attention is deployed out there, ready to see whatever Nicole puts there. You are only talking to Nicole to the side, with your attention out there, not on Nicole. You are doing what you are asking Nicole to do. You are ready to see anything. You are ready to be in any scene.

When you finish the opening instructions, you are peering ahead, all set to see whatever her words will evoke. Your insides are empty, drained. There are no thoughts, no notions, no executive removed part with its own stream of private thoughts. You are ready to let Nicole's words come in and through you, totally. Whatever Nicole does, whatever she says, will also be what you are doing and saying. You are thoroughly positioned to have the words be as if they are coming in and through you, and to see and be wholly attentive to whatever the words evoke before you.

Nicole starts. Her voice is high-pitched and strained, pressured and tight. Words rush out rapidly. "Um. Um. What is going on is panic! Panic! It's like a *pressure* in front of my face and in my head and arms and chest! I'm running out of breath and it's *panic* . . . (her voice rises even further) . . . and I don't know where panic goes if I give in to panic!!!"

These words are simultaneously reverberating in and through you: ". . . I don't know where panic goes if I give in to panic!!" You are enveloped in a maelstrom of whipped-up panic, caught in the vortex of high-energy, swirling panic, and the feeling is one of falling, sinking wholly into it, being totally caught up in it. What do you do?

In the first step, you are programmed to do two things: (a) Every time Nicole says something, you see whatever her words evoke. You see the image. You live and be in the evoked scene, whatever it is. You are to see the image as much as you can, and you are to live in the scene as much as you can. Invite Nicole to do the same. Nicole is to be riveted on the immediate image. She is to live fully in the immediate scene. (b) Every time Nicole says something, you are to have the accompanying feeling. You and Nicole are to be wholly receptive to having this feeling, to letting this feeling occur as strongly and fully as possible. If one image or scene opens into another, that is fine. Everything you do is to move toward attaining a level of very strong, very full feeling.

When she says, ". . . I don't know where panic goes if I give in to panic!!", you attend as much as you can to being caught in the enveloping maelstrom of whipped-up "panic," and you let yourself fully receive and have the accompanying feeling of falling into it, sinking into it. You say, "Well! Here's this feeling of letting myself fall into it, just sinking in. I'm falling! . . . It's all around! Like a whirlpool of panic, whipped up! . . . OK, here I go! . . . Ready to fall in and see what happens? Aaahhh, it's starting!"

In a much louder voice, higher-pitched and with sputtering words, she says, ". . . I feel *crazy!* It feels as close to crazy as I *ever felt!* . . . I don't really like this!!!" As these words come through you, there is a feeling of tightening up, holding back, not letting it happen, and your attention is drawn toward a vaguely defined inner craziness that is welling up in you. You say, "Right! There's this craziness inside! I don't like it! Uh . . . Let's get a grip on things. . . (With attention on the inner burgeoning craziness:) . . . I don't like you, and I'm not going to give in! No way! (And to Nicole:) . . . Hold tight! Fight it! We can do it!"

Nicole is crying, and this deepens into heartfelt sobbing as she mentions doll houses falling in on themselves and toy brick houses collapsing inward. While you see the doll houses and the toy brick houses, your feeling becomes that of screeching collapse, anguished falling apart. These images and this feeling continue for several minutes as Nicole is sobbing and you are undergoing and inviting her to see the images more vividly and to open up the increasing feeling.

Suddenly there is a shift. Nicole becomes clenched, grim and, through her sobbing, she hisses: "I am so ANGRY. DAMN YOU!" There is hard, wrenching sobbing. You are confronting an undefined person, and the feeling is a belting out anger: "Let it get STRONGER. I feel it! DAMN YOU! DAMN YOU! Oh yes! Here it comes!!!" Nicole continues the sobbing, interweaving hard staccato outbursts and prolonged softer moanings. Interspersed are anguished words: ". . . Oh Mother . . . Why did you? . . . I never could say anything . . . What was so wrong . . . I'll never understand." Your attention is fully on Mother, and the feeling is a pleading, hurtful anguish. You say, "Yes . . . Yes . . . I *hurt!* . . . Now I'm showing you and . . . there's more . . . Yes . . . All this HURT." The sobbing and moaning continue, and you invite Nicole to open up this awful feeling all the way: "SURE . . . NOW'S THE TIME . . . ALL THE WAY . . . ALL THE WAY . . . MOTHER . . . HERE IT COMES . . . YES!!"

Nicole's hard sobbing and moaning continue, deepen and intensify. Then there is an abrupt stop. A short pause, and it is as if a qualitatively different voice explodes. No sobbing. No moaning. No feeling of pleading, hurtful anguish. The new voice says, "I HATE YOU . . . I HATE YOU!!!"

Your attention is wholly fixed on the image of mother. Your whole body is charged with powerful sensations. In this moment, you and Nicole have attained the level of very strong and very full feeling. Inside you is a shimmering new quality that goes with these words, coming out in this way and in this immediate scene. You sense an inner, deeper experiencing of hardness, strength, power, toughness, an insistent standing up to, a solid defiance. You are receiving the precious inner experiencing, the deeper potential way of being and behaving. This is the culmination of the first step.

Step 2. Welcoming and appreciating the inner experience. Now that this inner experiencing is in you, you are geared toward welcoming and appreciating it. You do this by (a) letting it be here for a while, staying with it, just letting it remain; (b) accepting it, enjoying it, cherishing it, treasuring it; and (c) lifting it up and opening it up a little, bringing it forward a bit, giving it some form and shape, helping it to occur somewhat. You say, "Oh this is something! I'm still looking right at you, mother, and I got this thing inside me, a hardness, strength . . . wow . . . yes . . . a toughness, like being defiant . . . Just let me keep it around a little . . . in me . . . yes . . . Oh this feels good . . . really good . . ."

Nicole is still crying, but it is softer, and she whispers, "I never cried like that . . ." You are engaged in welcoming and appreciating this inner experiencing: "Yeah, and now I got this feeling in me . . . it's still here . . . I'm going to let it stay a while . . . it's nice . . . Like being tough and really strong, a standing up to her . . . I'm still seeing you, Mom, and oh this feels good (and to Nicole:) OK to just let it be here for a little? I want to . . ." There are still tears, but Nicole lightens: "I never felt this with her . . . or anyone . . ." For the next 5 minutes or so, you and Nicole welcome and appreciate this inner experiencing while keeping your attention on Mother, in this immediate scene. Finally, Nicole is almost playful: "I like this. It does feel good . . . (sighs) . . . Like a friend . . . (lightly laughing) I never was that way . . . Yes I was! . . . Not with Mom . . ." You and Nicole have welcomed and appreciated the inner experiencing.

Step 3. Being the inner experiencing in earlier life scenes. In the third step, your aim is to enable Nicole to have an opportunity to *become* this inner experiencing, to literally "be" a qualitatively new person who is this inner experiencing, and who feels good, even wonderful, being this whole new experiencing person. You aim at enabling this to occur within the context of some earlier life scene, incident, event. You and Nicole must work together to identify and locate some earlier life scene:

"If you can actually *be* this way—really feel what it's like to be firm and tough, hard and strong, we have to find some right time in your life. Let's see. We can go back and find one with the feeling, or maybe with some woman you're with . . . Let's use the feeling. . . . Are you ready to go back in your life? Is this OK now? (Uh-huh.) Good. So let's get ready. . . . You have to get ready. Back in your life, maybe being a little girl. Just let yourself sink into being a little girl . . . and you're seeing things . . . a little girl . . . like your room . . . the school. . . . See things already? (Nicole: I see the house on Sheridan Street . . . front yard . . .) Good. . . . Now I'm going to say words, slowly, and you'll see something. Whatever you see . . . whatever you see . . . It may have nothing to do with the words I say . . . You'll see something. Whatever you see is fine. So now get ready . . . OK? (Yes.) . . . I'm tough, strong, defiant, not going to stand for this . . . all right, what do you see?

Nicole's voice is hushed, low, a little squeaky. "She's in the bed . . .

They're bringing me to her . . . Just born, I mean . . . You never knew anything . . . Born, just born, being happy . . . (Now there is light crying) . . . I don't have a chance . . . Oh, oh . . . There's something wrong with me, like a birth defect . . . only I don't have one, but I have one, only it's not really . . . (You join with Nicole in clarifying these images to identify a moment, a scene, a vivid and real moment; you gently clarify along with Nicole. Then she continues.) . . . Babies got to be in the nursery till the mothers woke up, and they want the mothers to sleep . . . I am OK. I am happy (She cries) . . . (Then, a baby voice, she blurts out:) They *tricked* me! This one here! I mean she's gonna hurt me! She hurted me! I know it! They just show me! She doesn't want nothing to do with me!"

You have identified a vivid and alive scene. Now here comes the big change. Nicole is to "be" the inner experiencing in this moment. She is to be the inner experiencing fully and completely, with crashing pleasure and enjoyment. You are living in this scene, and you show her what to do and how to do it: "OK, you're already beginning to do it. Pretend that you're magically a 1-day-old baby who's already an accomplished tough guy, a defiant kid who stands up for her rights! (Nicole starts to laugh with gusto, and throughout the instructions she chortles and bellows with laughter). I mean this kid's got a mouth on her! Bring this kid into the room, and already she starts! 'They tricked me! She's gonna hurt me!' Where did this kid come from? You're already complaining about the management! (Nicole: "I don't want that one!") Right!! OK! Look at the Mother there! Waking up from this big ordeal! Make her confused! Stand up for yourself! Here's a born hard kid, tough and strong! 'Take me away! Not *that* one! I don't want her!' You're tiny, and the nurse is holding you, and the tiny thing belts it out: 'What? That one! No way!' Go ahead! This is you! Here's your chance!"

Throughout the next portion, Nicole and you galvanize each other in being this inner experiencing. Here are just a few selected highlights, with what you say indicated in parentheses): "They make mistakes! (Right! Check it! Check it! Look at the wristband! I demand a blood test!) I never saw this woman before in my life! (Look at her eyes! She's troubled!) Who was in the delivery room? Do you have any proof? I don't want this one! First of all, she's STUPID! . . . There's something wrong with you! I don't know what, but I DON'T WANT YOU! . . . You can't be trusted. YOU LIE . . . YOU FUCK AROUND AND YOU LIE! You have no right to have babies! YOU HAVE NO RIGHT TO BE A MOTHER AND SOMEDAY THERE'LL BE A LAW! (You never passed the Appropriate Parent Test! You FAILED) I hate you! I was inside you for nine fucking months! I know exactly what you think! You're EVIL. I HATE YOU. YOU DON'T DESERVE TO

HAVE A BABY, CERTAINLY NOT ME . . . I know you better than anyone, and you're gonna pull the biggest bullshit on me . . . Only I know. I DON'T WANNA BE YOUR BABY! . . . You listen to me. YOU JUST LISTEN! And you are gonna shut up and LISTEN . . ." Nicole continues, with lowered voice, but tougher and harder. She is thoroughly and enjoyably being hard, strong, powerful, tough, defiant, standing up to. The third step is achieved, and Nicole is fully and enjoyably being a person who is the inner experiencing.

Step 4. Being and behaving as the inner experiencing in the prospective extratherapy world. The purpose of this step is to enable Nicole to have a taste, a sample of what it can be like for her to be and to behave as this inner experiencing in ways that feel good, wonderful, and in the context of scenes and situations in the prospective extratherapy world. At the end of Step 3, Nicole is being and behaving as this new inner experiencing in the context of an earlier scene from her life. Now you show this new person how to be and behave as this new person in scenes from the extratherapy world of today, tomorrow, and from now on.

How do you do this? There are lots of methods of doing this (Mahrer, 1989a). Nicole may "really" be this new person, or she may just try it out for a short time on a kind of trial basis. The scenes and situations may be anchored in Nicole's actual extratherapy world, or they may be fanciful and far-fetched. The tone may be serious and reality-based, or it may be playful, silly, a little wild. Generating the scenes and behaviors may come largely from Nicole or largely from you. What you and Nicole do is guided by this question: What can you and Nicole do to provide this new person with a full and enjoyable taste and sample of what it can be like to be and to behave as this new inner experiencing in scenes and situations of a prospective, imminent extratherapy world?

One method is to address Nicole as this new inner experiencing and to invite this new Nicole to step into Nicole's world. "If you had free rein to do anything you want, when you leave here, if *you* were Nicole, what would you just love to do? Straighten out Nicole's world! Have fun doing whatever *you* want so you can be this great person who feels hard and strong, tough and powerful; you know, a defiant person who stands up to. Be playful. Make it all fantasy. Absolutely unrealistic. How would you *love* to be? Where? With whom?" Nicole even sounds just like the new Nicole, and she immediately pictures talking to her aunt who took care of her on and off throughout her childhood. "I never told her *anything!* Not what I really *feel!*" You show Nicole how to detail the prospective scene and to say it to her aunt. She throws herself into being hard and tough with her aunt: "This time you just sit down and *listen!* You're Mom's little sister, and you NEVER stood up to her! You're a *wimp!*

And so the hell am I! Well, now you listen. JUST LISTEN! I may let you talk later. Maybe!" Then she launches into defiant explosion. For example, "We were always scared mother'd feel bad and get depressed! Jesus Christ! We all collaborated! She died 4 *years* ago, and no one ever talked straight to her! No one! Not me or you or Dad or anyone! We were all scared of her! Well, no more! My God, remember when you . . ." Nicole was laughing as she recounts incident after incident, and as she joins with her aunt in recollecting times when they both should have stood up to Mother.

On her own, Nicole is still being this powerful, defiant person as she spontaneously comes up with things she'd love to do. She is going to direct her brother to give her Mom's wristwatch he took when Mom died. She is not going to play tennis any more with her husband. "Every week he drags me to the courts and makes me feel like an incompetent sheep. Yes, John! I'll try, John. Is this better, John? I HATE TENNIS!" In sheer playful fantasy, you show her how to make these scenes and behaviors vivid and actual, and to taste and sample being this new person as she lays it all out to her brother and to her husband. Sometimes she is booming and high-volumed, sometimes she is icy cool, but throughout she is actually being and behaving as this qualitatively new Nicole. When it is over, Nicole feels great: "Damn, this feels good . . . I feel like I just woke up. I was like a zombie with John, everyone, everyone! Half alive, dreaming."

You offer another avenue. "I'm looking at something, vague. You fill it in. OK? . . . It's the last place you'd ever really be this way. Strong and defiant? No way! Couldn't do it here. Huh-uh . . . All right, what are you seeing?" "My Dad! Yeah! . . . Oh this's hard . . . Oh, he'd die!" You fill in the scene and make it alive and real, and Nicole allows herself to be hard and tough as she barrels into her Dad. There is a rollicking energy as she exclaims how damned stupid they both were, how they co-conspired to exist under a veil of unfeeling throughout their lives, how she insists that the two of them will spend much more time together. And she goes on to other possibilities. She sees Marsha, her friend, and Nicole announces that she will not tolerate Marsha's running the lives of Marsha's two grown sons and their wives. Nicole wants to assemble these people and to command Marsha to lay off. In fact, Nicole is so detailed and alive in living this scene through that she declares her absolute intention to do this immediately.

Every session ends with the person identifying some behavior she is ready and willing to carry out, and with a good measure of intention and pleasant commitment. You wonder aloud if Nicole is really serious about any of these possibilities. "Yes! With Marsha! I'm *going* to do it! It's time! It's more than time!" All right, let's give it a dress rehearsal and try it out for real. You show Nicole how to make the scene exceedingly alive and immediate, how to be this inner experiencing fully and completely. Nicole tries it out and does very well. You check your body and invite Nicole to check hers. "See how it feels in the body to have done this. What's happening inside?" Nicole says, "Well, nothing. My stomach's a little tight. But OK I guess. Not bad . . ." You sense a little muscular tension in your chest, and you tell Nicole, "Yeah, well all I got is a little tension in the chest, and you don't have much better things inside, so let's drop it—or maybe you can change things a little, what do you think?" Nicole brightly deletes the sons and wives. "I want to tell Marsha. Just you." She returns to the scene, with Marsha alone, and keeps modifying what she says till it feels just wonderful: "Hey! Yeah! This feels great! . . . I'm buzzing all over! I got a little charge! Oh I'm gonna lay it on the line with her. One on one! That's better! Watch out Marsha, here I come! Don't get in my way, Marsha! (She chortles.) I'm ready! . . ."

Nicole has been the new person, tasted and sampled new ways of being and behaving as this new experiencing and has a reasonable degree of commitment to carrying out a given new behavior. The fourth step is accomplished, the "therapeutic charge" reduces, and you are ready to wind the session to a close.

Clinical Issues, Termination, and Follow-Up

How do you schedule another session? At the end of the session, you were quite satisfied with what was accomplished and you indicate that you would like to have another session: "I would like to have another session. Would next week at the same time be OK with you? Yes? No?" Nicole wants one in 3 days. You have no opening then, but the two of you agree on an appointment in 5 days.

Because the next session proceeds through the same four steps, Nicole's opening attention focuses on the warmly hilarious time she and her husband had with her father. One day after the initial session, she burst into his routinized life, brought him to her home for a few days, commanded him to tell stories about her early childhood, and enjoyed no longer honoring his characteristic overtures to avoid the least bit bothersome. Throughout the first step, she was briskly high-spirited as the level of strong, full feeling was attained, and what accessed was an inner experiencing of being cuddled, loved, intimately drawn close. But that is another story. Did she carry out the new behavior with Marsha? Yes, but in the second session other issues were central.

Nicole had 36 sessions. Each year she returns for short bursts of about 2 to 5 sessions. This is common.

In experiential therapy, each session is a complete minitherapy in that you proceed through the same four steps. Each session terminates the work of that session. In this way, even if there are many sessions and profound changes in ways of being and behaving, the usual issues of termination are essentially not constructed (Mahrer et al., 1992). In this approach, each session provides the follow-up data for the previous session. In the next session, is Nicole now a new and changing person who can be and behave on the basis of the inner experiencing accessed in the prior session? Was she able to be and to behave on the basis of the way of being and behaving tasted and sampled in the fourth step of the prior session? In virtually each subsequent session, the answer is yes.

OVERALL EVALUATION

A lot was achieved in this single session because both Nicole and the therapist were ready and willing to go through the four steps and because the therapist was reasonably skilled in guiding and accompanying Nicole through the four steps. Even if this had been the only session, it opened up significant depth and breadth of change in Nicole's ways of being and behaving.

Our clinical work and research suggest that this experiential psychotherapy can proceed through the four steps with any person whatsoever, provided the person is ready and willing. We respectfully invite you to be ready and willing to try out an experiential session. Use the manual as a guide, and please accept our invitation to correspond with us.

REFERENCES

Mahrer, A. R. (1978). The therapist–patient relationship: Conceptual analysis and a proposal for a paradigm-shift. *Psychotherapy: Theory, Research and Practice, 15*, 201–215.

Mahrer, A. R. (1986). *Therapeutic experiencing: The process of change.* New York: Norton.

Mahrer, A. R. (1988). The briefest psychotherapy? *Changes, 6*, 86–89.

Mahrer, A. R. (1989a). *How to do experiential psychotherapy: A manual for practitioners.* Ottawa: University of Ottawa Press.

Mahrer, A. R. (1989b). *Experiencing: A humanistic theory of psychology and psychiatry.* Ottawa: University of Ottawa Press (original work published 1978).

Mahrer, A. R. (1989c). *Experiential psychotherapy: Basic practices.* Ottawa: University of Ottawa Press (original work published 1983).

Mahrer, A. R. (1989d). *The integration of psychotherapies: A guide for practicing therapists.* New York: Human Sciences.

Mahrer, A. R. (1990a). *Dream work: In psychotherapy and self-change.* New York: Norton.

Mahrer, A. R. (1990b). Experiential psychotherapy. In J. K. Zeig & W. M. Munion (Eds.), *What is psychotherapy? Contemporary perspectives* (pp. 92–96). San Francisco: Jossey-Bass.

Mahrer, A. R., & Gervaize, P. A. (1983). Impossible roles therapists must play. *Canadian Psychology, 24*, 81–87.

Mahrer, A. R., Howard, M. T., & Boulet, D. B. (1991). A humanistic critique of psychoanalytic termination. *The Humanistic Psychologist 19*, 331–348.

13

Pathological Mourning in Short-Term Dynamic Psychotherapy

JASON WORCHEL

INTRODUCTION

The technique of intensive short-term dynamic psychotherapy (ISTDP) as developed by Davanloo (1978), which provides a direct view of the unconscious, has brought further evidence of the prevalence and toxicity of pathological mourning as a major source of psychiatric morbidity. Davanloo (1986) has further discovered that bypassing such unresolved grief reactions prevents successful resolution of other core neurotic conflicts. To increase the efficacy and shorten the duration of therapy, clinicians must maintain vigilance in detecting unresolved grief reactions. As the pathogenesis for this disorder resides within unconscious dynamic forces and because ISTDP provides a direct view of the unconscious, the diagnosis of pathological mourning (which heretofore has been based on presumptive evidence) can now be made conclusively. Many authors (Akisal & McKinney, 1975; Bowlby, 1963; Davanloo, 1990; Melges & Demaso, 1980; Siggin, 1966) recognized the importance of converting pathological mourning to normal mourning, in order to bring restitution and acceptance of the loss, but it was not

---

JASON WORCHEL • 1020 East Jefferson Street, Charlottesville, Virginia 21901.
Casebook of the Brief Psychotherapies, edited by Richard A. Wells and Vincent J. Giannetti. Plenum Press, New York, 1993.

until Davanloo developed his technique of ISTDP that a systematic method was available to achieve this goal. The success of ISTDP in the treatment of pathological grief results in part from its efficacy in overcoming the inevitable resistances that arise when attempting to convert pathological to normal mourning.

THEORETICAL CONSIDERATIONS

To better understand both the diagnosis and treatment of pathological mourning, an understanding of its metapsychology is important. The evolution of the metapsychology of pathological mourning reflects both the triumphs and failures of psychoanalytic theory itself. Freud's interest in mourning was preceded by his investigations into melancholia. It was his inability to discover a purely neurological basis for melancholia that led Freud to his discovery of a psychological (dynamic) etiology. His manuscript, dated May 31, 1887, a passage from which is quoted below, not only has formed the cornerstone for the metapsychology of mourning, but also the nucleus for the development of the Oedipus complex.

> Hostile impulses against parents (a wish that they should die) are also an integral constituent of neuroses. They come to light consciously as obsessional ideas. In paranoia what is worst in delusions of persecution (pathological distrust of rulers and monarchs) corresponds to these impulses. They are repressed at times when the compassion for the parents is active—at times of their illness or death. On such occasions it is a manifestation of mourning to reproach oneself for their death (what is known as melancholia) or to punish oneself in a hysterical fashion (through the medium of the idea of retribution) with the same states (of illness) that they have had. The identification which occurs here is, as we can see, nothing other than a mode of thinking and does not relieve us of the necessity for looking for the motive. (Freud, 1924a, pp. 254–55)

Freud (1924b) essentially dropped this line of investigation until 1914 when he wrote his paper on mourning and melancholia. Despite this paper being critical of his development of the theory of superego pathology, Freud and his successors minimized the importance of the superego pathology in the etiology of pathological mourning in favor of the disorders of narcissism and attachment (Bowlby, 1961, 1963a,b, 1969, 1973, 1980). Davanloo's method of ISTDP, which allowed for a direct view of the unconscious, has reinstated the role of the superego as the primary factor in the pathogenesis of pathological mourning. His successful treatment of a large series of patients having pathological mourning as one component of their core neurotic conflict has shown that it is unconscious guilt over sadistic impulses that is the primary form of the psychopathology. The identification with the deceased is with their negative qualities or with their physical suffering. This is further evidence for the role of superego pathology in unresolved grief. Furthermore, for successful resolution, patients have to experience their sadism toward the deceased before a normal mourning process emerges. The sadism that Davanloo helps the patient to work through is a reactive sadism. Its origins are in the disrupted libidinal bond. It is beyond the scope of this chapter to explore Davanloo's discoveries involving the metapsychology of the id, but they have been highlighted in his recent collection of papers (Davanloo, 1990).

Diagnostic Assessment

There are three fundamental steps in the treatment of pathological grief reactions: (1) diagnosis, (2) converting pathological mourning to normal mourning, and (3) facilitating normal mourning. Although acute grief is easy to recognize, its differentiation from pathological mourning is more difficult to ascertain and operationally define. To do so requires a working knowledge of the process of acute grief. Although many authors have addressed acute grief (Engel, 1960; Megles, 1982; Rees, 1975), the most detailed observations of the physical and psychological manifestations of acute grief are those of Erich Linderman (1979) following the Coconut Grove fire. Of particular importance to this chapter (in which the therapist strives to reactivate normal mourning) are the author's observation of the five or six pathognomonic components of normal mourning (Linderman, 1979, pp. 61–64): (1) There is somatic distress that occurs in "waves lasting from twenty minutes to an hour at a time, a feeling of tightness in the throat, a need for sighing and an intensive subjective distress described as a tension or mental pain. The patient soon learns that these waves can be precipitated by visits, mentioning the deceased . . . (p. 61)"; a profound sense of fatigue and exhaustion are almost universal. (2) There are often changes in sensorium that can include auditory and visual hallucinations. These are predominantly concerned with the deceased. (3) There is a preoccupation with feelings of guilt in which the bereaved believes he is somehow responsible for the death of his loved one. (4) There are hostile reactions, "[a] disconcerting loss of warmth in relationship to other people, a tendency to respond with irritability and anger and a wish not to be bothered by others . . . (p. 62)." (5) There is a change in activity that includes typical patterns of behavior; of particular importance is that "there is no retardation of action and speech; quite the contrary, there is a push of speech . . . there is restlessness, inability to sit still . . . [but] a painful lack of capacity to initiate and maintain organized patterns of activity (p. 63)." (6) Lastly, "there is the appearance of traits of the deceased in the behavior of the bereaved, especially symptoms shown during the last illness . . ." (p. 64).

Because normal mourning is reactivated by the therapeutic process, the therapist will observe these normal reactions within the therapy session. Many of these reactions are frightening to the patient, especially the emergence of intense hostility and the appearance of hallucinatory experiences. Unless the therapist recognizes these as normal, even necessary, in the mourning, he may, out of his own anxiety, disrupt the curative process that is taking place.

Once the clinician is familiar with the manifestations of acute grief, they are easy to recognize. Furthermore, because there is a recent loss, even bizarre symptoms such as hallucinations can be properly diagnosed as manifestations of acute grief. The problem with pathological mourning, however, is that it doesn't necessarily occur in proximity to an identifiable loss, and its presentation encompasses almost the entire spectrum of psychiatric disorders. Furthermore, even acute grief reactions can go awry and may be transformed into pathological mourning. Vulkan (1970; Vulkan & Showalter, 1968) have placed pathological mourning "in the middle spectrum between those on one end with 'normal' grief and those at the other end with full-blown neurosis or psychosomatic symptoms."

A variety of criteria have been proposed in an effort to differentiate pathological mourning from normal mourning (Hackett, 1974; Madison & Viola, 1986). One is the persistence, beyond an arbitrarily defined time, of psychiatric symptoms following a loss. Pathological grief should not be considered until after a "normal" time for acute grief has passed. Parkes (1972) noted that acute grief symptoms are present for around 8 weeks, but depressive symptoms are common throughout the first year of bereavement.

Another criteria that has been used to help the diagnosis of unresolved grief has been the presenting symptoms. Although depressive symptoms are a common presentation, Akiskal and McKinney (1975), in their review of the literature, confirmed the difficulty of differentiating between grief reactions and depressive disorders. Other common presenting symptoms include anxiety disorders, functional and psychosomatic disorders, and dissociative reactions.

Given the extreme variation in both the spectrum and duration of presenting symptoms in pathological mourning for unresolved grief reactions, the clinician must rely on other factors to help make the diagnosis. In the past, this information came from the developmental history section of the standard psychiatric interview, even though it was widely accepted that this information is distorted by unconscious mental mechanisms. When the developmental history reveals a significant loss, further investigation should be made into several specific areas that could suggest the presence of pathological mourning. Vulkan (1970) has divided these areas into the following categories: (1) specific events that occurred at the time of death that blocked normal mourning; (2) history of acute, morbid grief reactions following a death; (3) specific factors in the genetic history that increased the vulnerability to subsequent losses; and (4) a history of the subsequent development or reactivation of psychological and/or physical symptoms not evident prior to the loss.

There are a variety of unusual events surrounding death of a loved one that can foster the subsequent emergence of pathological mourning. Instances in which the body of the deceased could not be located, or tissue damage was too severe to allow viewing, promote unresolved grief. Ironically, medical technology can lead to pathological processes through the very methods used to save patients' lives. For instance, the author has seen several cases of unresolved grief in which the bereaved were prevented from being near their loved one during the terminal phase of the illness. This was due to the injection of radioactive isotopes used to treat specific cancers, oxygen tents, or isolation precautions due to immunodeficiency.

Pathological mourning should be suspected if there is a history that the bereaved was absent from the funeral and burial services. Unfortunately, this is common for children who are sent away to "protect" them from the emotional distress of the burial ceremony (Gareen & Solnit, 1964). Another event that can signal unresolved grief is a history of the patient having to terminate life support systems, or prohibit resuscitation efforts of their loved one. Although some authors have found a prevalence of sudden death of the loved one leading to pathological mourning, it is equally common to find cases where the terminal phase has been prolonged. This is particularly the case where the bereaved chose to be the primary caretaker. Death by suicide increases the incidence of pathological mourning among the survivors. When the death of a loved one leads to a dramatic change in financial status, either positively or negatively, there was a higher incidence of pathological mourning (Vulkan, 1970).

Although there have not been systematic studies confirming a vulnerability to unresolved grief reactions resulting from early childhood losses, the frequency with which this has been found has been commented upon (Engel, 1969; Siggin, 1966). That this should be the case comes as no surprise because loss of a parent in childhood often has a devastating effect on ego development and its subsequent ability to tolerate the painful and grief-laden affects that arise in working through any significant loss. The emergence of infantile neuroses often occur following the death of a family member. The child's attempts to resolve these neurotic conflicts frequently result in character pathology that secondarily becomes another barrier to normal mourning.

Other presumptive evidence for a pathological mourning reaction that can be obtained from the developmental history is the emergence or reactivation of specific symptoms following the death of a loved/hated one. During the acute grief phase, however, even brief psychotic episodes should not be considered indicative of a pathological process (Rees, 1975). When specific symptoms emerge beyond the time boundaries of normal mourning and the grieving process appears frozen, that is, not proceeding through the typical phases as outlined by Bowlby (1961) and Linderman (1979), then the clinician should actively investigate the possibility of an unresolved grief reaction. As in the case presented below, the onset of physical ailments or characteristics of the deceased often occur in pathological mourning. It is not uncommon that such symptoms exactly mimic the cause of death of the loved/hated one. Anniversary reactions, which typically emerge as discrete periods of dysphoria or major depressive episodes occuring on the anniversary of the death of the loved/hated one, are also evidence of unresolved grief reactions (Cavenar, Spaulding, & Hammet, 1976; Cavenar, Nash, & Maltbie, 1978; Pollock, 1961, 1971). The emergence of repetitive dreams in which the loved/hated one is in danger of dying, and the patient is engaged in a futile struggle to save him/her, is also further evidence for unresolved grief reaction (Vulkan, 1970).

Treatment Methodology

From the metapsychology of pathological mourning it becomes apparent that the moment a clinician attempts to initiate normal mourning, massive resistances that initially arise from the superego will emerge. Once these superego resistances are removed, then the instinctual resistances emerge and must be overcome to allow genuine grieving to take place. One of Davanloo's unique contributions to the field of dynamic psychotherapy has been his discovery of a systematic method of handling such resistances in an effective, immediate fashion. This technique has been adequately described in other publications and will only be outlined below to establish a frame of reference for its use in pathological grief. It must be emphasized, however, that there are critical differences in handling the resistances that emerge when patients are suffering from depressive disorders, psychosomatic disorders, developmental neuroses, and in ego-syntonic character pathology. Pathological mourning occurring in the context of these categories of psychopathologies can be treated with ISTDP, but it should not be attempted until the clinician has mastery over the treatment of these disorders. Davanloo has repeatedly demonstrated the importance of specific and extensive preparatory work to raise the ego adaptive capacity sufficiently in patients suffering from these categories of disorders, to allow the ego to tolerate the ensuring psychotherapeutic work without collapsing into devastating symptom formation (Davanloo, 1988).

Once the clinician has successfully restructured the ego's regressive pattern of defenses as described by Davanloo (1988), the technique of handling the resistances that emerge in the course of treating pathological mourning are not significantly different from those employed in the treatment of ego-dystonic character pathology. Briefly, the clinician must first identify the presence of such resistances and then clarify them for the patient. This is followed by systematic pressure and challenge to each defense until a breakthrough occurs into the defended feelings/impulses. These affective states can then be experienced by the patient's ego. Davanloo (1988) has called this sequence of interventions the Central Dynamic Sequence, and has described this process as follows:

Phase 1.
- (a) Inquiry, exploring the patient's difficulties; initial to respond.
- (b) Rapid identification and clarification of the patient's defenses.

Phase 2.
- Pressure, leading to resistance in the form of a series of defenses.

Phase 3. Clarification of Defenses.
- (a) Clarification, challenge to defenses, leading to rising transference and increased resistance.
- (b) Challenge directed against the defenses; recapitulation of the defenses and casting doubt on the defenses.
- (c) Challenge directed toward the therapeutic alliance.
- (d) To make the patient acquainted with his defenses so that he can see that they have paralyzed his functioning.
- (e) To turn the patient against his own defenses.

Phase 4. Transference Resistance.
- (a) Clarification and challenge to transference resistance.

(b) Head-on collision with the transference resistance with special reference to that maintained by the superego.
(c) Exhaustion of resistance and communication with the unconscious therapeutic alliance.

Phase 5. Intrapsychic Crisis.
(a) High rise in complex transference feeling, breakthrough of the complex transference feeling—the mechanism for unlocking the unconscious.
(b) Interpretative phase.
(c) The first direct view of the multifocal core neurotic structure.

Phase 6. Systematic analysis of the transference leading to resolution of the residual resistance with partial or major repression of current or recent past and distant past conflicts.

Phase 7. Inquiry, completing dynamic phenomenological approach to the patient's psychopathology, medical, psychiatric, and social history, and developmental history.

Phase 8. Direct view of the multifocal core neurotic structure and its relation to the patient's symptom and character disturbances and psychotherapeutic plan.

Davanloo uses basic psychoanalytic principles. He describes one aspect of the dynamic forces as the Triangle of Conflict. This shows the interrelationship within the unconscious between basic impulses/feelings (I/F), which give rise to anxiety (A), which are all under a system of defenses (D) (see Figure 1).

These dynamic forces were originally related to significant past (P)

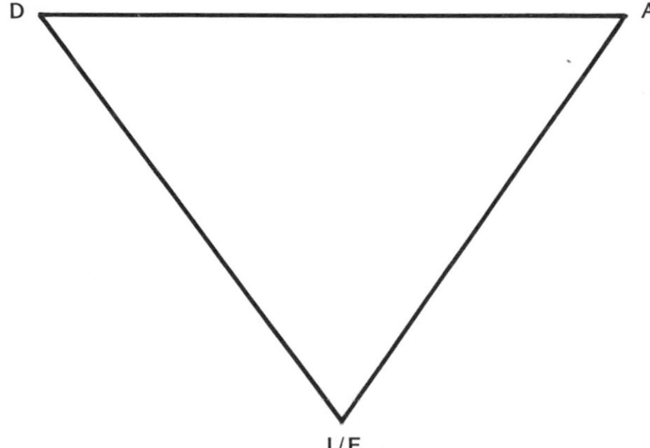

FIGURE 1. Triangle of conflict. D = defenses; A = anxiety; I/F = impulses/feelings.

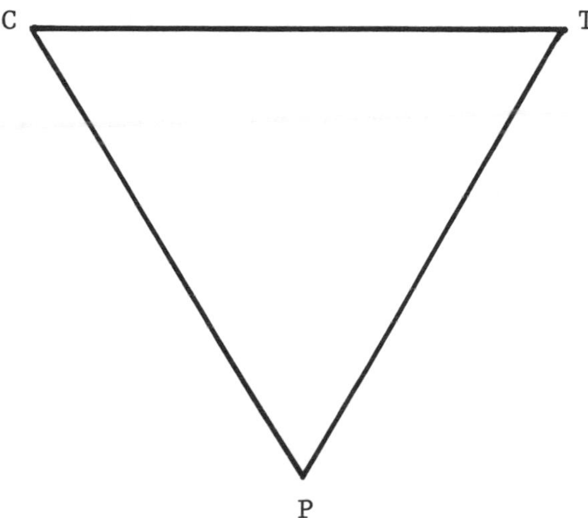

Figure 2. Triangle of person. C = current significant relationships; T = transference; P = postsignificant relationships.

persons, transferred to other current (C) figures, and are then manifested within the transference (T) relationship. This progression in time is diagrammed by a Triangle of Person (see Figure 2).

Davanloo has repeatedly demonstrated that a breakthrough into the unconscious occurs when a patient can experience repressed impulses and feelings within the transference (Davanloo, 1990).

The clinician must constantly monitor several factors simultaneously: (1) where the patient is in relation to the two triangles, (2) the degree of resistance manifested, (3) the type of defense present, (4) the immediate ego capacity, (5) the emergence of unconscious communications and genuine affect, and (6) the degree of unconscious therapeutic alliance in operation. Having all this information available, the therapist is then in a position to determine his next intervention, that is, further pressure and challenge to the defense, a shift from (T) to (C), clarification or ego restructuring, and so forth. These shifts will be detailed in the case analysis below.

Special Considerations in Treatment

Although the basic techniques of ISTDP as applied to character pathology are generally applicable to pathologic mourning, there are several aspects that require special attention. The first of these involves the *timing* regarding the initiation of the work on the pathological mourning process, vis-à-vis other core neurotic conflicts. During the descriptive, phenomenological history phase of the initial evaluation there often emerges evidences, as detailed above, that a pathological mourning process is a distinct possibility. Davanloo (1986) has demonstrated that such information should initially be "flagged" for both the therapist and the patient. Such a process can be as simple as saying:

> So your father died when you were 16 years old. It is important that we explore this further, but first, how would you characterize your relationship with men?

In such a way, the patient's ego recognizes that the therapist has discovered an important area for exploration, and this strengthens the unconscious therapeutic alliance. At the same time, the patient's unconscious ego appreciates the therapist's commitment to proceeding in a systematic fashion, with full knowledge, before such a major area is penetrated. Immediate penetration into this grief-laden and guilt-laden area would mobilize massive resistance requiring intensive confrontation within the transference relationships, without having a full survey of the current dynamism. The likelihood of "getting in the swamp" of an entangled transference reaction, with its attendant probability of misalliance, is high and should be avoided.

In describing such a procedure, Davanloo (1986) often uses the analogy of a surgeon examining an acute abdomen. When gentle palpitation produces pain and reflexive guarding, the surgeon immediately leaves that area to examine other areas of the abdomen. The practitioner knows that further examination of the painful area would result in a boardlike abdomen, and thus prohibit further exploration of other areas that might also have significant pathology.

Another aspect of the technique that is present in all types of ISTDP but that is especially significant in the treatment of pathological mourning is specificity (Davanloo, 1987). It is imperative that patients reexperience their life with the deceased in order to face the grief-laden and guilt-laden unconscious affective states. To do this first requires recreating one's life with the deceased in exhaustive detail. It is only after there has been a breakthrough into the unconscious in the fashion described in the Central Dynamic Sequence that an accurate picture of the past relationship emerges. Once the breakthrough has occurred, then the therapist must facilitate engaging the patient's ego with all the details of life with the deceased. If, during this process, resistances return—which is common—they are typically much less tenacious, and often of a "tactical" nature, rather than formal defenses (Davanloo, 1990). Some examples of these "tactical" defenses, designed to keep the therapist away from painful areas, are generalization, vagueness, and tentativeness. They can be gently overcome. Thus as details of the life with the deceased emerge, new affect-laden memories are evoked. It is through attention to detail that the systematic "piecemeal review" of the patient's past life with the deceased takes place. This affective review becomes the basis for the decathexis that leads to a final goodbye (Davanloo, 1986).

Once a breakthrough has occurred into the unconscious feelings for the deceased, the attention to specificity also serves the function for what Davanloo (1986) calls "intensification of the affect." For example, although there may be a moderate amount of sadness evident when discussing life with the deceased, when the therapist encourages further detail, for example, the smell of the deceased's pipe tobacco, the aroma of a favorite meal that was shared with the deceased, or a specific day fishing together, and so on, there is an outpouring of grief and sadness. Once this affective channel is entered, regardless of what affect emerges, the therapist should remain with that affect and not immediately jump to other affective states. The result of rapidly switching between the ambivalent feelings the patient had for the deceased tends to confuse the ego, resulting in a retardation of the therapeutic process.

In addition to this piecemeal review, it is often helpful to have the patient portray how the deceased would look and act if he/she were alive today. This facilitates the initiation of normal mourning as the ego has to further face the reality of the loss. This is particularly important when a parent has lost a child, or when the patient, as a child, lost a parent or sibling (Melges, 1982; Melges & Demaso, 1980).

It is important to remember that superego resistances prohibit the patient from establishing new, successful relationships. To address these resistances, Davanloo has developed a series of interventions. One technique he uses is asking the patient how the deceased would react to a successful relationship between the therapist and patient; moreover, one in which the goodbye to the therapist would be in an atmosphere of positive feelings. Such an intervention speaks directly to the patient's unconscious guilt over establishing new relationships and need to defeat the therapist's attempts to be an effective, important person in the patient's life. Such interventions may prophylactically dissolve transference resistances before they have crystallized.

The entire process of breaking through resistances to affectively relive the past with the deceased, through all its conflicts and triumphs, builds to a crescendo when the patient imagines standing beside the body of the deceased, ready to say a last goodbye. Now the therapist simply asks what is in the patient's heart to say. The patient, affectively engaged with the deceased, but within the context of the transference relationship, declares what had remained unresolved with the deceased and expresses the wish to bring a final resolution. Having experienced this with the therapist, most patients undertake at least one visit to the grave to make it final. The impetus to visit the grave, like all other aspects of the therapy, should come from the patient. For the therapist to make such a suggestion usually indicates the preparatory work has not been completed.

Following is a case analysis of segments of the initial diagnostic interview of a patient treated with ISTDP who manifested pathological mourning as one aspect of his core neurotic conflict. Davanloo's technique of ISTDP has been described in detail elsewhere (Davanloo, 1990) and will not be repeated here. The case analysis will show the progression of an interview, and particular technical interventions, as applied to pathological mourning.

CASE ANALYSIS

Patient Background

Bob is a 37-year-old cardiologist. He has a sister 2 years younger, and both his parents were immigrants. His father left Europe when he was 16 years old and never saw the rest of his family again; his mother immigrated with her family that included several sisters and brothers. Following their marriage, Bob's parents settled in a Jewish section of Chicago in close proximity to his mother's family. In his early years, Bob was close to many of these maternal aunts and maternal grandmothers.

Bob's father owned a small grocery store in which he worked 6 days a week. He was a small, affectionate man who suffered from asthma, chronic coughing, and aching feet. His pride in life was his only son, Bob, who was going to carry on the Jewish tradition, perhaps even become a rabbi like his grandfather. Bob's mother was an affectionate, devoted wife and mother who enjoyed visiting with her sisters and caring for her family.

Until his teenage years, Bob was close to both his parents and was a studious, obedient son. Following his Bar Mitzvah, however, he became openly rebellious, defiant, and nonreligious. In the midst of this turmoil, while he was on vacation with his mother and aunts, his father had a massive heart attack. The family immediately returned to Chicago where, with coercion from a friend, Bob visited his father in the hospital.

He initially did not believe the heart attack was serious and was angry with his father for disrupting his vacation. His father, in an oxygen tent, recognized Bob and whispered that he loved him. Within seconds, he was seized with chest pain and Bob, frightened, left the room while his father, holding his chest with his left hand, reached out toward Bob with his right hand. The medical staff rushed into the room, but Bob's father was dead.

In the aftermath of this death, Bob's relationship with his mother deteriorated, and he became progressively more dysphoric with periods of severe depression. Whereas he had once been a leader, he was now a follower, finding relationships where he ended up being used and abused. He was unable to make a commitment to a woman and, although he was sexually active, had a phobic reaction to looking at female genitalia. He married for 1 year but divorced his wife and then, around this same time, began to suffer from asthma. His present life consisted of working 6 to 7 days a week, unsatisfactory relationships with women, and helping out his male friends. Eventually his mother remarried, but he remained distant from her; similarly, he stayed distant from his sister and never returned to Chicago. Bob had a course of 4 years of psychoanalytically oriented psychotherapy, without result, before entering ISTDP.

Beginning the Interview

This initial interview took 3 hours. While outlining the areas of disturbance for which he was seeking help, the patient mentioned that his father died when he was 16 years old. This was acknowledged as an important issue that needed further exploration, but first a complete phenomenological history was obtained. During this process, when the focus was upon his sexual relationship with his girlfriend, resistance increased drastically. There was a head-on collision with the transference resistances and the patient experienced his anger at the therapist as a wish to beat him up and throw him out the window. He did not want the therapist to die, however, and when discussing his wish that the therapist should live, guilt and grief-laden feelings emerged. This was followed by memories in which he had protected his cousin as a child but felt that later in life there was no one to stand up for him. We pick up the interview at that point.

T: So you were there for your cousin, and all the other ones that got picked on, weren't you? Hmm?

P: Yeah.

T: So then you were the one who stood up for the Jew who was being humiliated, but who stood up for you?
P: Nobody that I know of. Although . . . now here's something. When I was in college this friend of mine, we were like this (*two fingers intertwined*) and, ah, there was another guy who started to pick on me . . .
T: You're fighting your feeling.
P: I'm just trying to tell a story.
T: I know, but the feeling comes, let's look at the feeling.
P: Well, Jim told the guy he'd kill him if he, . . . whatever, and I remember he may have grabbed the guy and threw him against a wall.
T: May have or did?
P: He did, and he got outraged that this guy was going to pick on me. (*Tears in patient's eyes.*)
T: This is very moving to you.
P: Yeah.
T: Why do you fight your feelings because it obviously brings a lot of painful memories from the past and . . .
P: Well, I don't know if it's painful . . .
T: But that doesn't help.
P: No.
T: You said the two of you were very close. Is he still alive?
P: Yes, he is in California.
T: The other side of the country, that would be painful too.
P: It is. (*Patient takes a deep sigh.*) Yeah, I really miss him. He was just here in September, and I hadn't seen him for a few years.
T: He was strong and willing to be there for you.
P: Right.
T: Uh hmm. It's obvious that you've missed such a person in your life.
P: Yeah. (*Breaks into deep sobbing.*) Yeah, I suppose the person could have been my father but wasn't.

By virtue of the partial breakthrough into the unconscious having taken place, there is relatively low resistance, and high unconscious therapeutic alliance in operation. As a result, in this vignette, the patient's resistances are primarily tactical in nature and easily pushed aside. Note there is little reference to the transference. The progression from transference to current life situations, to past life situations, shows how Davanloo's system of ISTDP validates Freud's economic concept of the mind. The transference, which is the patient's immediate experience, becomes the vehicle to open the unconscious. What then emerges is the next most accessible derivative of the core neurotic conflict, the current life situation with others. Finally, what originally was most distant and inaccessible (economically removed) becomes alive.

The patient momentarily resorts to the defense of externalization and victimization, but this rapidly gives way to further evidence that his father was there for him.

T: So obviously, there's a feeling that you wish you could have had a father like David.
P: Uh hmm, right. Instead, I just got . . .
T: You take a deep sigh.
P: Hmm. Instead I just got yelled at, unless I got good grades, and did this and did that, I got nothing.
T: You mean from him? (*Addressing the unconscious about the others in the patient's life who did give to him.*)
P: Yeah. Yeah, that was, once I was of age where I could be a bad kid, I was always good, good, good, you know.
T: Uh hmm. We can get to that change because it's important that we understand it, but what is clear is that you missed a person like David in your life, and that it could have been your father but wasn't. And now you are obviously feeling that. (*This is flagging that the change in the patient's life with his father is important, but now the affective channel must be maintained. Here rich and important content is used as a tactical defense of diversion.*)
P: Well, I'll tell you what! There was one episode when we were kids and my father, we were all driving to the beach and, ah, a policeman, a plain-clothed, ah, unmarked car, we were little . . . car was chasing us and my father didn't know who it was . . . the guy pulled up behind us, and he ran up the side of the car and started yelling and screaming . . . We were all crying, we didn't know who this guy was, like a bandit, or something. Even after he showed his badge, my father still laced into him for upsetting us.
T: Your father was protective of you?
P: Oh, yeah!
T: Exactly what did he say to this policeman? (*Increases specificity.*)
P: He said, "Look how you've upset these kids."
T: So then your father stood there, hmmm, and protected you, even in the face of the police?
P: Yeah. (*Tears rolling down his cheeks.*)

The patient has accessed a positive memory of his father protecting him, being strong and useful. This contradicts his earlier position that no one was there for him. It has been my experience that often patients will access a memory where the deceased defended the patient from the police or some similar agency.

T: So there was a wish he could have stood like that in your life and, ah . . .
P: Right (*still crying*). Instead, it seemed like it was turned around at me.
T: Uh hmm. (*Patient begins to address the ambivalence.*)

P: I always wished my father was somebody else, not always, but often. (*More tears*) Somebody bigger, you know, that played ball with me, we did a lot together, but all of a sudden that changed when I got older. When I left Jewish school, after that I was no good.
T: You mean he, in a sense, disinherited you?
P: Yeah, that's the way I see it. I know he had his reasons. (*Defense*)
T: But that doesn't help your feelings.
P: Right. So, like in the midst of the war between he and I, he died. (*More tears*)
T: But then he goes to his grave with so much unresolved between the two of you, and a craving that he could have been in your life in a different way. (*Intensification*)
P: Yeah. (*Long pause*)
T: Do you miss him?
P: Hmm? (*Patient preoccupied with internal feelings.*)
T: Do you miss him?
P: (*Patient is very choked up.*) Yeah. I wanted to, I wanted this stuff resolved, and he's not here to resolve it with, so I don't know if anything I ever do, you know, would be acceptable, because I never got approval.
T: But in the midst of the fight he died and, hmm?
P: Yeah, and, ah, yeah, it's not like he didn't love me, it's not that. It's just that it was over in the, in the middle of the unresolved fight.

Here the patient explicitly identifies the unresolved grief reaction over his father's death. He points to the intense ambivalence, specifically the battle between the two of them that never resolved, as the source of this pathological process.

Exploring Conflict

The next phase of the therapy consists of exploring the origins of the battle that erupted openly between father and son. This frequently leads to other aspects of the core neurotic conflict, and a reemergence of resistance within the transference.

T: So you say he never played ball with you, then who did you play ball with? (*Unconscious communication*)
P: It was my mother who taught me how to play baseball, and who was the den mother of our Cub Scout troop, and all that stuff. Yes, and I also see her, yeah, pitching baseball to me, and . . .
T: Uh hmm. So you were close to her . . .
P: Yeah, the thing that stands out the most was when he died, you see, I, she kind of tortured me with his death for a whole year. (*Tears welling into the patient's eyes.*)
T: Uh hmm.

P: I already felt bad but Jewish males, if their parents die, are supposed to say special prayers, morning, noon, and night . . . for a year. Well, I didn't want to go many times, and she would come in saying, "It's time to go," wake me up, "I don't want to go today." Well, then she'd start crying, and she made me feel like I killed him, that's the way I, I felt too many times, as if I were still killing him . . . I couldn't stand her crying, so I went more times than I didn't. (*Tearful*)

T: But still she cried.

P: She cried and wailed, wailed and, "Oh, he has no respect for his father," and this and that. You know, I mean it was just, you may as well have been shooting me, or hitting me with a baseball bat . . .

T: How do you feel when you say, "It felt as though I was still killing him?"

P: Helpless (*Defense*)

T: Feeling, how are you feeling? (*Challenge*)

P: She was wrong. (*Defense*)

T: How do you feel? (*Challenge*)

P: Kind of, you know . . . (*Defense*)

T: You still haven't declared how you feel. You said, "It was as if I was still killing him every morning." (*Clarification and challenge*)

P: That's how I felt. (*Defense*)

T: Again you are vague. What are you going to do with this vagueness? (*Challenge and pressure*)

P: Like it was something I was doing that was actually making him, whatever, I know he was dead, but even die worse. I used to think of it in terms of him going to heaven or hell, and I thought, maybe I was really causing him to go, you know, to hell.

T: But how do you feel?

P: Angry.

T: With whom?

P: With my mother.

T: What else do you feel? (*Here anger is used as a defense and is dismissed.*)

P: Some days I went. (*Defense*)

The therapist persists in challenging and pressuring the defenses, and eventually the patient declares a mixture of feelings, initially guilt over continuing to kill his father, anger at his father for "being him," and then sadness. Normal mourning, however, could not proceed until the patient faced all of his sadism toward his father, and this required further exploration into the triangular relationship between him, mother, and father.

T: You said that in the early part of your life your mother's very prominent, isn't it?

P: Yeah.

T: Teaching you to play ball and . . .

P: Den mother and all that.

T: But then where is your father?
P: Working 6 days a week, a couple of nights home at nine o'clock . . .
T: So it's as if he doesn't exist. (*Speaking to the unconscious*) What type of marriage did your parents have?

In response to this query, the patient becomes vague and is challenged by first asking for details. The interview continues:

P: Yeah, she ran the home, then when my father came home, I remember, she would bring him a thing of water to soak his feet in. . . . She waited on him.
T: She waited on him?
P: Oh, yeah. She would cook dinner for us, and then cook it for him, and often she knew what he liked so, you know, some of those Jewish dishes were tasteless to us kids, but he liked them, and we had to eat them. Like I remember the boiled chicken . . .

Therapist asks for more details and the patient goes on:

P: . . . He suffered from asthma his whole life that I know, it was awful, coughed and wheezed a lot.
T: During the night?
P: Yeah, he, you know, often I'd hear him getting up coughing . . .
T: So he couldn't do much because of the asthma.
P: Not really, Even, even, even laughing too much, you know, would get him into a wheeze . . . couldn't do anything.
T: When you talked of the asthma, and the physical, then he's crippled, isn't he?
P: Kind of, yeah, I think so. Yeah, I think so. (*Defense*)
T: I'm talking about your perception of him?
P: Fairly crippled, yeah.
T: So then your father is a cripple and your mother is waiting on him.
P: Yeah, she's being nice to him.
T: So then in that way, you end up in a fight with a cripple, isn't it?
P: Kind of. I mean, I used to get slapped around so, but I used to get, I used to feel guilty that I'd make him anxious.
T: And then he might start to wheeze?
P: And then he, yeah, he would, and then he'd hit me, and then he'd get excited, and I really did feel like I killed him when she used to lay there wailing . . . I could have been a better kid . . .
T: But then the idea is, if he starts to lash out at you, and you really go for him, hmm?
P: He'd die. I'd have killed him. (*Patient is crying.*)

Despite this wave of genuine, painful affect, the patient could only see the source of his anger at his father as stemming from the father's physical illness, his interest in business, his accent, small stature, and so on. The therapist continues to go deeper into the anger.

T: So you said he was useless to you, and you wanted to replace him. So then, obviously, you must have a certain feeling that the crippled, useless father comes home but then is treated like a king?
P: Well, he was king for her.
T: But you have said that she is there all day long, and all week long, playing ball with you, affectionate with you, involved with you, being there for you, hmm, isn't it?
P: Yeah. (*All choked up*)
T: But then this crippled guy comes home, and she goes and gives him every thing, hmm, isn't it?
P: Ah, I didn't really, you know, all I, I'm, I watched this go on . . .
T: I am questioning you about your feelings, that you look to your feelings, and be honest with yourself.
P: Yeah, kind of. I keep saying "kind of" as opposed to "Yes." (*Already the patient's ego has been turned against its own defenses.*) . . . Yeah, I was angry with him.

Continuing the Challenge

This situation was examined in more detail, and each round brought a certain amount of resistance. These were systematically challenged and pressured, as described elsewhere by Davanloo (1988, 1990). Fresh memories emerged regarding how the mother was serving both father and son, and the patient's rage at how his father had not only his feet soothed, his hunger quenched, but his sexual desires fulfilled by the patient's "queen."

T: Nine o'clock she's out serving him, and then making over him, hmm, this character who's useless to you in the first place, hmm?
P: Right.
T: And when she's serving him, where are you?
P: Watching TV.
T: So there's nobody there for you, is there?
P: I didn't need anybody.
T: Is that it? Again, you rationalize.
P: No. No, you're right—you're right, there's nobody there.
T: And then after supper, he's going to get more goodies, isn't he?
P: What do you mean?
T: You know it, and now you take a more crippled position, hmm?
P: My curiosity about sex, that is one thing I don't think they had much of.
T: She is a servant to his needs. She takes care of his feet, hmm?
P: Yeah.

T: Then who takes care of his penis?
P: Nobody else but her, but, ah, I don't know that they had a lot of sex.
T: Hmm? He is not her lover?
P: Not to my concept of lover. No!
T: Uh hmm. Who is?
P: Well, it's got to be me. (*Patient becomes anxious.*)
T: Then obviously there is a very intimate and close relationship, isn't there?
P: Yes.
T: But then you say in your fantasy that useless, crippled man is not her lover, you say that even laughing makes him wheeze?
P: Right.
T: So then he is not much of a lover to her, hmm?
P: Right.
T: But who is the strong one who doesn't wheeze?
P: Me. I don't want to think about it.
T: I know, but that doesn't help, because you want to take a crippled position, rather than to face things, hmm?

CONCLUSIONS AND SUMMARY

The patient goes on to recount many times he would hear his parents having intercourse in the next room. He believed his mother did not enjoy it but put up with her husband. He remembered his rage at his father and the wish to throw him out the second-story window. When he portrayed in his fantasy the way his father's broken body looked, he broke into waves of grief-laden and guilt-laden feelings and spontaneously moved to portray his last goodbye to his father. The therapist intensified the grieving process by focusing on the details of this last goodbye.

The patient remembered the train ride back from his vacation and the thoughts of wishing that his father would just go ahead and die. He recalled not going to the hospital that night but waiting until the next morning. He talked about not wanting to go to the hospital, what he had for breakfast, the location of the hospital, and the floor and arrangement of the Intensive Care unit. He described the oxygen tent, the IV tubes, his father's position in the bed, his dress, the smells in the room, and the sounds of the monitor. Waves of sadness burst out when he talked about how his father had waited for the patient's arrival, saving his strength to talk to his son, to say that he loved his son, and the final goodbye with his arm outstretched toward the patient.

With this active grief process now in operation, the therapist helped the patient with a piecemeal review of his past life with his father. Many tender moments were recalled, "for the first time in years," each with its attendant memories. The process of converting pathological mourning to normal was begun during this session but, as expected, there were many times resistance returned and had to be overcome to bring the process to completion.

To summarize, pathological mourning is a common cause of psychiatric morbidity that can be successfully treated utilizing Davanloo's technique of ISTDP. This chapter highlights those circumstantial evidences that can be found in taking a standard psychiatric history that suggest a pathological mourning process exists. The process and manifestations of normal grief, as detailed by Linderman (1979), were reviewed. Aspects of the historical evolution of the metapsychology of pathological mourning were described, together with specific contributions made by Davanloo. Those technical aspects of ISTDP that are particularly applicable to converting pathological mourning to normal mourning were described. This was followed by an analysis of the transcript of a patient suffering from pathological mourning who was treated in ISTDP. As Linderman so often said, one of the major tasks in life is to move "beyond grief." The process of ISTDP, as discovered by Davanloo, is a major step in that direction.

REFERENCES

Abraham, K. (1927). *Selected papers*. London: Hogarth Press and Institute of Psychoanalysis.

Akisal, H. S., & McKinney, W. T. (1975). Overview of recent research in depression. *Archives of General Psychiatry, 32*, 285–305.

Bowlby, J. (1961). Process of mourning. *International Journal of Psychoanalysis, 42*, 317–340.

Bowlby, J. (1963a). Pathological mourning and childhood mourning. *Journal of the American Psychoanalytic Association, 11*, 500–541.

Bowlby, J. (1963b). Process of mourning. *International Journal of Psychoanalysis, 47*, 14–25.

Bowlby, J. (1969). *Attachment and loss, Volume I: Attachment*. London: Hogarth Press.

Bowlby, J. (1973). *Attachment and loss, Volume II: Separation*. London: Hogarth Press.

Bowlby, J. (1980). *Attachment and loss, Volume III: Loss*. London: Hogarth Press.

Cavenar, J. O., Spaulding, J. G., & Hammet, E. L. (1976). Anniversary reactions. *Psychosomatics, 17*, 210–212.

Cavenar, J. O., Nash, J. L., & Maltbie, A. A. (1978). Anniversary reactions presenting as physical complaints. *Journal of Clinical Psychiatry, 39*, 369–374.

Davanloo, H. (1978). *Basic principles and techniques in short-term dynamic psychotherapy*. New York: Spectrum.

Davanloo, H. (1986). Core training program, International Institute of Short-Term Dynamic Psychotherapy. Montreal, PQ, Canada.

Davanloo, H. (1987). Fifth summer immersion course. Killington, VT.

Davanloo, H. (1988). The technique of unlocking the unconscious. Part I and Part II. *The International Journal of Short-Term Dynamic Psychotherapy, 3,* 99–159.
Davanloo, H. (1990). *Unlocking the unconscious.* London: Wiley & Sons.
Engel, G. L. (1960). Is grief a disease? A challenge. *Psychosomatic Medical, 22,* 326–327.
Freud, S. (1924a). *Collected papers, Volume 1.* London: Hogarth Press and Institute of Psychoanalysis.
Freud, S. (1924b). *Collected papers, Volume 4.* London: Hogarth Press and Institute of Psychoanalysis.
Gareen, M., & Solnit, A. J. (1964). Reactions to the threatened loss of a child: A vulnerable child syndrome. *Pediatrics, 34,* 58–66.
Hackett, T. P. (1974). Recognizing and treating abnormal grief. *Hospital Physician, 10,* 49–50, 56.
Linderman, E. (1979). *Beyond grief: Studies in crisis intervention.* New York: Jason Aronson.
Madison, D. C., & Viola, A. (1986). The health of widows in the year following bereavement. *Journal of Psychosomatic Research, 12,* 297–306.
Melges, M. T. (1982). *Time and the inner future.* New York: Wiley.
Melges, M. T., & Demaso, D. R. (1980). Grief resolution therapy: Reliving, revising and revisiting. *American Journal of Psychotherapy, 34,* 51–61.
Parkes, C. M. (1972). *Bereavement: A study of grief in adult life.* London: Tavistock.
Pollock, G. H. (1961). Mourning and adaptation. *International Journal of Psychoanalysis, 42,* 341–361.
Pollock, G. H. (1971). Anniversary reactions, trauma and mourning. *Psychoanalysis Quarterly.*
Rees, W. D. (1975). The bereaved and their hallucination. In B. Schoenberg (Ed.), *Bereavement: Its psychosocial aspects* (pp. 66–71). New York: Columbia University Press.
Siggin, L. D. (1966). Mourning: A critical survey of the literature. *Journal of Psychoanalysis, 41,* 14–25.
Vulkan, V. (1970). Typical findings in pathological grief. *Psychiatric Quarterly, 44,* 231–250.
Vulkan, V., & Showalter, R. (1968). Known object loss, disturbance in reality testing, and "re-grief work" as a method of brief psychotherapy. *Psychiatric Quarterly, 42,* 358–374.

III

Couple and Family Interventions

14

Brief Couple/Family Therapy

The Relationship Enhancement Approach

MARYHELEN SNYDER AND
BERNARD G. GUERNEY, JR.

INTRODUCTION

Relationship Enhancement (RE) therapies have been developed and empirically researched over the last three decades (B. Guerney, 1990). Their development began with the development of Filial Therapy, also called Child Relationship Enhancement Therapy, and then extended to couple therapy and family therapy with adolescents. In each instance, after the therapy had been developed and tested, a parallel problem-prevention/enrichment program was developed based on the same principles and methods (B. Guerney, 1988).

Many comparative studies of RE have been conducted. For example, RE has been compared to behavioral, gestalt, eclectic, and experienced marital therapists' own preferred eclectic approaches. Also, a meta-analytic study involving roughly 4,000 couples compared RE to about a dozen other systematic methods of enrichment and therapy (Giblin, Sprenkle, & Sheehan, 1985). A review of most of this research appears elsewhere (L. F. Guerney & B. Guerney, 1985). However, we

---

MARYHELEN SNYDER • New Mexico Relationship Enhancement Institute, 422 Camino del Bosque, Albuquerque, New Mexico 87114. BERNARD G. GUERNEY, JR. • Individual and Family Consultation Center, Department of Human Development and Family Studies, Pennsylvania State University, University Park, Pennsylvania 16802.

Casebook of the Brief Psychotherapies, edited by Richard A. Wells and Vincent J. Giannetti. Plenum Press, New York, 1993.

will provide a thumbnail sketch here. In none of these studies did RE show less favorable results than any other method. In all of them, RE showed significant superiority in client process or outcome variables or both. Possible reasons for its exceptional efficacy are:

1. Rather than emphasizing change at one or two levels of functioning over the others, RE promotes change synergistically at all levels—cognitive, affective, and behavioral (Snyder, 1991).

2. RE follows a skill-training, educational model as opposed to the medical model followed by most other therapies. A skill-training approach seems to greatly reduce resistance and induce strong motivation; in fact, clients usually considered to be unmotivated (e.g., court-referred wife batterers) generally are highly responsive to RE therapy.

3. RE is "gender-informed" and tends generally to empower the disempowered—factors that seem to enhance its motivating power and efficacy (Snyder, 1992a,b,c).

4. RE gives transfer/generalization a central role in the therapeutic process. Indeed, in RE, transfer/generalization is taught to the clients as a skill in its own right. This means that almost from the beginning, changes take place in the client's daily life.

5. The nine skills (L. F. Guerney & B. Guerney, 1985) taught in RE contribute to success in all the major aspects of living: family, friends, and work—and change is fostered in all of these areas, again producing a synergistic effect.

6. By teaching the clients how to elicit help and constructive interactions from others and also by directly teaching intimates how to act as psychotherapeutic agents, RE makes use of powerful therapeutic forces not harnessed in other couples or family therapies.

7. RE selectively integrates principles and methods from each of the major schools of individual psychotherapy—psychodynamic, humanistic, social-learning/behavioral, and interpersonal—so that, we believe, the advantages offered by each are available to clients, whereas the weaknesses of each are minimized (Snyder, 1991).

8. RE adds the advantages of a systemic approach to the change processes of individual therapy; by a systemic approach, we mean that RE makes direct changes in the usually not-conscious rules governing the interpersonal interaction between family members (Snyder, 1989).

To best illustrate both its educational goals (as well as some special techniques discussed later), we have chosen a case (seen by the senior author) that illustrates the "standard" form of RE as a brief therapy. Names and other identifying information have been changed for reasons of confidentiality.

CASE STUDY

Presenting Problems and History

Stan and Amy, married 4 years, had formerly been to two therapists for marriage counseling without making significant gains. Stan was referred by his cousin who had been seen for RE family therapy. During the week before the intake session, Amy had moved out for a period of 24 hours. Prior to that, they had had two month-long separations during the previous year, both instigated by Stan during periods of intense frustration over the issues described below. At intake, both Amy and Stan reported thinking that divorce might be inevitable. It is Stan's second marriage. He has a high-school-age daughter by his first marriage who spends every other weekend with Stan and Amy.

Stan felt so depressed at the time of the intake interview that he inquired about the possibility of a psychiatric evaluation for antidepressant medications; this was postponed and then considered unnecessary. Since the couple lived too far away to attend weekly sessions, it was decided to hold double sessions of therapy every 2 weeks. Therapy was completed after five sessions, totaling 10 hours.

Intake Interview

RE couple therapy has a specific structure for the intake interview. Each person speaks only to the therapist—never to each other—and only when invited to speak. (Among its many other advantages, this is a great time saver.) They are asked to speak about their relationship problems and goals, and each is given the opportunity to give his/her own perspective on whatever their partner has said. Each in turn is responded to empathetically in the same manner that is later taught to the clients.

Toward the close of every intake interview, the therapist used the RE technique of *Becoming*. In addition to deeply joining the therapist to both clients, Becoming accomplishes three important purposes, which are explained to the clients in this way:

Before I explain more about the nature of the therapy I will be doing with you, I would like to be you, Stan, talking to Amy. And then I would like to be you, Amy, talking to Stan. First of all, it will help me integrate and remember all that I have learned from you today. I particularly want to be sure that I've understood your deepest feelings and desires. Secondly, it will give you a way of checking whether I have understood what you most want me to understand. I'm going to take some risks in "reading between the lines," so to speak, so I really want you to let me know if I make any errors in doing this. And, finally, I will be speaking using some of the guidelines that I would like to teach you to use with each other that make it possible to be very honest about one's feelings without putting the other person on the defensive. After I'm finished being you, Stan, I'll check with you so you can add or change anything that I don't get quite right; you can also interrupt me if I get off base. And I'll also check with you, Amy, about whether you felt at all defensive listening to me as Stan. Then I'll switch and be you talking to Stan.

Although the five guidelines of the RE Expresser skill are not explained yet, it is their consistent use by the therapist now that makes it possible for the therapist to speak authentically while minimizing the likelihood of the client's feeling defensive. These guidelines include (a) subjectivity; (b) the expression of deep positive or negative feelings; (c) reference to specific problematic events and behaviors rather than generalizations about behaviors and/or blaming language; (d) the expression of the positive feelings, attitudes, or goals that are responsible for or underlie the negative feelings; and (e) assertion of what one wants from the other person and the benefits that would accrue to both parties if these wants were met. The following reconstruction of the therapist's Becoming statements are based on notes written immediately after the session.

THERAPIST [TO AMY AS STAN]: *Well, first and most important, I don't want to lose you. This last year, and even before, have really been painful for me, even though I've been the one to leave you the first two times, and I'm usually the one to threaten it. I do that because I get really scared that you don't care about me the way I want you to. And I get really angry, too. You know, I lived alone for 5 years, and I took care of our daughter on alternate weekends, and I did okay, but what I longed for was someone to really share my life with, to talk everything over with, and to lean on when I needed to. And when we got married 4 years ago, it seemed to me that you were that person.*

I guess what I want most is to be a priority in your life, and what that would mean is that you would really want to know how I'm feeling about things and that you would want to be with me more than it feels like you do. I get scared when you have so many activities outside the home—your school job and your sales job—and then lots of friends on top of that. I also get scared that you might have an affair with one of the men you know at work. Part of me knows that you're not like that, but I also know how wonderful and attractive you are, and especially when you have a couple of drinks with people after work, I worry. At that corporate conference last year in Boston, I felt almost out of my mind the night you stayed out until 2:00 A.M. *with friends. I know you'd invited me to come with you, and I'd been the one to say "No." But I wanted you to come home early and be with me. I want you to belong to me, to be my wife and to be happy about that. Like when we go to a bar with your friends from work and you dance with other people, it just feels like you're not announcing to the world like I want you to that you and I are a couple and that we belong to each other. It's hard to say these things. They sound possessive, but I think the possessiveness is there just because I'm not sure that you really want to be with me.*

You know I try to talk myself out of these feelings; they seem so dependent. But at the same time, I feel like I deserve more from you. Intimacy is really important to me, and you're the one I want to be intimate with. It's not just sex I'm talking about or touching each other. I think we do that okay. It's talking about our feelings and wanting to be with each other. That's what I miss from you.

The therapist then checked with both Stan and Amy about their feelings as the therapist had done this. Stan was crying. He said that it was accurate and that he would like to speak this way, but more often it came out angry or he just gave up. Amy said that she didn't feel at all attacked, but that the feelings she'd expressed in the interview kept coming up strongly.

THERAPIST [AS AMY TO STAN]: *You know, I really like it that you love me, but sometimes I feel so strongly that I have to pick between you and me! Sometimes I feel like I can hardly breathe in this relationship. And then I want to make room for myself, to be really free—not divorced, not unfaithful—just free. For instance, I love my job, and my second job, too, and I love being active in company activities. And I love traveling to conferences. And I love seeing friends. And, although I love your daughter—and I do love you—I lived alone for 13 years before I met you, and I got really used to being independent, and I know I don't want to give that up.*

What's hard for me is that you seem so suspicious, and you don't seem to trust me. I've gotten so I feel really hopeless about that. When you threaten to pack up and leave, I feel mistreated. And when you get really glum, I feel mistreated, too. From my point of view, I'm a trustworthy person. I'm not a quitter, and I'm not somebody who has affairs.

When I came back after leaving you for a day, I really liked it that you talked in a calmer way about what you'd been feeling. You tell me that you want us to talk more, but what's hard for me is that I feel like you slip in insults, or you're so gloomy about things, that I just get defensive and want to be left alone. Like the other day: Right before I left, the incident with you fixing my car seemed like just a lot of miscommunication and misunderstanding, but I felt like the way you saw it was me not respecting you, and then it seemed to me that you got depressed and insulting. I begin to feel like nothing I say will make any difference.

> *I guess the deepest thing is that I want the right to make mistakes and the right to be my own person. And I want you to trust me. I want you to know that I love and respect you without my having to prove it in ways that limit my spirit. I think you like my free spirit and I like it, too. I really believe that I can't give up that independent spirit and still be a loving person.*

Again the therapist checked with Amy and Stan about the accuracy of this *Becoming* and about the effect on the listener. Both of them expressed feeling moved. Stan said, "Can you come home with us and just *be* us?"

One of the benefits of using this comprehensive Becoming technique at the close of the intake interview (as well as at other times in the therapy process) is that it joins the therapist deeply to both clients. In addition to overcoming clients' deficiencies for them, as mentioned earlier, it is useful to become a client when you are confused about his/her position, or when you begin to find it difficult to accept his/her ideas or feelings; putting yourself so completely and forcefully in his/her place and subjecting yourself to corrective feedback tends to overcome the confusion and disaffection and rekindle the compassion and equality of understanding toward each party that, in our view, is so necessary to being a maximally effective couples therapist.

As usual in RE, at the close of the intake interview, the partners were briefly coached in how to avoid hostility-inducing actions between sessions, and a homework assignment was negotiated. That assignment was to read Chapter 1, to complete the Relationship Questionnaires in the *Relationship Enhancement Manual* (Guerney, 1987), and to listen to two *Relationship Enhancement Demonstration Audiotapes* (B. Guerney & Vogelsong, 1981) that contrast the typical way in which couples discuss problems and conflicts of various sorts with the way they are discussed using the basic RE skills.

The first therapy session began with teaching the clients Empathic skills with the Identification (I) method. A nonconflictual topic is generally used here. The senior author suggests a particular topic that seems especially effective because it enhances bonding of the clients with each other and with the therapist. She suggests that the clients talk about a *very significant* event from their lives—one that has affected their childhood, friendships, or work values pleasurably or painfully. Then, in a manner similar to Becoming, the therapist models the process of identification, the all-important component of the Empathic skill, by putting himself/herself in the place of the person who has spoken and, using the pronoun "I," expressing the important thoughts and feelings of the person who has spoken. In doing so, emphasis is placed on what the person was thinking and feeling but did *not* say. In order to discover the unspoken thoughts and feelings, RE therapists and clients, while listening, are prompted to ask themselves certain questions that are part of the guidelines of the Empathic skill—questions that aid in the identification process, for example, "If I were the other person, what would I be feeling?" The accuracy of the "identification" is always checked with the client.

After this exercise in identification, which promoted significant catharsis for both Amy and Stan and after which both reported the mutual satisfaction of this level of listening, the therapist taught them the henceforth-used "You" form of Empathic Responding. In instruction, the topic, as usual, was the positive qualities/behaviors of their partner as listed on their Relationship Questionnaires.

The therapist explained the five elements of the Expressive skill and role played, speaking without, and then with, these elements. Although the teaching of the Expressive skill usually begins with noncontroversial planning about ways to strengthen the relationship, it was decided instead to begin with a "minor conflict" because the couple were already engaging in a number of satisfying shared activities and because they were eager to begin using the skills with tougher problems.

We chose the issue of sharing in the housework, which both Amy and Stan listed as "minor conflicts" on their Relationship Questionnaires. We then stayed with this issue through the explanation and practice of the next two skills (Discussion/Negotiation and Problem Solving).

At this session, several comments were made by Amy and/or Stan that are typical occurrences when a couple is initially experiencing the RE approach. Stan commented about a "sudden shift" in his viewpoint as he was empathizing with Amy. Amy commented that at one point she was "boiling," and she thought she might not be able to empathize. But then she noticed she could do it anyway, by just setting the "boiling" aside. She observed that two things happened as a result. One was that the boiling seemed to lessen as she empathized, but the other was that after being empathized with, Stan arrived at the awareness on his own that she was angry at him for not seeing that asking her to remind him about chores that needed to be done was burdensome to her. Several times during the course of therapy, either Amy or Stan noted with some amazement that such shifts resulting from the empathic process (whether one is in the Empathizer or the Expresser role) feel almost magical.

Following standard RE procedures, the couple held weekly audiotaped sessions at home using the skills. The therapist provided brief supervision of segments of these sessions.

The second therapy session was a difficult one for the couple. Amy's upcoming attendance at a work-related conference had evoked Stan's fears. By now the couple had read about and practiced the first four skills, but the topic was in many ways their most emotional issue. The therapist permitted them to deal with so difficult an issue at this early state of their skill development, because this issue seemed to be primary in their ambivalence about whether or not they could stay together and the upcoming conference therefore had some crisis elements. The therapist did a great deal of Becoming and Laundering. (In Laundering, the therapist, following a set of guidelines—in addition to the usual RE guidelines—alternatively becomes both parties in a problem/conflict-resolving dialogue while alternately also receiving input from both parties.) The session ended with Stan expressing uncertainty about whether he could stay in the relationship.

The third session saw the issue resolved as shown below. (This and future excerpts are transcriptions from audiotapes of the sessions, with minor editing for clarity and space saving.)

> STAN: *I just realized that I could say "I'm not going to leave you, Amy" and that would be very scary, because I've used it as a threat to make you do it the way I want you to; and, if I didn't have the threat, I'd have to figure out another way to deal with the intense emotions I get when you're going to a conference, for instance, or when you're late getting home, or when I feel like you're ignoring me or not respecting me. And somehow I felt calmer after I made this decision—like in one sense it was scarier, but in another sense it made everything safer, like we'd just have to keep working this stuff through because I wasn't going anywhere.*

Amy cried while Stan spoke to her in this way. Amy and Stan carried this session without the therapist having to use Laundering or Becoming responses. However, as is standard in RE, the therapist did frequently use the techniques of Modeling and Prompting for the Expresser and Modeling for the Empathizer to help them recognize and express their own and the other's deeper, underlying thoughts and feelings. (In Modeling, as the term is used in RE, the therapist presents the exact words that the Expresser or Empathizer may use to express his/her deepest thoughts and feelings if he/she so chooses. In "Prompts," as the term is defined in RE, ideas or types of responses, rather than exact wordings, are suggested.) In this session, the clients also were taught the Facilitation skill (to use in coaching each other at home) and Self-Changing and Other-Changing skills.

The following transcript from an audiotape of the first part of the fourth therapy session (with some omissions to save space) shows the clients' use of the Expressive and Empathic skills and labels some of the RE techniques used by the therapist.

AMY [AS EXPRESSER]. *I tried to think about what I could have done differently. Like maybe I could have apologized sooner. But when you picked up your boots and left the room, that was really hard. I mean, I thought if you were just going to go in the other room, you would have left your boots. To me that was like "I'm leaving."*

STAN [AS EMPATHIC RESPONDER]: *It was like implying to you that I was going away. You thought maybe you could have apologized sooner. But in any event, when I picked up my boots, you got upset because you thought I might be leaving.*

AMY: *Yeah.*

THERAPIST [TO STAN; MODELING FOR THE EMPATHIC RESPONDER]: *Try adding something like this in your own words: "It means a great deal to you that I've made a promise to myself and to you not to leave. It's a tremendous relief to you to know that when I'm upset or scared or angry I'm not leaving it as an option to walk out. It helps you to feel safe and feel like you're not going to get abandoned or treated like you're bad. (Amy starts to cry as the therapist says this.) When I picked up my boots, you wondered for a moment if I really meant that promise."* (Stan does say this in his own words and then, in the Expresser Mode, says he's not sure why he picked up his boots. Amy gave him an Empathic response.)

THERAPIST [TO STAN, PROMPTING FOR THE EXPRESSER]: *I'm wondering if, when you picked up your boots, you were thinking for a moment that you might leave the house, like an old habit that you're changing, just like Amy is changing her old habit of not apologizing after she's been grumpy with you. Or whether maybe it was just a way of showing Amy what was going on with you. Could you talk to her about that?*

STAN [TO AMY]: *I was feeling really disempowered by what was going on between us, and I got up out of the bed maybe feeling "pouty." I felt, like really—in my bare feet—I felt disempowered, and I grabbed my boots to feel empowered, I guess. I think I knew what it would do. I didn't have any intention of leaving the house.* [Amy empathizes.]

THERAPIST [PROMPTING TO THE EXPRESSER]: *And perhaps you could talk about what you might have done to feel empowered instead of what you did. I remember last session you spoke, I think, about having said to Amy, "I feel like you're being mean to me," and that felt good to you, as I recall.*

STAN: *Yeah. I guess I could have said, "I feel mistreated, and I'm going to go watch TV in the other room."*

AMY [AFTER EMPATHIZING]: *I like it when you tell me what you're doing and why. You've done that a few times, and I really like it. And I like that we have a different way of dealing with things now. I really thought about that last night as I was lying there. What first came up for me when you left with those boots is "I'm really pissed." Then I, we really have learned new ways to do things—*

and it hit me early enough to realize I really was being awful to you. I had no business treating you like that. And I just sort of know that I have from you your commitment and that you're going to be here through good times and bad. I want that. I suppose what I want from you is to be patient, because I'm just beginning to really deal with things. (After Stan empathizes, Amy looks very pensive.)

THERAPIST [PROMPTING THE EXPRESSER]: *I'm wondering what you're thinking, Amy.*

AMY: *I think maybe I doubt the part that you feel your commitment totally.* (She starts to cry a little.) *I don't tell you how much I like to know that you're there and that I can reach over and grab your hand and hold on. I love you even when I'm acting like a bitch.*

STAN: *Sometimes when you reach over and we're laying there, it feels real warm and loving. And you love me and sometimes you don't say it as often as you recognize it. And you're still scared about my keeping my commitment to you.*

AMY: *[Yeah.]*

STAN [SWITCHING TO EXPRESSER MODE]: *Well, I'm committed, I know that—but I think maybe each of us is only human and we make mistakes. I was thinking, actually it just came to me, maybe we can say, "Time out; I need half an hour." It would feel like there's not going to be any quick resolve, but just accepting that each of us is only human, and we need some time to think it out before we talk about it. I'm not saying it would be easy for me to say, "OK, Babe, I understand, but I think it would be more honest and up front if you would say, "I'm feeling cranky and like being mean, and maybe we should take a break." Same for me, sometimes I'm cranky and I've had a bad day, and I think sometimes I tell you that and sometimes I act it out.*

AMY [AFTER EMPATHIZING]: *Well, I think those are good ideas. And I don't want to have to talk in the middle of the night. Like, let's say we call time out at 8—until 9. I don't want to talk then until 12 or 1 or 2 in the morning, like maybe have a time limit on how much talking is done, even if we don't resolve it.*

STAN [AFTER EMPATHIZING]: *This may surprise you, but I agree with you. How about the idea of calling a truce and saying, "I love you even though I'm mad at you."* [Amy empathizes, switches modes, and agrees with Stan.]

THERAPIST [STRUCTURING AND THEN MODELING FOR EXPRESSER]: *I want to make sure that the details of this are enough in place that you're very, very likely to do it. You remember, with the Problem-Solving skill, one important step is looking at what situations might come up in which your solution would be difficult to apply. Does it seem to you that in any situation that you can imagine at this point, it would work fine to say, "We're tired now and we love each other, and even though we're still angry we can talk about this whenever we agree to, and we can go to sleep loving each other." Talk to Stan about that.*

AMY [TO STAN]: *I can't think of any situation, an extreme situation, where it wouldn't work. I think we've made the situations extreme with our own behaviors. There are types of things that come up for us again, and we may not have them resolved. But I feel the ideas we've come up with so far, owning it, taking time out, and going to bed with the understanding that we'll deal with it and that we do love each other—I think those are good ideas and I could make them part of me.*

STAN: *The ideas that have come up about time, owning our stuff, time limit, and the understanding that things will be dealt with the next day—you feel like you can commit yourself to do that.* [Switching to Expresser Mode]: *I have one more thing to say that's important to me. Each of us has a right to have his or her thoughts about what's important to them, even though it might seem trivial to the other person.*

AMY: *You're feeling that what either of us feels is a problem or a concern that we should be able to express it and it be okay, rather than the other person saying it's not a problem or judging whether it's something worth discussing or not. Did I get it?*

STAN: *Very good.* [With mutual laughter they agree to discuss all issues deemed a problem by either party.]

Termination and Follow-Up

Before the close of the fifth therapy session, we discussed the final two RE skills of Generalization (which they had already been doing to a large degree) and Maintenance. In regard to the latter, time set aside on at least a weekly basis to practice RE skills is desirable. Amy and Stan had been doing this and promised to continue it.

We had tentatively decided at the previous session that this fifth session would be the last, partly for economic reasons, but mainly because Stan and Amy felt confident in their skills and because they and the therapist agreed that their skills, level of commitment, and intimacy had improved dramatically. At the time of the 2-month date, Stan and Amy reported that everything was going well and decided they did not need to come in. This was also the case in two follow-up calls, made at 4 and 6 months past the last session. Recently, Stan's cousin said he thought the couple could use a skill-refresher session, but confirmed that they were getting along much better and that their commitment to each other was very evident.

CLINICAL ISSUES

If brief therapy is defined as a therapy that always sets goals that, though not immutable, are clear at the outset to both therapist and clients; focuses treatment around those goals; uses systematic, replicable methods that can be easily related to specific needs, problems, and behaviors of the clients; and may often be completed successfully in a matter of hours when that is what is called for, then RE certainly is a brief therapy. If, on the other hand, one defines brief therapy as a therapy that *never* extends beyond *X* number of sessions, such as 10 or even 20, then RE is not a brief therapy. RE uses a number of different time formats depending on the needs of the clients and their life circumstances. As these differ, so do the priorities assigned to the various goals of RE therapy. How this adjustment process works requires some background about the philosophical–strategic orientation of RE in relation to the delivery of mental health services.

RE therapy is the first holistic couple/family therapy. *Holistic* therapy has been defined by Guerney, Brock, and Coufal (1986) as including the goal, when feasible, of bringing clients to a *high* level of functioning rather than simply restoring equilibrium or bringing clients to the level of normalcy. We view holistic therapy as the most cost-effective way of delivering mental health services, whether the cost-bearing unit is the family, an organization, or a society. The idea is to equip couples/families not only to overcome a current crisis or pressing problem, but simultaneously to teach them how to deal with future problems and, most important, how to prevent future crises and serious problems from developing.

With respect to time formats, in line with the above-stated views, the RE therapist's preference is to teach the clients the skills necessary to resolve their conflicts and problems *before* tackling their problems. When this sequence is followed, the clients then apply the skills in the office and, generally, in tape-recorded sessions at home to accomplish conflict/problem resolution under the supervision of the therapist. This not only gives family members the skills they need to prevent and resolve their present problems, it significantly promotes generalization of therapeutic changes to permanent use in everyday life, and it gives the clients the experience and the confidence that they need to prevent and resolve future difficulties. To do therapy in this sequence means asking the clients to put their most serious problems on hold for 3 to 6 hours of therapy (by scheduling lengthier sessions, and/or seeing clients more frequently, this can mean as little as 1 or 2 days). Most therapists learning RE are very surprised to find that the majority of clients are quite amenable to waiting, even when the delay is weeks rather than days. But there are circumstances in which delay is not feasible. It is then that RE crisis intervention methods are called into play.

One such instance is when there is an outside deadline, that is, one not under the family's control. An example would be a daughter's unwillingness to have the abortion her parents want her to have, with the time for a legal abortion rapidly running out. Another example would be a deadline imposed by a family member: For example, a husband has just discovered that his wife is having an affair and demands that she terminate any contact with her lover instantly, or he will immediately move out and divorce her. RE crisis intervention methods also are called into play if and when the therapist concludes (e.g., during one of the routine inquiries about the subject) that someone would be very unhappy about continuing to delay work on heavy problems. In special circumstances, such as an imminent move, a time-limited format may be used.

Generally, however, the format developed for RE therapy, called "time-designated" (B. Guerney, 1977), is used. We believe this format best incorporates the advantages and minimizes the disadvantages of open-ended and time-limited formats. In the time-designated format the therapist tells the family the estimated number of sessions necessary to accomplish the goals set by the family after discussion with the therapist. If the couple or family is unwilling to contract for the length of time the therapist estimates it will take to accomplish the desired goals, a negotiation process takes place in which both the goals and number of sessions are pared down until an (informal) contract can be reached. When that targeted session is reached, an evaluation is held. Both the therapist and the clients use a form to indicate the level of goal attainment. Any differences of opinion among family members, or with the therapist, are discussed, and if necessary negotiated and, accordingly, the sessions either are terminated, or a new future session is set as the target session, at which time the procedure is repeated.

The RE techniques used in the sort of crises described above are often used in the course of routine RE therapy. They are especially called into play when clients are unable to perform at the level the situation demands because they as yet lack the level of skill required, because they are overcome with emotion, or because of built-in insufficiencies such as those stemming from youth, limited intelligence, mental illness, or neurological damage. In all these situations, the therapist's assistance extends far beyond routine supervision; it involves great skill in entering the phenomenological world of the client. The assistance may also involve speaking for the client at levels of sensitivity, understanding, and problem-solving ability of which the client is not capable momentarily, temporarily, or permanently. The technique of Becoming used in the case material earlier presented illustrates one of the RE techniques offering that type of therapeutic assistance.

In crisis intervention and time-limited formats, these special RE methods, plus a minimal educational role, may almost entirely replace systematic skill training and supervision. But, no matter how short the therapy, the Educational Model also always plays *some* role in the treatment process. At the absolute minimum, this consists of explaining to the clients how the behavior of the therapist adheres to certain principles and practices that they could learn to apply to their own lives if and when their needs and circumstances permitted.

REFERENCES

Giblin, P., Sprenkle, D. H., Sheehan, R. (1985). Enrichment outcome research: A meta-analysis of premarital, marital, and family interventions. *Journal of Marital and Family Therapy, 11*(3), 257–271.

Guerney, B. G., Jr. (1977). Should teachers treat illiteracy, hypocalligraphy, and dysmathematica? *The Canadian Counsellor, 12*(1), 9–14.

Guerney, B. G., Jr. (1987) (Ed.). *Relationship Enhancement Manual*. P.O. Box 391, State College, PA: Ideals.

Guerney, B. G., Jr. (1988). Family relationship enhancement: A skill training approach. In L. A. Bond & B. M. Wagner (Eds.), *Families in transition: Primary prevention programs that work* (pp. 99–134). Newbury Park, CA: Sage.

Guerney, B. G., Jr. (1990). Creating therapeutic and growth-inducing family systems: Personal moorings, landmarks, and guiding stars. In F. Kaslow (Ed.), *Voices in family psychology* (pp. 114–138). Beverly Hills, CA: Sage.

Guerney, B., Jr., & Vogelsong, E. (1981). Relationship enhancement demonstration dialogue (Audiotape). Individual & Family Consultation Center, University Park, PA 16802.

Guerney, B. G., Jr., Brock, G., & Coufal, J. (1986). Integrating marital therapy and enrichment: The relationship enhancement approach. In N. Jacobson & A. Gurman (Eds.), *Clinical handbook of marital therapy* (pp. 151–172). New York: Guilford Press.

Guerney, L. F., & Guerney, B. G., Jr. (1985). The relationship enhancement family of family therapies. In L. L'Abate & M. Milan (Eds.), *Handbook of social skills training and research* (pp. 506–524). New York: John Wiley & Sons.

Snyder, M. (1986). Love and trust as decisions: Applications to relationship therapy. *Psychosynthesis Digest*, 3:24–48.

Snyder, M. (1989). The relationship enhancement model of couple therapy: An integration of Rogers and Bateson. *Person-Centered Review, 4*, 358–383.

Snyder, M. (1991). The relationship enhancement model of family therapy: A systematic eclectic approach. *Journal of Family Psychotherapy, 2*, 1–26.

Snyder, M. (1992a). A gender-informed model of couple and family therapy: Relationship enhancement therapy. *Contemporary Family Therapy, 14*, 15–31.

Snyder, M. (1992b). The co-construction of new meanings in couple relationships: A psychoeducational model that promotes mutual empowerment. In B. J. Brothers (Ed.), *Equal partnering* (pp. 41–58). New York: Haworth.

Snyder, M. (1992c). The meaning of empathy: Comments on Hans Strupp's case of Helen R. *Psychotherapy, 29*, 318–322.

15

Two Cases of Brief Therapy in an HMO

Michael F. Hoyt

> I think the development of psychiatric skill consists in very considerable measure of doing a lot with very little—making a rather precise move which has a high probability of achieving what you're attempting to achieve, with a minimum of time and words.
>
> Harry Stack Sullivan (1954, p. 224)

Introduction

More than 100 million Americans are now covered by HMOs and other forms of managed care such as IPAs, PPOs, EAPs, student health services, and armed forces psychiatric services (Austad & Berman, 1991; Bennett, 1988; Boaz, 1988; Feldman & Fitzpatrick, 1992; Goldman, 1988; Zimet, 1989).[1] Although there are important differences within and between these different approaches to regulating the costs, utilization, and/or site of services, psychotherapy provision arrangements in managed health care settings all have as their ideal the principle of optimal use of time and resources. Brief therapy is the backbone of these ap-

[1]For any latecomers, this alphabet soup denotes Health Maintenance Organizations, Independent Practice Associations, Preferred Provider Organizations, and Employee Assistance Programs (see Austad & Hoyt, 1992).

Michael F. Hoyt • Department of Psychiatry, Kaiser-Permanente Medical Center, 27400 Hesperian Boulevard, Hayward, California 94545-4299.

Casebook of the Brief Psychotherapies, edited by Richard A. Wells and Vincent J. Giannetti. Plenum Press, New York, 1993.

proaches, the way to provide some services to many rather than many services to a privileged few. Therapists working within HMOs and other managed care settings know the challenge of our Sullivanian epigram through daily experience.

The essence of good HMO therapy is that it is *short-term, eclectic,* and *effective.* The goals of most therapy in an HMO involve enhancing coping skills, reducing distress, restoring function, promoting growth, and practical improvement rather than mythical "cure." Therapists work to assist patients in getting "unstuck" (Hoyt, 1990; Hoyt et al., 1992). To do this, a brief therapy "credo" or set of pro-brief therapy values and working assumptions are instrumental and essential. These may include such items as the belief that it is the patient who has the ultimate power and control over treatment progress, the desire to be "time sensitive" and not to prolong treatment beyond what is truly necessary, and the willingness of the therapist to be active and to forego the emotional and financial pleasures of long-term treatment (Budman & Gurman, 1988; Hoyt, 1985; Talmon, 1990).

ESSENTIAL CHARACTERISTICS OF HMO THERAPY

Cutting across various systems and specific brief therapy technical approaches and extending beyond the single parameter of "short-term" are a series of principles that characterize what Austad et al. (1988; Austad & Berman, 1991; Hoyt & Austad, 1992) have called "HMO therapy." The application of the following principles will be illustrated in the two cases to be presented later in this chapter.

1. *Rapid setting of clearly defined goals, with an orientation toward brief therapy and specific problem solving.* The effort is to implement specific treatments for specific problems rather than taking a broad, "exploratory" (i.e., unfocused) approach. A rapid, accurate assessment leads to an effective and comprehensive treatment plan.[2] In many cases, assess-

[2]The term *diagnosis* derives from Greek and Latin words (*via gnossis*) meaning "the way to know or distinguish," precisely what a good functional diagnosis should do: provide information that helps point the way (Hoyt, 1989). The HMO therapist, like any clinician hoping to work efficiently, needs to go beyond conventional psychiatric diagnostic issues to find the patient's useful strengths and resources. Three heuristic questions (Hoyt, 1990) are often useful: (1) Where/how is the patient "stuck" (the problem or pathology)? (2) What is needed to get "unstuck"? and (3) How can the therapist facilitate or provide what is needed? Being able to conceptualize and intervene from multiple perspectives (Gustafson, 1986) allows the clinician many more degrees of freedom in which to work parsimoniously.

ment and intervention are intertwined, with test interventions used to clarify the assessment.

2. *Crisis intervention preparedness,* with rapid response so that problems can be dealt with before they get entrenched or produce avalanches of secondary problems.

3. *Clear definition of patient and therapist responsibilities,* with an explicit understanding (sometimes called a "contract") of the purpose, schedule, and duration of treatment. The therapist is responsible for appropriate structuring of therapeutic contacts, recommending and conducting particular interventions, and involving significant other people as needed. The patient is encouraged to assume much of the initiative and responsibility for the work of therapy, including actively participating in sessions, carrying out "homework" assignments, and implementing behavioral changes outside of therapy sessions.

4. *Flexible and creative use of time,* for example, appointments need not occur on a once-a-week basis or last for the conventional 50 minutes (Hoyt, 1990). The frequency, length, and timing of treatment varies according to patient needs, with the ideal being the "least intensive, least expensive, least intrusive" intervention that would be appropriate and likely to have positive effects in a given situation.

5. *Interdisciplinary cooperation,* including the use of concurrent psychotherapy and psychopharmacology when needed. In the context of a primary care HMO medical setting, medical and psychological involvement may blend into a more holistic view of the patient.

6. *Use of multiple formats and modalities,* with treatments sometimes involving concurrent or sequential combinations of individual, group, and/or family therapy. Frequent referrals to community resources are made, and participation in various 12-step, self-help, and support groups is vigorously encouraged when appropriate.

7. *A "family practitioner" model* that replaces the notion of definitive once-and-for-all "cure" with the idea that patients can return for intermittent treatment throughout the life cycle (Cummings, 1986, 1990). Therapy may be "serial" or "distributed." The therapist–patient relationship may be long-term although frequently abeyant. The therapist encourages autonomy and independence rather than regression and dependence; as soon as the therapist is not needed, he or she recedes into the background of the patient's life until needed again.

8. *Utilization review and quality assurance.* The former involves procedures to monitor and insure that services are being delivered in the most cost-effective manner possible for purposes of cost containment. The latter is complementary and assesses what care the patient received. The two procedures may need to be kept separate to avoid conflicts of interest

(Chestnut et al., 1987). As in the field of psychotherapy private practice, there is a clear need for standards and regulations in the emerging field of managed-care mental-health services.

TWO ILLUSTRATIONS OF BRIEF THERAPY IN AN HMO

Case One

A 67-year-old man was sitting in a wheelchair next to his wife in our HMO Psychiatry Department waiting room when I met him. At the suggestion of his internist, he had scheduled an intake appointment and had waited about 2 weeks for our meeting. The receptionist's brief note succinctly indicated, under Reason for Seeking Services: "Referred by M.D. Post-stroke. Fear of falling."

When I introduced myself and shook hands I could see that he was a pleasant and engaging man. He had not shaved in a few days and was wearing casual clothing and (somewhat crookedly) an Oakland A's baseball cap. When I asked "How shall we go to my office?" his wife offered, "Sam (a pseudonym) can walk but he's afraid. He came into the building on his own, slowly, with me helping. We got that wheelchair downstairs." Although she was pleasant and trying to be helpful, I sensed it would be useful to have some time with the patient alone, and so I asked him: "Do you want to walk or ride to my office?" He replied: "I'll take a ride, at least this time."

As I pushed him around the corner and down the corridor, we talked baseball. "What do you think of the Hawkins' trade?" and "How'd they do today?" got us talking and connected. He made a few remarks that showed a good knowledge of the game, and I asked intelligent questions.

At my office door I stopped and asked him if he could take a couple of steps into my office and use a regular chair because the wheelchair was bulky and awkward. He obliged. When we sat down I asked: "So, what's up? What brings you here? How can I be of help?" I learned that he was a retired mechanic and printing pressman. He had suffered a stroke 3 years earlier, with a residual partial paralysis of one arm and leg. He had grown "too damn dependent" on his wife, he said, but could no longer drive and had considerable difficulty walking. "I sure miss Dr. Jarrett," he added, referring to his former internist who had retired himself a few years earlier. "He was a great doctor. Did you know him?" I had and said so and asked what he thought Dr. Jarrett might say to him about his current situation. "I know what he would tell me now.

He'd tell me I just have to get going and do it. He'd give me a pep talk, get me going. Just give me a good boot if I needed it." I replied: "Took the words right out of my mouth. Dr. Jarrett and I would sure agree."

The patient nodded. "Yeah. I just need a push. You know, my two sons want to take me to an A's game next month. I've got to get over this fear. I know I can do it, but I'm not. I'm frustrated. But I get so worried and down that I freeze up."

"Now, what's this about falling?", I asked him. He was very fearful of falling. Physical therapy rehabilitation had taught him, among other things, how to fall safely (protecting his head, softening his landing as best he could), but he was scared to go out of the house or be on his own: "I'm not sure what would happen to me if I fell and no one was around. I might not be able to get back up."

I could see his predicament. He was a practical man. (And just the night before, by coincidence, I had read my 4-year-old son a story [Peet, 1972] about a series of animals that each gets stranded, culminating with an elephant stuck on his back until an ant he befriended rescues him with the help of an ant hoard.) "Well, that makes sense to me," I responded. "You know, there are only three reasons to fear falling: (1) You might get hurt falling, but it sounds like you know how to fall safely, and you're not worried about falling down stairs or in front of traffic or anything like that. (He shook his head indicating, "Nah, no problem.") (2) You might be embarrassed, but you don't look like a man that's prissy or worried about that. (Again he indicated not.) Or (3) you might not be able to get up once you fall. (Sam nodded affirmatively.) I'll tell you what. Let's do a little experiment. I'll be you, you be the coach, and teach me how to get up." I then proceeded to sort of throw myself on the floor in front of him. He got right into it, advising me, "No, turn the other way, get up first on three points," and so forth. I said, "Let me try it with my arm not working" and held it limply against my side. For the next 8 or 10 minutes or so I repeatedly got down on the floor and Sam instructed me on how to get myself up again.

Back in my chair, I asked him if he wanted to "try it" here in my office or wait until he got home. He chose to wait until he was home, but sitting in his chair he showed me some of the "exercises I still can do." I was interested and watched, and then asked him to "stand and do a little walking just so I can see how you do." I opened the door, and we slowly proceeded into the corridor outside my office. "Take your time, but let me see how you do walk," I repeated. We slowly but steadily made our way up and down the hallway. A couple of times I remarked, "Oh, good," "Fine," and "Nice, better than I expected." As we got going in the hallway, I switched back to baseball, asking him about the game he was planning to attend with his sons. "Where are you going to park? Which ramp will you take?" I learned that the Oakland Coliseum has handicap access, but there were a couple of long ramps to be negotiated. Knowing the stadium fairly well, I painted aloud a vivid picture of entering the baseball park as we made our way up and down the hallway a couple of times.

Back in my office we sat down. "You know, I'm worried about my wife. She's trying to help me all she can, but she's getting tired. It's not good for her, or me, to have her watching me all the time. Maybe you could talk with her, too." I replied, "I'll be glad to, and when you begin to do more walking on your own then I'll really be able to convince her." He understood and agreed to practice his falling and getting up. I indicated he should fall and get up "at least four times a day to get good at it." That seemed to him too much to start with. We playfully bargained, and he agreed to do it twice a day for the first 3 days, then three times per day until I saw him in 2 weeks.

Before leaving my office I said: "You know, I think it's really important that you go to that game with your sons if you can. I know you want to go, but I think it will be even more important for them. Someday they will look back and remember going to the game with you, you know what I mean?" Sam didn't know exactly how baseball was in my blood and that one of the last good times I spent with my (now deceased) father was in San Francisco's Candlestick Park,[3] but he knew I was saying something heartfelt and important. Fathers and sons. It spoke to him. "I'm sure going to give it my best."

Follow-Up

Two weeks later Sam was sitting in the waiting room, in a regular chair. He proudly walked into my office, slowly. He had been practicing and was eagerly anticipating going to the game with his sons in another week or so. He reviewed the good work he had been doing. I then, with

[3]The Cubs lost the National League playoffs to the Giants that day, breaking my father's heart along with those of most Chicagoans. But this brings up another story. My father, a salesman by trade, was a keen observer of human behavior and something of a brief solution-oriented therapist himself. Once at a ballgame some years ago, an intoxicated fan sitting not far from my father was threatening and cursing about one of the ballplayers, and revealed that he was carrying a pistol. Needless to say, the situation was alarming. My father, something of a gun fancier, began to talk to the man, got him engaged, offered him cash, and actually bought the pistol from the man on the spot. The police never came. The next day my father took the weapon to a gunshop and sold it, for a profit. When I heard this story and asked him why he sold the gun, he replied: "Hey, you've got to get paid for this kind of work!"

his permission, brought his wife into my office. We talked about ways she could help by doing things and ways she could help by not doing things. Two weeks later I saw him (and them) again. He had gone to the game and was planning to go to another. He expressed the desire for more activity, and I suggested attending our Older Adults Therapy Group. He gladly accepted the referral. Several months later, I still see Sam (and his wife) in the waiting room before his therapy group, wave, and sometimes visit for a couple of minutes. I am also available if and when he may again request my professional services.

Comments[4]

The office intervention with this patient was essentially a case of single-session therapy (Hoyt et al., 1992; Rosenbaum et al., 1990; Talmon, 1990), a one-meeting piece of work that promotes the patient's self-empowerment and facilitates his finding a useful solution to the problem that brought him to therapy. It is not intended as a "cure" and does not obviate the possibility of additional useful therapy.

There are a number of technical points to note. There were obvious strategic and hypnotic qualities to the work (Rosenbaum, 1990, 1993). The approach was highly pragmatic, quickly getting the patient walking. Language and therapeutic interventions were constructed to make things happen. The therapist was able to use his own personal experiences constructively, to employ what might be termed *countertransference* to make a feelingful human connection. The essential notion is not to throw oneself on the floor in front of stroke victims nor to talk baseball with father figures, but to be alert to and use what resources are available in the service of the patient's therapeutic needs. This is what I take Erickson and Rossi (1979, p. 276) to mean when they suggest: "To initiate this type of therapy you have to be yourself as a person. You cannot imitate somebody else, but you have to do it in your own way."

It was helpful and felt natural to temporarily "reverse roles," Sam becoming the teacher/coach rather than the humbled stroke patient. This change in "story" (White & Epston, 1990) was morale restoring and opened possibilities for change that would not have been available if we pursued "cure." Part of effective brief therapy is deciding what paths *not* to take. Expanding Sam's discouragement or grief and exploring his concerns about failing powers and limited mortality were issues that might be worthwhile, but first helping Sam regain his confidence in

[4]Grateful acknowledgment is made to Eric Greenleaf and the members of our hypnosis study group for their helpful comments on this case.

walking and being able to get up when he fell enhanced the quality of his life and put him in a stronger position to realistically appraise his future options. This is what Sam and his wife wanted. The multimodal use of group therapy focused on older adults' developmental issues (Hoyt, in press), the combined individual and systemic perspective, and the "family practitioner" model of the available psychotherapist are features of an HMO approach.

Case Two

Sue Smith (a pseudonym), a 38-year-old woman, was brought to our HMO Psychiatry Department by her parents late one afternoon on a walk-in crisis basis. She and her husband had not been getting along for the past year, with his becoming increasingly angry and critical and her becoming increasingly timid and incompetent. Many of their quarrels focused on how poorly she managed their household and how she "failed to control" their two children. A former alcohol abuser who had been through an outpatient alcohol treatment program and had been abstinent for several years, Sue had recently resumed excessive alcohol consumption to calm and numb herself. Two days before, the husband had taken the kids and moved out. Sue's parents became alarmed when she did not answer their repeated phone calls, so they went to her home to check. They found her huddled in a corner of the house, quite anxious, fearful, and overwhelmed.

A staff psychologist in our Chemical Dependency Program initially met with the patient. He recommended that she actively participate in the Chemical Dependency Early Recovery Treatment Group, to begin the next week. He also determined that her current level of alcohol abuse did not present any medical risk for detoxification. It was also clear that her level of psychosocial dysfunction went beyond her alcohol problem, with her degree of fear and dysphoria making him consider the possible necessity of a short-term psychiatric hospitalization. I was called for consultation.

Entering my colleague's office, I saw a timid, somewhat beaten-down-looking woman. The psychologist began to "present" the "case" to me, but I quickly interrupted him and asked the patient why she was there. She hesitated—and I had to ask the other psychologist not to talk for her—and then somewhat haltingly at first, but with increased fluency, she told her story with some prompting. "I can't do anything right, at least that's what Jim says, and he took the kids," she cried. With lots of active questioning and supportive listening, we soon learned that she felt "stupid," that she had been working as a clerk, and that she desperately wanted to see her kids (ages 8 and 2). Careful questioning revealed no psychotic thinking and no suicidal ideas, impulses, or history.

I told her that I didn't know yet what would happen with her and the kids, but "a first step will involve you and your husband. Obviously, you've been having lots of troubles—maybe we can help you there. Has he said anything about counseling?" She responded: "He said he was leaving until I get help. He said he doesn't want a divorce, but he's had it with all the hassling and the kids running all over me and me being so upset." I then asked where her husband was right then. "Probably at his sister's, with the kids." With her permission, I called the sister. Jim wasn't in, but the sister offered to phone Jim at work and have him call me. About 10 minutes later, Jim called. I told him: "Sue is here. She's pretty stressed out, but she's OK, and she wants help getting things back together. Are you interested in counseling to help your marriage and your family? I have an appointment open in 2 days, at 6 P.M. Do you want it, for you and Sue?"

He accepted the appointment. Sue asked if he would bring the kids over later that day, and he agreed to.

Sue also asked if she could have "something to help me sleep—I've hardly slept for several days." The on-call psychiatrist was called in, evaluated her, and prescribed two nights worth of sleep medicine, enough to last until our conjoint appointment.

We then asked Sue's parents, who were in the waiting room, to join us. Her father appeared a bit gruff and her mother somewhat anxiously overprotective, although they were both genuinely concerned and distressed by the crisis in the family and the obvious unhappiness of their daughter. I explained to them, with Sue listening, that we had carefully evaluated the situation and had several recommendations: (1) Sue, while "unhappy and demoralized," did not need to be "locked up" in a psychiatric hospital; (2) Sue had agreed to stop all alcohol use and would be following up in our Chemical Dependency Program the next week; and (3) I had spoken with Sue's husband, and she and Jim would be coming in for marital counseling beginning in 2 days. I conveyed to all present my belief that there was some hard work ahead, and that with everyone's effort we would see what could be done. The parents were relieved, promised to be very available especially during the next few days, and offered a little homily about "everyone having problems," and how sure they were that Sue and Jim could, with counseling, "be as happy as they used to be." I had Sue repeat the plan, reinforced the importance of both her and Jim attending the upcoming session, and reminded her that she could come or call back sooner as needed. They left.

Two days later Sue and Jim were sitting in the waiting room at the appointed hour. Once in my office, I asked Jim what his understanding was about why they were there. He started by saying it was "to learn how to get along better," but he soon refocused his energy on describing his wife's faults. She began to sink visibly. I halted the discussion, noted that "when you point a finger at someone, there are three pointing back at you," and asked him to talk about his role in the problems they had. He acknowledged his being a "perfectionist" and "getting real upset and angry" and asked several specific questions (mostly for his wife's edification) about how to manage the kids, set limits, etc. Sue entered into the discussion and said that she didn't try to do much disciplining with the kids anymore "because no matter what I do, it isn't good enough, and Jim tells me so right in front of them." This led us into a discussion of what professionals might call "systemic logic" or "circular causality": "So you're saying that you don't stand up to the kids and then Jim criticizes you and they see they don't have to respect you and so they act worse and then Jim gets mad and you feel bad and do even less and then the kids walk over you and Jim blows his top and undermines you and the madder Jim gets the sadder you get and the badder the kids get, and around and around it goes, right? What are you going to do?" Their mouths dropped open; they stopped arguing and looked at each other. Jim, to Sue: "He's right. It sounds like he's been watching in our house!" Sue, to Jim: "We both need to stop it!" Jim, to me: "We'd like help, but we've been doing this so long I'm not sure we can really change. Can we?" Me, to them: "It is a mess, but if you're both serious and really willing to learn and do something different, there's hope. I've seen bigger messes. I'd say there's more chance of you guys getting it together and growing up then there is, say, of the Communist Party getting thrown out of Russia!" They both seemed to "get it" (fortunately) and laughed.

Follow-Up

This launched us into the nuts-and-bolts work of helping them to improve their communication and parenting, with both needing to strengthen certain skills and make considerable changes. This process has not been without its challenges and difficulties, with Jim struggling to accept Sue and feel useful without being dominating or undermining and Sue learning to assert herself without collapsing or self-sabotage. Both have been hopeful and well motivated, however, and good movement toward their goals has been achieved.

This is a "work in progress." We have had several conjoint sessions, with an agreement to meet eight times and then reevaluate. The approach has been truly "eclectic," including psychoeducational enhancement of parenting skills, communication training, some family-of-origin work, lots of cognitive/behavioral emphasis, a dip here and there into the psychodynamics of warded-off guilt and anger, some support and friendly confrontation. Sue completed her Chemical Dependency Program and has abstained from alcohol. She is on a waiting list for a time-limited 12-session Women's Therapy Group (which usually has themes of assertiveness and avoiding codependency), and Jim is considering a possible referral to a Men's Therapy Group. Our conjoint sessions were initially held weekly; we continue to meet, now every 3 weeks.

Comments

This episode, while not yet completed, illustrates some of the strengths of a comprehensive and integrated full-service HMO mental-health program, including individual, group, and marital/family therapy as well as chemical dependency treatment, psychopharmacology options, and appropriate inpatient services when indicated. It is important to note that such synergistically interdigitated arrangements are usually much more available in a staff or group model HMO, where clinicians are centrally located and cooperatively aligned, whereas clinicians in IPA- or PPO-style arrangements tend to be more scattered geographically and are more likely to operate in a traditional one-on-one private practice model (Austad & Hoyt, 1992; Bennett, 1988; Hoyt, in press; Hoyt & Austad, 1992).

A number of technical points may be noted. Rapid (and accurate) assessment identified individual and family resources that indicated Sue could be maintained as an outpatient through the family crisis (see Pittman et al., 1990). Indeed, hospitalization would have further invalidated her: Her self-image ("stupid") and her husband's view of her ("incompetent") might not have recovered from the stigma of psychiatric hospitalization. Following the suggestion of Budman and Gurman (1988, p. 252) that "rather than emphasizing, for example, the depression and anxiety experienced by those dealing with strained relationships, it is the nature of the relationships *themselves* that is examined," the initially identified patient's problems were construed as interpersonal, and she and her husband were seen together for marital/family therapy.[5]

[5]This case is somewhat reminiscent of one reported by Boaz (1988, pp. 36–39) of a woman who went to her HMO with symptoms of "agoraphobia" that were treated successfully with marital therapy and parenting classes to resolve the primary areas of her stress and conflict.

For therapy to be as efficient ("brief") as possible for the Smith family, multiple interventions have been used concurrently to impact several interrelated problems. This is consistent with the idea of Budman and Gurman (1988, p. 6) that treatment be "time sensitive" and rationed in a manner likely to "achieve maximum benefit with the lowest investment of therapist time and patient cost, both financial and psychological." In the case presented here, the effort has been first to stabilize and support and then to engage Sue and Jim in experiences that would help them cope more skillfully and successfully with their problems in living. From initial contact, the approach has been to respond quickly to avoid further regression, to set clearly defined goals and engage in specific problem solving, and to foster the patients' sense of hope, competency, and responsibility for the course and "outcome" of their therapy (and lives).

CONCLUDING REMARKS: TOWARD THE FUTURE

The two cases presented here illustrate some of the methods and principles of psychotherapy in HMO settings. There is no single approach, method, or theoretical school of therapy that is appropriate for all situations. To be effective and efficient, the good HMO therapist needs a variety of perspectives and skills, with the search being for a conceptualization that will allow a viable and parsimonious solution. The therapist needs to be versatile, innovative, and pragmatic, asking "What will help this patient today? Nothing works all the time, but what might work this time?" (Hoyt et al., 1992).

The demand for brief therapy is growing everywhere, not just within HMOs and managed care settings (Austad & Berman, 1991; Austad & Hoyt, 1992; Bloom, 1992; Budman et al., 1992; Wells & Giannetti, 1990; Zeig & Gilligan, 1990). Society is responding to both tremendous economic pressures and to advances in treatment methodologies. With the rapid and continuing expansion of the managed care movement, we can expect HMOs to increasingly serve as areas for brief therapy training (Hoyt, 1991), research, and development.

ACKNOWLEDGMENT

Support for this project was partially provided by the Sidney Garfield Memorial Fund, administered by the Kaiser Foundation Research Institute. The opinions expressed here are those of the author and do not necessarily reflect any policies of Kaiser-Permanente.

References

Austad, C. S., & Berman, W. H. (Eds.). (1991). *Psychotherapy in managed health care: The optimal use of time and resources*. Washington, DC: American Psychological Association.

Austad, C. S., & Hoyt, M. F. (1992). The managed care movement and the future of psychotherapy. *Psychotherapy, 29*, 109–118.

Austad, C. S., DeStefano, L., & Kisch, J. (1988). The health maintenance organization—II. Implications for psychotherapy. *Psychotherapy, 25*, 449–454.

Bennett, M. J. (1988). The greening of the HMO: Implications for prepaid psychiatry. *The American Journal of Psychiatry, 145*, 1544–1549.

Bloom, B. L. (1992). *Planned short-term psychotherapy*. Boston: Allyn & Bacon.

Boaz, J. T. (1988). *Delivering mental healthcare: A guide for HMOs*. Chicago: Pluribus Press.

Budman, S. H., & Gurman, A. S. (1988). *Theory and practice of brief psychotherapy*. New York: Guilford Press.

Budman, S. H., Hoyt, M. F., & Friedman, S. (Eds.). (1992). *The first session in brief therapy*. New York: Guilford Press.

Chestnut, W. J., Wilson, S., Wright, R. H., & Zemlich, M. J. (1987). Problems, protests, and proposals. *Professional Psychology, 18*, 107–112.

Cummings, N. A. (1986). The dismantling of our health system: Strategies for the survival of psychological practice. *American Psychologist, 41*, 426–431.

Cummings, N. A. (1990). Brief intermittent therapy throughout the life cycle. In J. K. Zeig & S. G. Gilligan (Eds.), *Brief therapy: Myths, methods and metaphors* (pp. 169–184). New York: Brunner/Mazel.

Erickson, M. H., & Rossi, E. L. (1979). *Hypnotherapy: An exploratory casebook*. New York: Irvington Publishers.

Feldman, J. L., & Fitzpatrick, R. J. (Eds.). (1992). *Managed mental health care: Administrative and clinical issues*. Washington, DC: American Psychiatric Press.

Goldman, W. (1988). Mental health and substance abuse services in HMOs. *Administration in Mental Health, 15*, 189–200.

Gustafson, J. P. (1986). *The complex secret of brief psychotherapy*. New York Norton.

Hoyt, M. F. (1985). Therapist resistances to short-term dynamic psychotherapy. *Journal of the American Academy of Psychoanalysis, 13*, 93–112.

Hoyt, M. F. (1989). Psychodiagnosis of personality disorders. *Transactional Analysis Journal, 19*, 101–113.

Hoyt, M. F. (1990). On time in brief therapy. In R. A. Wells & V. J. Giannetti (Eds.), *Handbook of the brief psychotherapies* (pp. 115–143). New York: Plenum Press.

Hoyt, M. F. (1991). Teaching and learning short-term therapy within an HMO. In C. S. Austad & W. H. Berman (Eds.), *Psychotherapy in managed health care: The optimal use of time and resource* (pp. 98–107). Washington, DC: American Psychological Association.

Hoyt, M. F. (in press). Group psychotherapy in an HMO. *HMO Practice*.

Hoyt, M. F., & Austad, C. S. (1992). Psychotherapy in a staff-model health maintenance organization: Providing and assuring quality care in the future. *Psychotherapy, 29*, 119–129.

Hoyt, M. F., Rosenbaum, R., & Talmon, M. (1992). Planned single-session psychotherapy. In S. H. Budman, M. F. Hoyt, & S. Friedman (Eds.), *The first session in brief therapy* (pp. 59–86). New York: Guilford Press.

Peet, B. (1972). *The ant and the elephant*. Boston: Houghton Mifflin Company.

Pittman, F. S., III, Flomenhaft, K., & DeYoung, C. D. (1990). In R. A. Wells & V. J. Giannetti (Eds.), Family crisis-therapy. *Handbook of the brief psychotherapies* (pp. 297–324). New York: Plenum Press.

Rosenbaum, R. (1990). Strategic psychotherapy. In R. A. Wells & V. J. Giannetti (Eds.), *Handbook of the brief psychotherapies* (pp. 351–403). New York: Plenum Press.

Rosenbaum, R. (1993). Heavy ideals: Strategic single-session hypnotherapy. In R. A. Wells & V. J. Giannetti (Eds.), *Casebook of the brief psychotherapies* (pp. 109–128). New York: Plenum Press.

Rosenbaum, R., Hoyt, M. F., & Talmon, M. (1990). The challenge of single-session therapies: Creating pivotal moments. In R. A. Wells & V. J. Giannetti (Eds.), *Handbook of the brief psychotherapies* (pp. 165–189). New York: Plenum Press.

Sullivan, H. S. (1954). *The psychiatric interview.* New York: Norton.

Talmon, M. (1990). *Single session therapy: Maximizing the effect of the first (and often the only) therapeutic encounter.* San Francisco: Jossey-Bass.

Wells, R. A., & Giannetti, V. J. (Eds.). (1990). *Handbook of the brief psychotherapies.* New York: Plenum Press.

White, M., & Epston, D. (1990). *Narrative means to therapeutic ends.* New York: Norton.

Zeig, J. K., & Gilligan, S. G. (Eds.). (1990). *Brief therapy: Myths, methods, and metaphors.* New York: Brunner/Mazel.

Zimmet, C. N. (1989). The mental health care revolution: Will psychology survive? *American Psychologist, 44,* 703–708.

16

She'll Cook It Herself

Brief Family Therapy with an Elderly Couple

WILLIAM I. COHEN AND KATHLEEN REED

INTRODUCTION

The Brief Therapy Center model of the Mental Research Institute (MRI) proposes a bare bones theory of change. In contrast to a psychodynamic framework, which constructs problems based on unsolved issues from the past, this model proposes that the distress people experience in their lives results from the current interaction between the problem they are trying to solve and the solutions they choose—solutions that inadvertently maintain the problem. Therefore, a therapist, wishing to interrupt this recursive pattern, devises an intervention that stops the attempted problem solving by substituting a different behavior that breaks the pattern. Most novices using this model find it relatively easy to describe an intervention that is likely to interrupt the ever-escalating cycle. The challenges arise in presenting the task to the family in such a way as to induce them to engage in this new behavior.

This model has been extensively described in the literature (Fisch et al., 1982; Keeney & Ross, 1985), and its roots trace back to the contact between MRI and Milton Erickson, the gifted psychiatrist and hypno-

---

WILLIAM I. COHEN • Child Development Unit, Children's Hospital of Pittsburgh, 3705 Fifth Avenue, Pittsburgh, Pennsylvania 15213. KATHLEEN REED • Pittsburgh Action Against Rape, 81 South 19th Street, Pittsburgh, Pennsylvania 15203.

Casebook of the Brief Psychotherapies, edited by Richard A. Wells and Vincent J. Giannetti. Plenum Press, New York, 1993.

therapist. As described in *Change,* Watzlawick and his coauthors were struck by the way in which Erickson was able to influence his clients to undertake some unusual behaviors in order to achieve their goal (Watzlawick et al., 1974). At the same time this team was absorbing Erickson's ideas, the evolving work of Gregory Bateson provided another framework for understanding human problems. He observed that the therapist and family joined to form a new system (Hoffman, 1981, p. 5). By questioning the family system, the therapist forms hypotheses about its structure and function and generates an intervention that is presented to the family. This intervention can be thought of as new information introduced into the system. The family's response confirms or discredits the hypothesis thereby leading to a new hypothesis, which is tested with a new intervention. Haley has remarked (personal communication) that the therapist only understands the case when it is finished. This contrasts dramatically with the standard psychiatric practice of a short diagnostic phase of treatment preceding a lengthy treatment phase. For the brief therapist, the initial 'diagnosis' is merely a description of how the system appears to be stuck.

CASE IDENTIFICATION AND PRESENTING COMPLAINT

Ms. A. was a 75-year-old married white woman who was admitted to an inpatient geriatric psychiatry unit for evaluation of her inability to swallow solid foods. Her eating difficulty began 9 years prior to this admission. At that time, 6 months after her retirement, she went to the kitchen to get a glass of milk at 3:00 A.M. Unknown to her at the time, burglars were in her basement. Following this incident, Mrs. A. became "nervous" and reportedly did not want to leave her house. Six months later, there was another burglary. It was following this second burglary that Mrs. A. first had trouble eating. This inability to eat was accompanied by her withdrawal from most family members and staying in bed. At times, she expressed the belief that her son had killed someone. On other occasions, she was reported to hallucinate situations from her childhood.

Within 2 years of the beginning of these problems, Mrs. A.'s family sought professional treatment. She had three psychiatric inpatient admissions where she was treated for psychotic depression. However, she did not comply with tricyclic antidepressant and neuroleptic treatment as an outpatient. Four years prior to the current and fourth psychiatric admission, she had a medical admission where she was diagnosed with gall bladder problems and anorexia. She weighed 80 lb. and a gastrostomy tube was inserted. She was discharged to a nursing home and, for financial reasons, 7 months later was transferred to another long-term care facility located 45 minutes from her family. She remained in this facility for the 2 years prior to her current hospital admission. During the most recent placement, she did increase her ability to perform self-care, and the gastrostomy tube was removed. Her diet consisted primarily of ice cream and milk. Although she claimed to be unable to swallow solid food, candy wrappers were found in her room. Her weight was fairly stable at 78 lb.

During the 2 years at the long-term care facility, she made frequent phone calls to her husband, pleading that he take her home. Both Mrs. A. and her husband of 43 years were unhappy with her living in a nursing home. The oldest son, Henry, was responsible for providing his father with transportation. They frequently made the 90-minute round-trip drive to bring Mrs. A. home for overnight visits, adding 200 miles to the son's weekly driving. Mr. A. had chronic, moderately severe health problems, and Henry was concerned that his mother's demands were killing his father. During the home visits, Mrs. A. would typically refuse to eat the meals her husband prepared and often insisted that the food in the refrigerator was poisoned. Frequently, she threw out fresh food.

Within the first week of admission to the geriatric psychiatric unit, a medical evaluation was completed that included geriatric medicine, dietary, neurology, and orthopedics assessments. Mrs. A. was unable to walk independently and generally ambulated in a wheelchair. There were no medical problems identified that could account for Mrs. A.'s complaint that she was unable to swallow solid foods. An extensive occupational therapy evaluation was ordered to assess Mrs. A.'s ability to perform activities of daily living in her house. The treatment team on the unit consisted of the attending psychiatrist, resident psychiatrist, primary nurse, physician assistant, occupational therapist, and social worker (KR), who was the primary clinician. Other ancillary services were available by consultation from the University Medical Center. Shortly thereafter, the treatment team decided to consult with a strategic family therapist (WIC) in order to develop strategies for family intervention.

Background Information

Mrs. A. completed the twelfth grade and married at the age of 32. She had two sons, and early in her marriage, she went to work as a secretary for two elementary-school principals. Her husband, who worked the evening shift as a stationary engineer, was primarily responsible for raising the children with the help of the grandparents. Mrs. A. worked for 33 years, retiring at the age of 65. Although she liked working, there were several conflicts during the last few years of her career, so that she was glad to retire.

Both sons became secondary-school teachers and were married with children. The oldest son was in daily contact with his father, whereas the younger son was quite distant in his relationship with his parents.

Mr. A., who was 73 years old, was involved in a serious automobile accident 2 years prior to Mrs. A.'s current admission. Although he spent 2 months in the trauma unit of a teaching hospital, he had a good recovery. His only major restriction of activity was that he could not drive a car.

THE HYPOTHESIS

On October 1, 1984, 6 days after Mrs. A. was admitted, the strategic family therapist met with the staff at a team meeting and learned in detail about the problems that the family had been experiencing. His role would be to find an intervention that would break the cycle.

In reviewing the history, we decoded a number of patterns. First of all, Mr. A.'s intense preoccupation with his wife's eating was not matched by a corresponding interest on her part. In fact, her interest appeared to be inversely related to his. His insistence that the food was not tainted led her to believe even more strongly that something was wrong. Mr. A.'s stubborn insistence on not throwing out food seems to have been met by Mrs. A.'s insistence that it had to go. As Mrs. A. refused to eat, she would lose weight, and then, after much threatening, she was sent to the nursing home. However, at the nursing home she had been able to maintain her weight for reasons that were not readily apparent.

Another pattern was the cycle of movement from the family home to the nursing home and back again. Mrs. A. would call up and cry about how miserable she was. When Mr. A. was unable to tolerate her unhappiness any longer, his son would drive out to pick her up. Once she arrived home, the eating battles would begin, and because they had no other way to deal with this problem, she would often end up again in the nursing home.

The attempted solution of demanding that she eat, threatening her with going back to the nursing home, and reassuring her that the food was not tainted ironically led to a refusal to eat. Mr. A. was taking full responsibility for her health and well-being. Her only autonomous response could be to refuse him, which inadvertently led to the disasters recounted above. Our goal would be to remove Mr. A. and Henry from the loop and allow Mrs. A. to take full responsibility for her eating. Mr. A. showed his love when he prepared food and sought to care for his wife. However, their fights were anything but loving. We would seek to allow him to show his caring in a different way. Having analyzed the recurrent pattern, the family therapist knew that his intervention needed to prevent Mr. A. from taking responsibility for his wife's eating because no one can successfully take control of another person's physiological processes, be they eating, or sleeping, or sexual.

The Interview

The family therapist had only one interview with the family, 4 days after he met with the team. Initially, he met with Mrs. A. alone for about 5 minutes and then invited Mr. A. and Henry to join the session. Also present were the primary nurse, the resident psychiatrist, and the social worker. Because all the diagnostic information had been gathered by the inpatient treatment team prior to the consultation, the family therapist used the interview to set the stage for the intervention that was to follow.

The family therapist told the group that Mrs. A. was the only one who knew what she could eat. He knew that families look to outside consultants for dramatic improvement, as unlikely as that might be. In order to lower their expectations and respect the innate desire for stability, he predicted that her eating and weight problems were not going to get much better. Nevertheless, the next statement made was that the team thought that they could make things a lot better. "The weight of my experience makes this clear to me," he said, injecting a hopeful note and an embedded metaphor. This related to the team's belief that the family's emotional well-being could improve dramatically, with Mrs. A. living at home and maintaining a stable weight. In order to accomplish these goals, it was also necessary to address Henry's role in the recursive pattern. Therefore, the team expressed appreciation for the important job that Henry had been doing in driving his mother back and forth to the nursing home. However, in order to change the situation, Henry was about to be fired from the job.

The health care team's short-term priorities were to assure that Mrs. A.'s health issues were no longer to be the responsibility of the family: If she did not eat, she would go back to the nursing facility. Her husband would no longer be involved in cajoling and coaxing her to eat. The central dilemma of this case was focused on blocking her husband from encouraging her to eat because this was the way he showed his loving and caring.

During the interview, Mr. A.'s distress was as noteworthy as Mrs. A.'s boredom. There was no evidence of any delusional thinking on Mrs. A.'s part. The family therapist joined with Mr. A.'s distress and caring about his wife, and Mr. A. agreed to do something different in order to help her. The interview lasted 30 minutes and closed with an appointment for a subsequent family meeting 5 days hence. The family therapist was to be present to clarify the details.

After the meeting, the social worker went back into the room to set up the next meeting with Mr. and Mrs. A. She found the son to be very angry with the family therapist's intervention. The social worker quickly aligned with the son on a feeling level, responding that experts can be wrong. By relying on the strong premise that the son cared very deeply for his father, the social worker gained the support of the son by continuing to frame the request for the son's disengagement as a way to care for and support his father.

TREATMENT

The family therapist did not attend the next meeting. Having consulted with the social worker by telephone, it was decided that his presence was not needed to proceed with the intervention. Several points were negotiated with Mrs. A. and Mr. A. regarding transportation and Mrs. A.'s food. A local senior citizens transportation service would be used in place of the son's driving. The application form was completed during this meeting. Regarding food, Mrs. A. and Mr. A. agreed that they would keep separate food in their home. Mrs. A. would have a specific shelf in the refrigerator, and although she could decide when to throw out her own food, she could not touch her husband's food. Mrs. A. agreed to write a list each day for the food she wanted. Mr. A. agreed to make a trip to the grocery store each day and would only buy the food that she requested for that day. Mrs. A. also agreed to begin working with a dietitian during the remainder of the hospitalization to choose her own foods. She also agreed to work with the occupational therapist to see what foods she could prepare for herself.

The next day, the dietitian suggested that Mrs. A. try baby foods, and the following day Mrs. A. received nutritional counseling. On the third day, the nursing staff changed their strategy regarding a nutritional supplement between meals. Instead of automatically providing it, she was to request it as desired. That same day, the social worker held a meeting with Mr. A. and Mrs. A. Mr. A. agreed to purchase a selection of baby foods within 3 days so that Mrs. A. could work with the occupational therapist to prepare a meal. Preliminary plans were made for a pass home to see if Mrs. A. could prepare a meal for herself at home. A discussion began regarding a maintenance range for Mrs. A.'s weight following discharge.

Three days later, Mrs. A. prepared her first meal in the hospital. The only difficulty she experienced occurred when attempting to remove the lid of the jar of baby food. The following day she prepared another meal with further occupational therapy evaluation. At the suggestion of the resident psychiatrist, Mrs. A. agreed to continue preparing all her meals while she remained in the hospital. Within 4 days, she made a visit home and prepared two meals there without difficulty. In the family meeting 2 days later, Mr. A. voiced his surprise and pleasure that Mrs. A. had done so well.

At the time Mrs. A. began preparing her own meals in the hospital, the social worker placed an initial call to the mental health center that would be responsible for providing follow-up care. The follow-up care was limited to weighing Mrs. A. If her weight fell below the acceptable cutoff, they would then call the nursing home and request that she be placed on the waiting list for admission. The inpatient social worker explained that there was a behavioral contract being developed that Mrs. A. and Mr. A. would be using for their discharge plan. A copy of that contract was promised to the mental health center along with another phone call from the social worker closer to the day of discharge, in order to make final plans for outpatient follow-up.

CLINICAL ISSUES

A distinguishing feature of this treatment model is utilization of Mrs. A.'s belief that her food was poisoned. Standard psychiatric practice might well choose to focus on this delusional system and perhaps attempt to dissuade her from this idea. Her husband's seemingly benevolent attempts to help might be explained, so that she could come to allow him to prepare her food and look out for her best interests. In distinction, we constructed an intervention that respected her beliefs and placed her alone in charge of food preparation.

The Brief Therapy Center model identifies the complainant in the system and seeks to intervene primarily, if not solely, with this person because that individual has the greatest energy for change. Mrs. A. was the identified patient but hardly a complainant. Mr. A. and his son were both complainants, and therefore, the interventions were designed to interrupt their behaviors, even though they surely expected the clinicians to focus on their wife and mother.

The most important factors that led to success in this case involved building in the support structures to insure the shifts in responsibility that were prescribed. This occurred when the outpatient mental health center was actively involved in the unusual follow-up. Their task was limited to weighing the patient at biweekly intervals and contacting the nursing home for readmission if her weight fell below 78 lb. The outpatient therapist was also expected to work with the couple if other relationship problems were identified as interfering with their daily lives. The local senior citizens' organization was also contacted to provide inhome assessment and ongoing transportation services.

The team's intervention gave Mrs. A. total responsibility for where she lived. The function of monitoring her weight was transferred from the family to the outpatient mental health center, which, theoretically, had little interest in the outcome of the weighing. Because Mrs. A. had demonstrated in the hospital her ability to eat a variety of foods that would maintain her weight, we were confident that she would be able to take care of her dietary needs. The consequence of her weight loss was made clear, but without threats: it was simply a statement of fact.

As the case moved toward closure, we discovered that we had failed to attend to a very important issue in this case, the role of psychiatry in a psychiatric hospitalization. Most geriatric patients who are hospitalized are frequently treated with psychotropic medications. Indeed, the psychiatrist suggested a trial of neuroleptic medication, but because of Mrs. A.'s refusal and pattern of previous noncompliance, psychopharmacological treatment was not pursued. The obvious interactional nature of the problem led to the early involvement of the family therapy consultant. At this point, there appeared to be no place for the central involvement of the psychiatrist. The major therapeutic modalities included occupational therapy, which assured that Mrs. A. was able to prepare her own meals, and the family therapy that blocked the family's attempted solutions that had failed. This systemic error, which did not affect the outcome of this case, had significant subsequent consequences. The resident psychiatrist assigned to the case made the offhanded remark to the attending physician that psychiatry was not needed at all: just simply occupational therapy and social work. We failed to find a way to make this intervention palatable or creditable to the attending physician and neglected to include her as an active participant in the case. Subsequently, the attending physician refused to involve the family therapy consultant in any future cases.

TERMINATION

The transition from inpatient treatment to outpatient follow-up was initiated when the social worker had both Mrs. A. and Mr. A. sign the behavioral contract outlining each of their responsibilities regarding Mrs. A.'s eating behavior and weight maintenance. Copies of this contract were given to each of them, and an additional copy was sent to the follow-up therapist at the mental health center. Additionally, the initial appointment for Mrs. A.'s weigh-in at the mental health center was scheduled.

In a phone conversation held 6 months later between the social worker and the outpatient therapist, it was learned that Mrs. A. was still living at home and had been keeping her weight within the contracted acceptable range. There were no further attempts to attain ongoing post-treatment evaluation data. Given the nature of the presenting problem, however, it is evident that the strategic family therapy interventions were successful in interrupting the family patterns so that the goals identified by the husband and son, and agreed to by Mrs. A. could be achieved: living in her home and maintaining an acceptable weight.

OVERALL EVALUATION

The authors believe that the successful outcome was directly related to the fit between the model used and the particular circumstances of the case. Because Mrs. A. did not meet DSM-III diagnostic criteria for either psychotic depression or anorexia, the team was seeking alternative treatment. It was easy to identify the recurring pattern that needed to be interrupted, and we were fortunate enough to come up with an intervention that used the outpatient resources in a way that maintained the desired change.

The more a patient's symptoms fit standard psychiatric diagnoses, it is understandable that standard psychiatric therapies, such as psychopharmacologic agents, electroconvulsive therapy, group and individual psychotherapies, are more likely to be employed, whether or not they achieve the desired goal of treatment. Psychiatry faces the challenge of incorporating the contextual understanding of human dilemmas into its standard frames of reference. The rapid attainment of the patient's and family's goals attest to the value of including systemic thinking in developing treatment strategies.

REFERENCES

Hoffman, L. (1981). *Foundation of family therapy.* New York: Basic Books.
Fisch, R., Weakland, J., & Segal, L. (1982). *The tactics of change.* San Francisco: Jossey-Bass.
Keeney, B., & Ross, J. (1985). *Mind in therapy.* New York: Basic Books.
Watzlawick, P., Weakland, J., & Fisch, R. (1974). *Change.* New York: Norton.

17

A Brief Family Therapy Model for Child Guidance Clinics

Daniel J. Hurley and Stuart G. Fisher

Introduction

When the first child guidance clinics were founded in the United States, they were primarily devoted to diagnosis and short-term interventions (Parad, 1971). Under the influence of psychoanalytic theory, these clinics were gradually transformed into providers of long-term individual therapy for both children and parents (Witmer, 1946). With few exceptions, it was not until the 1960s that we saw widespread experimentation with brief therapy in child guidance clinics (Fisher, 1978). The idea of brief treatment has found greater acceptance among family therapists than among other therapists. So, it is perhaps no coincidence that this rising popularity of brief therapy has been accompanied by phenomenal growth in the use of family therapy in child mental health settings.

Even more radical changes in public mental health are being precipitated by reduced government funding and an increasing reliance on third-party reimbursements with limited outpatient coverage. Clinics are being forced to limit the amount of treatment provided at the very time that cases are becoming more complicated, characterized by signifi-

Daniel J. Hurley and Stuart G. Fisher • Worcester Youth Guidance Center, 275 Belmont Avenue, Worcester, Massachusetts 01609.

Casebook of the Brief Psychotherapies, edited by Richard A. Wells and Vincent J. Giannetti. Plenum Press, New York, 1993.

cant issues of protective care and substance abuse. In order to stay afloat, child guidance clinics are demanding higher levels of productivity from their staff, while asking them to treat extremely difficult and emotionally demanding cases.

The treatment model described here has as its goal making treatment maximally effective within a brief time by improving the initial assessment and case planning and by providing collegial support and guidance to the treatment of one family. The therapeutic model integrates Family Systems theory with Object Relations family theory (Scharff & Scharff, 1987). The treatment program began with a Milan Systemic orientation (Tomm, 1984) and has drawn on constructs from the Structural, Strategic, and Bowenian approaches. More recently, we have become interested in the relationship between intrapsychic and family systems levels of analysis. The Wachtels' (1986) notion of "cyclical psychodynamics" and the Object Relations concept of "projective identification" have helped us to think about the way that the dynamics of individual family members weave together to maintain the relationship patterns of the family system. We have also found it useful to focus on the "holding capacity" (Scharff & Scharff, 1987) of families, the ability of family members to empathize with, care for, and support each other.

Based on this theoretical framework, the treatment model involves a time-limited initial phase of assessment/therapy: four family sessions, each of 1½-hour length, held every 2 weeks. These sessions are conducted by a family therapist assisted by a team of one or more clinicians. In the case presented here, the team observed behind a one-way mirror and periodically communicated with the therapist by telephone. The team provides at least one other vantage point (more frequently, two competing theses) from which to understand the family's problems and strengths. The team can also help the therapist to intervene quickly, keep focused, and set in motion some therapeutic change. We consider this crucial for any effective brief treatment of the complicated problems of the families that often present themselves at child guidance clinics.

Following this first phase of the intervention, a decision is made in the fourth session with the family what the next step in treatment should be. One direction is to stop treatment. In this case, the problems for which the family sought treatment have improved sufficiently so that the team and the family are comfortable with the family trying on their own for awhile. It is important to note that our model assumes that the great majority of families will return at some point. This framework is consistent with other models of brief intermittent treatment (Cummings, 1986) in which families may have several episodes of brief treatment over a period of years. Thus *termination* is viewed as a pause or practice/implementation period, rather than an end point.

The second option after four sessions is follow-up monitoring. The family continues to be seen for a period of 3 to 12 months by a member of the original treatment team with the team available for consultation. The goal is to provide continuity and support for maintaining the work that the family has begun. We prefer follow-up with those families in which the members seem to have insufficient confidence that the positive changes will be durable. These families have difficulty attributing therapeutic changes to their own efforts, but rather to the team's efforts or to luck. A major goal of follow-up is to empower the family to continue to recognize and rely on their own strengths. The case described here followed this course.

The third option is a recommendation to engage in long-term treatment for the family, the marriage, or individual members in the appropriate teams in the guidance clinic. These teams all have access to the team's process notes and videotapes, as well as the availability of the team for a consultation. Generally, the families that follow this treatment course are ones in which the team has not seen evidence of the capacity to provide the basic essentials of a safe and nurturing holding capacity for the children.

CASE IDENTIFICATION AND PRESENTING COMPLAINT

The client family selected for discussion in this chapter is a family of four members: father (30 years old), mother (30 years old), brother (10 years old), and sister (7 years old). The family lives together in a small, older house that they own in a white, working-class, urban neighborhood. The father is employed full time as a day-shift plant worker at a large manufacturing plant in a nearby town. The mother works a part-time (30 hours per week) evening shift as an aide in a special education program for children. The parents had been married for almost 11 years at the time treatment began, with no separations in what is the first marriage for both partners. The parents reported that there were no significant financial problems. The children both attend the local public school, where the brother is in fifth grade and the sister in second grade. Neither child is involved in special school programming. Parents report that their daughter is more successfully involved with friends and activities. Their son has only one friend (whom they dislike) but mostly stays home.

The intake interview was conducted by a staff psychologist with all of the family members participating in the session. The clinician's report defined the family's presentation of problems as a "seemingly isolated pattern of severe combative relationship between the children, with brother as 'aggressor.'" Parents criticized the son for name calling and "unprovoked" hitting of sister. Parents described concern about community acts of "vandalism" (e.g., throwing rocks at cars and at neighbor's van) and about an incident in which son threatened to kill himself by holding a knife to his throat.

The referral of this family originated with the Department of Social Services (DSS). Approximately 1 month earlier, authorities at the son's school had filed a protective petition with DSS when they observed bruises on son's face. Upon questioning, son reported that he was slapped by his father. In the intake interview, father reported that son had become "mouthy" and oppositional when confronted about his misbehavior. This defiance provoked father to "smack" his son, leaving a "red mark" on his face. The parents expressed a desire for help for the family in dealing with their son and for individual therapy for the son. The only other service system involved at the time of intake was DSS. Parents noted that they had tried Parents Anonymous, but felt that they were very different from those parents and stopped attending. The intake record included the clinician's diagnostic formulation of the son as Oppositional Defiant Disorder (313.81), with questions about possible Attention Deficit Disorder and Conduct Disorder (Mild). The intake session concluded with parents contracting to engage in brief family therapy to be followed by a subsequent decision on the appropriate follow-up option to pursue.

BACKGROUND INFORMATION

In this treatment model, background information available to the therapy team prior to treatment is used in several ways: (1) to help formulate alternative working hypotheses in order to begin treatment with multiple perspectives on individual and family dynamics; (2) to highlight particular components in the family system (themes or processes) that will be sensitive processes or "hot spots"; and (3) to find existing dynamics in the client system that will serve as strengths upon which to build treatment interventions. In this case, the sources of information were the Clinic Intake Summary, the DSS assessment report, and a short telephone report from the principal of the son's school.

For this case, there were several alternative hypotheses contained in the record. The bulk of evidence located the problem within the individual child. Parents presented hitting of his sister as "unprovoked." His repeated conflict with her was presented as an "isolated" pattern. Consistent with this working hypothesis, parents blamed the son for any conflict and moved quickly and necessarily to protect the daughter and control/confront the son. First, the mother proposed that the attention sister received at birth after John had been "spoiled" for 3 years might be the problem. Mother had reported to DSS that her mother believed that the parents "favored" the daughter. Also, the DSS report contained one anomaly. In the medical history section, mother noted one serious injury to John, stitches from splitting his head open on the radiator when his sister pushed him. There was no report of such injuries to the daughter in the report or of her ever being hit. The mother's description of the son as "fine" other than hating his sister allowed for an alternative hypothesis: that there was something about this brother–sister dyadic interaction and its family context that might be maintaining the "problem." Finally, the reason for referral—father's hitting his son—offered the hypothesis of a family dynamic of intensely escalating aggressive interactions, not simply an individual problem.

In terms of highlighting sensitive dynamics, or "hot spots" in this family system, the background information indicated several warnings for potential difficulty or resistance in the upcoming treatment. One issue was mother's sensitivity to the critical evaluation of herself and her family by outsiders. The presenting complaint of son's hitting was described as an isolated dynamic, not only "in" the son, but not indicative of any other problems in the system ("otherwise, fine"). The mother had been sensitive to disclosing her place of employment and actually refused to do so in the intake interview. The team hypothesized that this action might have been motivated by the mother's embarrassment that a special education aide would be judged even more critically for having trouble with her son. Mother made a clear effort to describe her son as an "excellent" student, even providing standardized test results at the intake meeting. However, in the school principal's telephone report, he noted difficulties at school and the possible need for a core evaluation. This manner of reporting family information indicated that the treatment team would need to be sensitive to mother's perception of the team as devaluing or critically judging her or her family. A final signal to the team was mother's calling prior to the first meeting and asking to meet the observation team "before they made their judgments about us."

A second issue of note in the records was mother's disclosure very early in the intake session of her being physically abused by her brother throughout her childhood. The prominence of this report made the team attentive to the possible dynamics of (1) mother's identification with daughter and the projection onto her daughter of her own sense of victimization; (2) the need to quickly assess and then establish the safety and security of the daughter in this family; and (3) the need to establish alternatives to the explanation of son's behavior as hating his sister and wanting to hurt her. The third issue evident in the background information was the documentation of how little time and energy the parents have to work together to develop a supportive family environment. The records indicated that the father worked a full-time day shift and part-time carpentry jobs, and was renovating their house, while mother worked evenings. It would be a critical goal in treatment to focus on the parent's capacity to work together as a team to nurture the children and their marriage. The final issue highlighted in the archival data was the focus in the DSS evaluation on the family dynamic of control versus the individual developmental dynamics of this family's preadolescent. Parents made clear their dislike of son's choice of friends and employed extensive grounding not only to punish misbehavior, but also to keep son away from these bad influences. Father described to the DSS worker his need to escalate to "smacking" as provoked by son's increasing "mouthiness and independence." One product of the DSS evaluation was a contract containing nine (sure-to-fail) rules to be followed if the son wanted to live with the family. Included in the contract (signed by son) were such items as when at the table, just sit and eat; when told to do something, just do it the first time told; do not do anything to Becky, tell us; sit and keep mouth shut and listen when being spoken to; and so forth. It was clear that the treatment team would also have to quickly resolve this confrontation between the parents' need for and focus on control and son's developmental need for growing independence within the context of more secure, supportive attachments to his parents.

Consistent with its model, the team searched the available information for evidence of positive dynamics. In the DSS report, father described a major life event as his recent bonding with his estranged sister. Also, father reported that he had been in therapy to help with the death of his father, and had found it helpful. The team found both events as potentially helpful. The first dynamic might prove useful as a reference for the successful rapprochement of feuding brothers and sisters. The second piece of information showed capacity to work and trust the therapeutic process in at least one family member, as well as some historical success with the resolution of loss—a dynamic that would be tested again in son's growing independent.

TREATMENT PROCESS

First Session

There were three main goals to accomplish in the first meeting with the family: (1) to make the family comfortable with the team format and to understand their presenting problem; (2) to construct the family's hypothesis within an interactive, more systemic framework; and (3) to test alternative hypotheses generated from the background information. As the family entered the room, the parents told the children to sit down. The son lay down on the floor and began to play noisily with a truck. The daughter remained standing next to mother, quietly playing with her hair. The parents sat across from each other in the circle of chairs. At the request of the therapist to bring the team up to date, the father launched into a detailed description of son's noncompliant behaviors that had escalated into his hitting his son. He presented the parents' case that the school had overreacted, but that the DSS investigation was "fine." Maintaining the family's commitment to an "isolationist" thesis, father noted that 90% of the problem was son's treatment of his sister, and concluded, "other than that I have no complaints." Mother added quickly that she did not like the way that son treated her, either. Mother described feeling increasingly disempowered by her son's defiance, which she saw as increasing "since DSS and everyone else has been involved." Father indicated a level of deterioration to the point where son wanted to go to a foster home. Mother concluded with an emphatic, "I told him to go." When asked what the family wanted from the clinic, mother indicated individual therapy for son "to find out why he acts the way that he does."

Throughout this initial formulation of the problem, the therapist was committed to joining with the family in the parents' frustration, despair, and confusion. The therapist's first strategic move to construct an interactionist hypothesis came as the father noted that when his sister was not around, the son is "the greatest kid that you ever want to meet." The therapist turned to the daughter and asked how she had such a powerful effect: her mere presence there turning the "greatest kid" into a monster. Mother thwarted the reformulation with the defense that her daughter could be just sitting there, and her brother would go by and hit her. Mother continued with further evidence of son's noncompliance. In a second attempt to reframe, the therapist turned again to the daughter to ask about her not complying with parents' request to sit in the chair. As daughter made a face of scorn, mother protected her again with the statement that "she is good, though"—a process that highlighted for the team a protective mother–daughter alliance, perhaps a result of mother's projective identification with daughter. The therapist processed the different styles the two children had exhibited in not complying with the parents' command to sit down at the beginning of the session: one loud, one quiet. The therapist asked if this process was parallel to what might happen at home. Parents described spiraling conflict with their son: tell him "no" five or six times;

then, screaming and yelling back and forth between son and mother, then son and father (if home); then, son being sent to room; and finally, "nothing accomplished." Sister summarized the results, "He gets nothing, I get what I want."

When the therapist responded with sympathy for son's "losing" all the time, the team telephoned their directive—a third interactional redefinition of this process as one of engagement. The message was that this might not be a matter of losing, but of the son's engaging parents in an intense game or contest. The son agreed spiritedly, "I can take them all on." For the remainder of session, the family explored the dynamics of the family ritual that draws first sister, then mother, then father into intense engagement with the son.

Following the team discussion, the therapist met with the family and delivered the team's observations and homework assignment for the family. The assignment called for the mother to engage in the above contest once a day with their son, but with the parents clearly in control. The mother was instructed to play for four "moves" (e.g., son's refusal, mother's yelling or chasing, etc.), and then, the fifth move would be for mother to stop the game with a clear message to son (e.g., "knock it off!" or "your father and I will discuss this!"). The son was assigned the task of frustrating all four moves by mother, and then to stop. The team gave the parents the job of being judges. Should son not stop, parents were to sit down together and decide what the punishment would be. Father and son were given the task of thinking of other good games that they liked to play together.

Second Session

The goals in the second session were twofold: (1) to review the assignment within the context of parental control and family members engaging positively with each other; (2) to connect current family dynamics to mother's historical sensitivity to hitting from her family of origin; and (3) to begin to assess parents' capacity to establish a safe and nurturing holding environment.

Mother began immediately with a report on the family's success in doing the assignment. She related that over the 2 weeks since the first session, there had been only three instances of conflict. Even the duration of conflict decreased. Mother reported that when she played to a point (even laughing a couple of times as she did it), then declared "it's over," son stopped. Mother confessed that she was somewhat disappointed with this success because she "could not take away what I wanted." The therapist acted first quite pleased and complimentary, then became visibly perplexed, and finally dismayed. He expressed his sadness that (1) mother and son would no longer have a "game" to play together; (2) son might be sad with the loss of such an exciting, intense interaction that got his whole family involved together; and (3) this conflict ended so quickly that mother and father never got to work together. The therapist mused that, had the team known that the family would have been so successful, they might have held off the assignment. The son reminded the therapist—with a coy look—about the rest of the assignment. As assigned, father and son had come up with an exciting game: a 25-minute game of baseball.

Mother redirected the meeting to the fact that nothing had changed with son's treatment of his sister. This remark seemed to cue father to provide a detailed account of how he had seen the son causing trouble in the neighborhood. Both parents then began to document son's wrongdoings—one process that they seemed to do together. In the midst of this, father mentioned that son "knows that he will pay." The therapist focused on how son pays, in order to explore parents' ability to hold son accountable. Parents described a system whereby son pays for any damage that he causes from a savings account. The understanding and use of such a consequence system by the parents allowed the team to refocus on the attachment/relationship dynamics of this system.

The team intervened at this point with a directive to discuss the parents' two families of origin and how their families had found time to work and play. Mother started with a description of not having a father and of having a mother who was unavailable due to full-time work. Parenting was left to her older sister (who was "out a lot") and to her brother. This brother would beat her about once a day ("sit on me and keep pounding . . . not even stop when I cried"). The therapist asked the family to think about what this must have been like.

MOTHER: "I just see Uncle Fred (her brother) all over again when he (her son) hits his sister."

SON: "I'm not Uncle Fred."

THERAPIST: "Your mother feels the pain that Uncle Fred gave her."

MOTHER: "When he hits his sister, it brings back memories and feelings that I do not want to remember . . . as if I am getting hit."

THERAPIST (TO SON): "Do you understand what your mother is saying?"

SON: "When I hit her (his sister), I am hitting both of them."

MOTHER: "You can feel it. I can feel Uncle Fred hitting me."

After a long, silent pause, father took the initiative to establish the generational difference: their son does not hit his sister to the same extent as Uncle Fred, and their daughter has parents to help and protect her. It was clear that all of the family members had a much more sensitive context for relating to mother's reaction to hitting in this family.

The message from the team was about an internal debate. One half of the team saw the family's success as too quick—a fluke—and predicted that next week would be worse. The other half was amazed that this family went beyond expectations and suggested that they should continue to replace the old game with new ones. The final assignment was for the parents to meet and come up with a list of consequences for the children's noncompliance.

Third Session

In this model, the third session is designed to be a "practice/implementation" of the themes constructed in first two sessions. For this family, the goal of the session was to deal with specific events of the week within the frame of positive engagement. The first task was to review and discuss the list of consequences made up by the parents. The team expressed their concern that in families where one sibling is so loud and constantly engaging the parents in conflict, the quieter sibling can lose his or her place in the family. Mother lamented that daughter was always out at activities or with friends. The therapist engaged the mother and daughter in strategizing about ways to build connectedness. Son volunteered that he had a game of Scrabble with mother, and games of wrestling and baseball with father. Both parents complained that they were often too busy or tired to have time for such play. For both diagnostic and practice purposes, the team instructed the family to enact a game using the toys available in the session. The therapist observed and processed with the family their roles and dynamics. The team assignment was to maintain this focus of struggling to build a safe, secure, and playful environment in their home.

Fourth Session

For this final session, the team had established the goals of: (1) highlighting differences in the family's dynamics over the 8 weeks of treatment; (2) focusing on the maintenance needs of the marriage; (3) deciding with the family what the next treatment direction should be. Mother opened the meeting by praising her son's success at school. Father told how he took the family out and entertained the children while mother shopped. It was clear that the family enjoyed talking about their success. When mother asked why she was so tired, she answered herself that it was because she was more relaxed at home. The team observed that the parents had created a new dimension for the family game statement like "We're proud of you!" The therapist commented that they all may have been so caught up in conflict before that they could not feel positive feelings or relax. The team observed the more benevolent nature of the children's play in the session. The therapist used this process to discuss the parallel one between mother and father. The mother compared herself to her son for the first time, "We both like to be alone and stay home a lot." The therapist explored with parents how they could enjoy themselves in ways that would make the family more relaxed.

Building on this discussion, the therapist introduced the team's proposal for follow-up. The team recommended family meetings as opposed to individual therapy because of their confidence in parents' growing ability to provide a safe and nurturing environment for both son and daughter. The therapist concluded the sessions with the team's compliment to parents: how they had begun to overcome some deep, past hurt to give their children a different kind of family environment. Mother added that this was what they had always swore to do.

TERMINATION AND FOLLOW-UP

An important part of this model is that follow-up be provided by a member of the observation team. This strategy allows the therapy to maintain the same positive focus developed by the team and allows the "new" therapist to draw on dynamics/strategies that have already been effective with this family. For example, in the first follow-up meeting, the parents began with son being the only problem again and dismissed the "game" idea as not helpful. Having seen the family, the therapist wondered what had made the parents so different, so discouraged. The key event was a negative report from the son's principal questioning the effect of treatment. Attuned to the mother's sensitivity to critical outside judgments, the therapist was able to redirect the parents' focus and bolster their confidence. For this case, follow-up consisted of two sets of four monthly sessions. The second group occurred 5 months after the first and focused mostly on the parents getting time for themselves.

CLINICAL ISSUES

There are several critical developments that seemed to determine the effectiveness of such a brief intervention. First, the investment in researching available background information and communicating with other service providers was critical to the treatment's efficiency. Preexisting data offered important alternative hypotheses that gave clear direction to early treatment. The team was also forewarned of potential sources of resistance and "hotspots" for this particular family, and planned accordingly. A second critical process was the team's ability to expand the family's understanding of the problem: from the son's individual problem to one dyad with sister, to a second dyad with mother, to the systemic focus on control and positive engagement. The original symptoms could then be dealt with as an intense effort by the identified patient to generate and maintain more intense, constant attachments within the family. A third critical development was the family's ability to synthesize the individual dynamics of mother's projective identification with daughter into the systemic dynamics of the family's conflict. This integration cultivated a sensitivity among the members, particularly the son, that made a significant positive change in the family environment. The final important development was the evolution in focus from control to attachment. This change allowed the team to assess both the parents' experience and understanding of constructing a supportive holding environment in their families of origin, and the marriage's ability to generate support and caring for each other and the children. It is the team's assessment that the family's ability to move at both a conceptual and experimental level through these processes enabled the therapy to be so constructive in a brief time.

REFERENCES

Cummings, N. (1986). The dismantling of our health system. *American Psychologist, 41,* 426–431.

Fisher, S. (1978). Time-limited psychotherapy: An investigation of therapeutic outcome at a child guidance clinic. (Doctoral dissertation, University of Illinois, 1978.) *Dissertation Abstracts International.*

Gurman, A. (1981). Integrative marital therapy: Toward the development of an interpersonal approach. In S. H. Budman (Ed.), *Forms of brief therapy* (pp. 415–457). New York: Guilford.

Parad, L. (1971). Short-term treatment: An overview of historical trends, issues and potentials. *Smith College Studies in Social Work, 42,* 119–146.

Scharff, D., & Scharff, J. (1987). *Object relations family therapy.* Northvale, NJ: Jason Aronson.

Tomm, K. (1984). One perspective on Milan systemic approach. *Journal of Marital and Family Therapy, 10,* 113–125.

Wachtel, E., & Wachtel, P. (1986). *Family dynamics in individual psychotherapy.* New York: Guilford.

Witmer, H. (1946). *Psychiatric interviews with children.* New York: Commonwealth Fund.

18

Solution Focused Therapy

Elam Nunnally

Introduction: The Practice Model[1]

Solution focused therapy originated with a group of marriage and family therapists in Milwaukee, Wisconsin (de Shazer, 1985, 1988; Nunnally et al., 1986). In the mid-1970s, this group of researcher clinicians began experimenting with the brief therapy approach originated at the Mental Research Institute in Palo Alto, California (Watzlawick et al., 1974). The influence of the MRI model was initially noticeable in the Milwaukee group's attention to problem formulation, goal setting, and the uses of homework assignments (de Shazer, 1982). Some influence from the Milan group of therapists (Selvini-Palazzolli et al., 1978) can be discerned in the early 1980s in task construction and use of timing (Nunnally & Berg, 1983). Influence from the Milan group can also be found in the Milwaukee group's evolving uses of "systemic questioning" (Lipchik & de Shazer, 1986). By 1980 the Milwaukee group's model of brief therapy had evolved to the point where it was distinctly their own although still rather close to the MRI brief therapy approach, as can be seen in a major work by de Shazer (1982). Probably the major innovations in the Milwaukee model at that time were the uses of positive feedback or "compliments" and a view of the problem pattern as a system with multiple points for intervention.

[1]This portion of the chapter draws from a paper presented at the World Conference on Family Therapy, Finland, 1991 (Nunnally & Tuovinen, 1991).

Elam Nunnally • School of Social Welfare, University of Wisconsin–Milwaukee, Milwaukee, Wisconsin 53201.

Casebook of the Brief Psychotherapies, edited by Richard A. Wells and Vincent J. Giannetti. Plenum Press, New York, 1993.

A revolution in the Milwaukee model occurred in the mid-1980s when the group shifted from a focus on problems and how they change to a focus on solutions and how they fit the "exceptions" to the problem. The Milwaukee group began studying the nonoccurrences of problems and the behaviors and contexts that promote or expand the nonoccurrences (or exceptions).

In contemporary solution focused practice, therapists seek to uncover effective behaviors that clients already are using to some extent to deal with their problems. Therapists do this by inquiring closely about exceptions to the complaint that brought the clients for help. For example, a couple who complain that they quarrel too much about money matters will be asked if they sometimes discuss money without quarreling. If the answer is yes, the next step is to explore the conditions under which they peacefully discuss money and examine with them how these conditions differ from the times when they quarrel. After identifying those elements that seem to make a difference between quarreling and not quarreling, clients are encouraged to expand upon these and report back in subsequent sessions on progress achieved in reducing the degree and/or frequency of quarreling. In subsequent sessions, their progress reports are carefully explored and recognition given for movement in the direction of goal. Therapists may also offer some suggestions on how to "fine tune" the exception behaviors further, but usually interventions consist of identifying and encouraging effective behaviors already in use.

Goals

Solution focused therapy is goal driven. Clients' goals determine the direction of therapy, and therapy usually ends when client goals are reached or when clients feel that they are well on their way and no longer need therapy. Therapy is usually brief, perhaps because focusing on strengths rather than deficits generates hope, confidence, energy, and creativity in both therapists and clients. Successful therapy typically requires four to eight sessions, with significant change occurring by the third session. However, there is no time limitation inherent in this practice model, and a small proportion of cases may continue for a much longer period.

In every case, therapists clarify client goals before attempting any major intervention. The term *goal* here refers narrowly to goal of therapy and not to some general, much less utopian, wishes for a better life. Therapists inquire closely about indicators of goal achievement ("How will we know when the goal is reached?") and also how clients expect to be better off as a result of reaching their goals. In the example above, the couple's explicitly stated goal was to be able to discuss money matters without quarreling.

Other Exceptions

After clarifying clients' goals, therapists search for other exceptions to the complaint. (Goals constitute "future exceptions," a time in the future when a complaint is eliminated or substantially reduced.) These include:

1. "New exceptions." Exceptions that have only recently begun to happen. Therapists often speak of these behaviors as pre-session change and as between-session change. Example: "We quarrel all the time, every day—except we've had no quarrels for the last few days."
2. "Recurrent exceptions." These occur periodically in the present. Example: A couple report that they quarrel every day, Monday through Friday, but usually not on weekends.
3. "Past exceptions." These occurred in the past but do not occur at the present time. Example: A couple report that they have been arguing every day for the past 6 months, but prior to 6 months ago had no more arguments than most couples.

New and recurrent exceptions usually offer the best clues to what needs to be done to resolve the problem. When new or recurrent exceptions are not found, exploration of past exceptions may turn up useful ideas for solution (as in Case 2 in this chapter). When therapist and client are unable to uncover any usable exceptions to the complaint, the therapist may help a client to view the complaint or problem in a new way and/or experiment with new behaviors in order to create exceptions related to the goal. After the client has begun to produce exceptions, the therapist encourages further effort in the same direction expanding on the new exceptions.

Integrative Framework

Solution focused therapy can be viewed as an action system composed of three elements: (1) exception behaviors, (2) problem behaviors, and (3) intervention behaviors. As in any system, each element affects and is affected by every other element in the system. The four kinds of exception behaviors are defined above. The other elements of this action system are defined as follows: (a) "Problem behaviors" constitute the

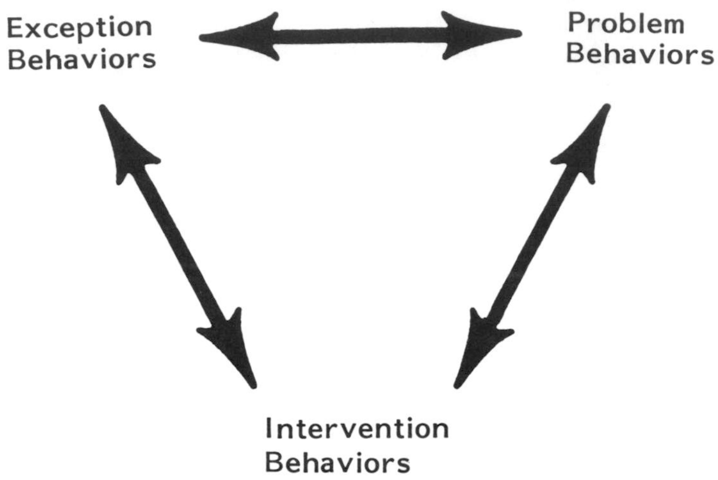

FIGURE 1. Solution focused action system.

complaint that brings the client(s) to therapy. Behaviors may be overt, such as "I drink too much" or covert, such as "I'm constantly thinking about what I did wrong." The complaint may refer to the client's own behaviors, as above, or to another's behaviors, such as "My son doesn't do his homework," or may refer to interactions between client and others, such as "My wife and I are quarreling too often" (see Figure 1). (b) "Intervention behaviors" typically include (1) questions to elicit data on exceptions and change, (2) positive feedback or "compliments," (3) educative comments, and (4) task directives or "homework."

Intervention behaviors initially focus on a search for exceptions, for example, asking questions about when the problem doesn't happen or is reduced in scope or degree, or, another example, giving a homework assignment to notice what happens during the next week (with reference to the problem situation) that the client would like to continue happening. A therapist may also collaborate with clients in constructing genograms, family sculpting, making home visits, or any other activity the therapist believes may help in uncovering usable exceptions to the problem behaviors. Therapists support and encourage exception behaviors with positive feedback about what the client is doing that is working or has potential to work in direction of goal. They also support exceptions by means of task directives of the general type "do more of what works." Example: "You seem to be on the right track. Keep using those listening skills and continue to notice the changes."

Intervention behaviors designed to create exceptions include task directives of the general type "do something different." The assignment may be as simple as "try moving your next argument to another room" and as complex as a set of instructions to study one's family of origin, with particular attention paid to, for example, how members expressed affection to one another. (Most solution focused therapists favor use of the simplest task directives and use complex ones only when the simpler ones are not productive.)

Educative comments may be used to create exceptions or to support existing exceptions. These may serve to change meaning, for example, "your quarrels represent your efforts to redevelop your marriage and are temporarily necessary," a change of meaning that may help to reduce the emotional impact of quarrels. They may serve to change expectations, for example, "As your child improves, you can expect her to be less helpful at home and more interested in going out with her friends," a comment that may help the parents respond appropriately to changes in their troubled preteen daughter. Educative comments may also provide useful new information for clients, for example, "Kids typically respond poorly to 'why' questions. It works better with most kids just to tell them what you are sore about and what you want them to do." This comment may help a parent to change some of his/her disciplinary behavior. Educative comments are intended initially to change client thinking and ultimately change client behaviors or support existing exceptions.

Intervention behaviors designed to create exceptions may be focused directly on exception behaviors such as "between now and next week, take one behavior from your picture of the future with the problem solved and do it at least once and notice the result." Alternatively, intervention behaviors may focus directly on the problem behaviors, as in the use of directives intended to interrupt or disrupt a problem pattern, for example, "Instead of explaining, just give your child an order in a firm voice" (to a parent who was trying too hard to achieve cognitive agreement and failing to achieve behavioral compliance). A skilled therapist may encourage existing exception behaviors and at the same time act to encourage new exceptions when additional exceptions are needed for achievement of goal.

Solution focused therapists tend to be direct with clients and very active in interviews, keeping focus on goals and other exceptions and holding discussion of problems or complaints to a minimum. Positive feedback or compliments are data-based, derived from therapist observations of clients and/or clients' reports of events. Solution focused therapists provide as little intervention as possible, consistent with achieving the goal, and they typically resist the temptation to try for extraneous goals.

Therapy Session

In a typical first interview rather little time is spent in exploring the problem or complaint. After ascertaining which problem the client wants to resolve first (when there is more than one), a therapist usually shifts the focus to an exploration of goal and other exceptions. Toward the end of the session the therapist takes a "consultation break" to consult with team members, if working with a team, or to consult his or her own notes if working alone. The session concludes with an intervention message from therapist or from therapist and team. The message usually includes positive feedback and task directive(s) and often includes educative comments as well.

In subsequent therapy sessions, therapists typically focus with clients on between-session change, carefully exploring how the change(s) occurred and what the client and others need to do to continue the change. When substantial change has occurred, the intervention message consists mainly of positive feedback and task directives are minimal, for example, "Just continue along the same line as you've described in our session today."

Therapists' Skills

The structure and underlying premises of solution focused therapy are basically simple, but doing solution focused therapy requires all the skills of interviewing and all the knowledge of people, relationships, and environments that one needs in most other approaches. In addition, therapists using a solution focused approach must acquire a mind set of looking for what works rather than looking at what is wrong, a mind set not easily acquired by therapists trained in other approaches. Success with solution focused therapy also seems related to a therapist's ability to view complaints/problems from alternative perspectives, for example, viewing conflict between a couple as part of a process of redevelopment of their relationship. A therapist's presentation of alternative perspectives can often help clients to share in a view of the problem that is more conducive to problem resolution. Finally, considerable creativity may be needed by therapists in devising ways to initiate and to support clients' changed behaviors.

Outcome Study

In an outcome study designed to determine the effects of solution focused therapy with a broad spectrum of clients and problems, 164 clients at an outpatient clinic were telephoned at 6, 12, or 18 months posttreatment and asked if therapy had accomplished their goals or if substantial progress had been made toward goals. About 80% reported goals met or substantial progress achieved (Kiser, 1988). Controlled outcome studies involving this practice model have not been undertaken.

Three Case Examples

The case examples presented here differ substantially from case examples found in much of the professional literature. Typically, solution focused therapists gather only enough data to intervene and to assess whether their interventions are productive. The focus of a therapist's assessment is on goal and other exceptions, not on origins of the problem, although some attention to history may enable the therapist to better understand the meaning of the problem to the client. In assessing the data, the most salient questions are: Is there a goal? Are there exceptions to the problem? Are goal and/or exceptions clearly and concretely specified? Who does the client think had a role in producing the exceptions? Is the client able to describe the behaviors that contributed to the exceptions? Is the client(s) likely to do homework assignments? In addition to exceptions (above), what other strengths of client and client situation can be identified, and which of these would be helpful to incorporate in positive feedback to the client?

In Case 1 below, the focus is largely on new or recent exceptions. In Case 2 the focus is on past exceptions. In Case 3 the focus of intervention varies across family members: expanding the teenager's ongoing exception behaviors and changing the parents' behaviors to increase and support the teenager's exception behaviors.

Case 1: Recent Exceptions

Mary (not her real name) has a history of more than 10 years treatment for anxiety. She had been on tranquilizers for most of that time, more recently placed on beta blockers. At time of the initial consultation with the solution focused team she had been on medical leave for 3 months. She complained of tiredness and a need for greater energy so she could return to work (full-time secretarial position). She was 43 years old, mother of two preteens, and married about 15 years to Larry (not his real name), who is an engineer. She attended the sessions alone.

The therapist began the session with a question about recent change. Mary described how she had gone off medication entirely 2 weeks previously. She found the days going quickly, and she was thinking of going back to work. She didn't have as much energy as she needed, and she still got nervous too quickly, but she felt better than when she was taking medication. She was sweating less and not having to shower as often and had more energy than before. She went jogging every evening, and she thought the exercise helped her. She had some trouble getting to sleep at night but was no longer taking sleeping pills. Despite trouble getting to sleep, she was not feeling stressed in the evenings; in fact, evenings were the most peaceful time, and she was calmest then. In response to the therapist's question, she said that she was avoiding stressing herself in the evenings by reminding herself that night was coming and then another day and she could leave things to the next day. She didn't try to go to sleep earlier or force herself to sleep. She would go to bed late and read in bed if not sleepy.

The therapist asked how the team would know that her goals in therapy were achieved. She gave several instances: She would enjoy again caring for flowers; she would get new clothes, she would be active socially, as before, without being tense; she wouldn't be grinding her teeth; she would be more open and direct with Larry and the children. (Getting these details required some prompting questions from the therapist, e.g., "What else?")

The therapist asked if any of the above imagined improvements were beginning to happen, just a little. Mary replied that there were some little things. She was getting out a little, and she was generally more active. How did she get herself to be more active? She told that she tried to get up earlier in the morning, go for a walk, do normal morning things, get her housework done and then take a shower. She wasn't getting nearly so tired as before and that was very different. The therapist asked how she had gotten all this change started. She emphasized that she had been thinking about what was good for her and what wasn't and she was noticing the results of making changes, for example, going off meds. She reminds herself that she has to do it (do what is good for her), and it works.

In the intervention message from the team, the therapist complimented her on developing strategies for herself that were working and on clearly noticing the steps she was taking toward her goal. Comments were also made about her courage in dealing with her anxiety state and willingness to try something different. The homework assignment from the team was to continue using the strategies that were working for her and continue to notice small changes. As an afterthought, one team member suggested (through the therapist) that she experiment with jogging earlier in the evening to see if this led to her being able to go to sleep more readily.

In subsequent sessions with the therapist, meeting biweekly and then monthly, Mary continued to report improvements and was able to return to work full-time.

Commentary: The intervention in this case was to help the patient identify what she was doing that was working and then validate her efforts and encourage her to continue. The suggestion about jogging earlier rather than later in the evening was a very minor addition, a suggestion for a small change that could facilitate her getting to sleep more easily. When patients or clients are already making substantial changes, solution focused therapists typically do not add homework assignments that appear to ask for still greater effort or for more change.

The therapist and team were aware that in situations like this the client's family members may be able to add to the solution; however, in this particular case it seemed unnecessary at this time to work with other family members, and this is consistent with a philosophy of "do as little as need be" to reach the goal. Finally, the reader should not infer from this case that solution focused therapists are opposed to medication. Simply, at this point in time, when the team met the client, going off meds was part of her goal and she had the concurrence of her psychiatrist.

Case 2: Past Exceptions

Matti and Leena (not their real names) are a Finnish couple the author counseled during a sabbatical in Finland. Married almost 30 years, the couple have two grown children ages 21 and 23, who have been gone from the home for 2 and 4 years respectively, continuing their education in another city. Matti and Leena are employed full time, Matti in his own business and Leena holding a managerial position in a manufacturing concern.

Trouble between the two began about 3 years prior to the intake therapy session. Over the 3 years, relations between them steadily worsened, and at the time of the initial session they had been separated for about 3 months. They were extremely critical of each other, frequently quarreling, no sex for months, and Matti sometimes drinking excessively. Difficulties between them seemed to have been precipitated by severe financial setbacks in Matti's business leaving the couple with heavy indebtedness. Leena believed Matti handled the indebtedness badly, although she was not critical of his handling his business. They had begun divorce action, and one of their attorneys, who knew them both, suggested that they consult a marriage therapist.

Therapist and team were not able to discover any new or concurrent exceptions to their marital complaints. Neither could find a good word to say about the other's behavior. Each of them seemed to have as a goal for therapy reaching a firm decision about whether or not to divorce.

Past exceptions surfaced when asked what had kept them together for 30 years. In speaking of their earlier years they told of enjoying many activities together, both as a couple and with the children: hunting, fishing, camping, gardening, and especially going to the horse races. In season, they had attended horse-racing events most weekends, sometimes with children and sometimes without. Matti's occasional drinking was not viewed as a problem then. They had few disagreements. They usually agreed on child rearing and on financial matters. The children did well in school and were generally well behaved. They both enjoyed their sexual relationship. Each thought the other a good parent who had good relations with their grown children.

Following a consultation break, the therapist delivered an intervention message to the couple complimenting them on their ability to recall the positives in their years together despite their recent very unhappy years. So many couples seem unable to do this. The therapy team validated their persistence in continuing through 3 hard years rather than quickly giving up. The team thought that it was consistent with their prudent approach to problems and with their Finnish *sisu* (a special Finnish term for toughness sufficient to do the impossible). The team acknowledged that people change over time, and it might be that they had had all the good years together that they were going to have. The team didn't know about that. The couple were invited to try a small experiment that might help them to reach their goal of making a firm decision, and they agreed to try it. The therapist suggested that sometime during the following 2 weeks, between the present and the time of the second therapy session, they bring one small piece of the past back into the present, something that was not *too* difficult to do. The therapy team didn't know what this might be. The couple recalled rather quickly, and with smiles, that the racing season was to begin that same week, and they decided to go once to the races together.

In their second session, they told of attending races on two weekends without any quarrels. They weren't sure how they had managed to not quarrel, but perhaps they just stayed away from talking about problems. They were clearly pleased with what happened but unsure how much confidence to place in this development. The therapy team agreed they should not get their hopes up too high and also complimented them on their courage to risk the experiment and on their managing to find a way to be together without big quarrels at least some of the time. They recommended that the couple continue the experiment and, when they felt like it, add one more small piece from their past and see what happens.

In the third session, 3 weeks after the second, the couple reported further outings to the races and also going dancing after the races (another former activity, one they had not recalled in the first therapy session). Furthermore, they had had sex for the first time in nearly a year. They were thinking of moving back together but also were afraid the improvement would not last. Therapy team agreed they should go slow and expect some ups and downs, normal in any relationship, and also suggested they continue the experiments.

In the fourth session, three weeks after the third session, the couple reported more trips to the races, dancing afterwards, having sex, and also enjoying a late spring ski vacation in Lapland. They were making plans to try living together. They also had reached an understanding about how to deal with each other around their debt problems. Matti was no longer drinking excessively, and his drinking had not been an issue between them since the initial session. The team openly and honestly admired what they had been able to accomplish and also cautioned that they were in a process of redeveloping their relationship, and this could take some time yet. The couple and therapist agreed to leave further appointments on an "as-needed" basis. Occasionally, over the following year, one of the team encountered one or the other of the partners socially and was assured that the couple were continuing to get along well.

Commentary: This case illustrates the potential utility of drawing upon past exceptions and is fairly typical of the way solution focused therapists focus on usable past exceptions when new and recurrent exceptions are not available. The therapy team's intervention was tailored to fit the couple's presentation of the exceptions. The couple were specific and detailed in presenting past exceptions, and the team were also specific about what the couple could do. Some clients, of course, offer neither new, recurrent, nor past exceptions. In such cases, a therapist may be able to interest a client in bringing into the present a piece of a future exception, if the client is able to provide a detailed picture of a future in which the problem is solved and the client is behaving differently. Alternatively, the therapist may opt for some other way to get the client to do something different in order to create exceptions, as in Case 3 below.

Case 3: Recurring Exceptions

Mr. and Mrs. A. and their 16-year-old daughter, Rachel (not her real name) presented with a problem of frequent and intense arguments between father and daughter, beginning a little more than 2 years ago and escalating to the point where Mr. A. feared he could become physically abusive. The arguments included shouting and name calling and occurred any time Mr. A. corrected Rachel and almost any time they were in the same room together. Mrs. A. tried to keep peace between them and smooth things over and felt very much caught in the middle. Mr. A. thought that their 13-year-old daughter, not present in the session, might emulate Rachel if they did nothing about the situation. Rachel had recently begun skipping some classes at school, but the problem they wanted to resolve first was the conflict between Rachel and father.

When asked how important it was to each of them to resolve the problem, the parents promptly said 10 (on a scale of 1 to 10). The therapist was surprised by Rachel also saying 10. She had said little and looked angry up to this point. Therapist asked what would be the benefit of reaching their goal. All agreed there would be less yelling and shouting, mother said she would not feel pulled two ways between them, father would feel less upset, and Rachel said the house would be more peaceful, and she would be grounded less and able to see her friends more.

The therapist asked how confident each was that they could reach the goal, on a scale of 1 to 10. The therapist was again surprised when each of them said about 9 or 10. Asked to explain why they were so confident, the parents began to list the good points about Rachel: She was generally a responsible person who did her share about the house, had good friends, was good to her sister, was not into drugs, was a very good worker last summer in a fast food restaurant, was a good student except for recently skipping some classes, and Rachel and father had been close until the last 2 years. (As is typical, this list was not produced in one breath but required prompts from the therapist, e.g., "and what else.") Mother added that father had always been a very conscientious and caring father, for example, more often than mother making trips to school to deal with school issues, and so forth. Rachel evaded the question as to why she was so confident with a typical teen "I don't know" and shrug, and at this point the therapist made a mental note to see Rachel alone before the session ended. No family member seemed to be able to point to times recently when the problem was less (current exceptions), but parents told that during the summer, when Rachel was working full time, things had gone rather smoothly at home (a recent past exception), even though Rachel was at home just about as much as she was during the school year.

The therapist requested some private time each with Rachel and the parental couple. In the individual session with Rachel, the therapist again inquired about Rachel's confidence that she could resolve the problem with father. Rachel now told that sometimes she avoided arguments with father, and she knew how to do it, by just keeping her mouth shut. She didn't mean by this that she could pointedly ignore him. She would look like she was listening and say something like "okay" or "I'll try" and that would head off an argument. It annoyed her that her parents didn't realize that she sometimes acted so as to avoid arguments with him. In response to therapist's question, she told that she got herself to do this by reminding herself that she didn't want to be grounded again or telling herself that arguing does no good. She thought she could do this pretty much anytime she decided to, except not if he were really unfair and not if he started asking "why" questions, for example, "Why did you do that?" or "Why didn't you do that?" It really got her goat when he asked "why" questions, and she couldn't resist the urge to give it back to him. She also stated that the only reason she was skipping some classes was because she wanted to spend some time with friends, and she had been grounded so much lately that there was no other way of seeing them. She thought her parents were okay for the most part, just hard to get along with lately, especially her father. She had "no beef" about her mother.

Following a consultation break, the therapist delivered the following message to Rachel: "You seem very clear of your goal, and I'm impressed with how much you've already done about finding some ways to begin to make progress. I also think it's really neat that you're able to see what's okay about your parents even while you're in the midst of a lot of difficulty with them. I think you have reason for your confidence that you and your parents can work this out, not that it's going to be smooth. There'll be ups and downs. Between now and next week I'd like you to continue to notice whenever you resist the temptation to "get into it" with your father and notice how you manage to do this. Can you do that?" Rachel agreed to do the homework.

In the private time with Mr. and Mrs. A. the therapist again sought data about any recent or recurring exceptions to the parents' complaint about Rachel's verbal combativeness, but without success. Following a consultation break, the therapist told Mr. and Mrs. A. that he was reasonably sure that the difficulty related to a normal developmental process of growing toward self-sufficiency and independence. In this process it often happens that children who have been close to a parent or parents must find some way to increase their distance until they feel comfortable. Teens do this in different ways, and Rachel is doing it by being verbally combative with her father. Some of the evidence for this lies in the fact that when Rachel was working full time, she was much easier to live with, an indication that she was feeling more independent and thus could give up some of the unpleasant behavior. They could expect the behavior to diminish as Rachel began to feel easier about her distance from father, and when she is older and more truly independent she will be able to be closer again, as an adult. In the meantime, could Mr. A. turn over to Mrs. A. at least 50% of the disciplining he is now doing? Even though it wouldn't be easy? Mr. A. thought he could do this and that it made sense, and on leaving inquired with a laugh if it would be okay to give up 75% of it. In response to therapist's inquiry, Mrs. A. said it would be no burden on her to take over more of the disciplining because that would be easier than being caught in the middle, but Mr. A. would have to be content with her doing it her way in her own time and that might be hard for him because she is more easy going. Mr. A. acknowledged that was true but was sure he could manage to keep out of it whenever he leaves something for his wife to deal with.

The therapist added that, of course, he didn't mean for Mr. A. to give up all disciplining with respect to Rachel, and when he does correct her it might help to just tell her what he is concerned about and what he wants her to do about it, briefly, rather than asking her for an explanation of why she did or did not do something. This seemed to make sense to him, too.

The educative comments and homework assignments above were preceded by positive feedback to the parents: Rachel has a lot going for her and that, among other things, indicates that the parents have been doing a lot of things right. The situation is painful for all and not easy to work out quickly, but the therapist believes they have reason for their confidence that it can be worked out. They seem to be a very close family with basically very positive relationships.

In the following three sessions, at weekly and then every-other-week intervals, Rachel and the parent couple were seen in individual sessions for about a half-hour each. In Session 2 Rachel reported diminishing her arguments with father substantially and had come up with a couple of new strategies for avoiding arguments. She reported that he was trying, too, not getting after her so much and not asking her "why?" The house was more peaceful. She was still grounded but that would end soon, if she watched her step. The parents reported that father was succeeding in turning much of the disciplining over to mother, but it was harder to do than he had expected. and it was also hard to not nag mother to act more quickly or firmly. However, Mrs. A. thought he was doing pretty well on both counts. They both thought Rachel had improved substantially, keeping her temper on the few occasions she had been corrected by father or mother. The therapist gave Rachel and the parents positive feedback about their efforts and shared in their pleasure in the results they were getting.

Sessions 3 and 4 were basically reports of further signs of change and small celebrations of their progress. The homework assignments for everyone in Sessions 2 through 4 were to keep up the good work, that they appeared to be on the right track. In Session 4 the therapist thought they might be ready to interrupt treatment, but all members were still feeling insecure about their progress and thought it would be helpful to continue a while longer. A fifth appointment was scheduled for three weeks later.

In the beginning of Session 5, Rachel and the parent team were again seen separately and agreed that their goals were reached. The therapist called them all together to end the session and to terminate therapy with his acknowledgment of how well they had worked on dealing with their issues and how much progress they had made. He also pointed out that they could continue to expect the normal ups and downs that any parents and teens might expect in a loving family.

Commentary: This case illustrates a situation where the therapist was able to build on recurring exceptions offered by one family member (Rachel) and work with the other family members (Mr. and Mrs. A.) by getting them to do something different. Solution focused therapists tend to be rather flexible: In a single case they may use new exceptions, recurrent exceptions, past exceptions, and also make suggestions for adding something new and different, although it's true that they prefer to keep things as simple as possible and do as little as possible consistent with achieving the treatment goal. This case also illustrates a therapist's use of his/her knowledge of human development and family development in offering educative comments to the parents that diminished some of the excess emotionality and enabled them to accept some suggestions for change. It worked. If it hadn't worked, the therapist would have had to do the same thing he/she advocates clients do when what they are doing doesn't work: Do something different.

The author believes that the successful outcome of this case, and most other successful solution focused cases, can be attributed in part to the use of positive feedback to the clients. People need to know when they are doing something right, and they need validation of their efforts.

In each case, solution focused therapists are initially like investigators assigned the task of ascertaining what works or is salvageable. Having found something that can be built upon, they shift to a coach role, helping the client to make the most of whatever they have going for them. Finally, they become a sort of cheering section affirming the client's successes. More than one person has commented that this treatment seems to be a "therapy of hope."

REFERENCES

de Shazer, S. (1982). *Patterns of brief family therapy: An ecosystemic approach.* New York: The Guilford Press.

de Shazer, S (1985). *Keys to solution in brief therapy.* New York: W. W. Norton.

de Shazer, S. (1988). *Clues: Investigating solutions in brief therapy.* New York: W. W. Norton.

Kiser, D. (1988). Follow up study conducted at the Brief Family Therapy Center. Unpublished Master's thesis, University of Wisconsin-Milwaukee.

Lipchik, E., & de Shazer, S. (1986). The purposeful interview. *Journal of Strategic and Systematic Therapies, 5*(1), 88–89.

Nunnally, E., & Berg, I. (1983). We tried to push the river. *Journal of Strategic and Systemic Therapies, 2*(1), 63–68.

Nunnally, E., & Tuovinen, L. (1991). *Training Finnish diaconate workers in solution focused brief therapy.* Paper presented at the World Family Therapy Congress, Jyväskylä, Finland, June 1991.

Nunnally, E., de Shazer, S., Lipchik, E., & Berg, I. (1986). A study of change: Therapeutic theory in process. In D. Efron (Ed.), *Journeys: Expansion of the strategic-systemic therapies* (pp. 77–96). New York: Brunner/Mazel.

Selvini-Palazzoli, M., Checchin, G., Prata, G., & Boscolo, L. (1978). *Paradox and counterparadox.* New York: Jason Aronson.

Watzlawick, P., Weakland, J., & Fisch, R. (1974). *Change: Principles of problem formation and problem resolution.* New York: W. W. Norton.

19

The Case of Oppositional Cooperation

Phillip A. Phelps

Introduction

Problems of behavior or conduct in school-age children are quite common in both mental health and medical settings. Specific presenting problems often include defiant behavior, temper tantrums, hitting siblings and/or parents, impulsivity, short attention span, and other socially frowned-upon actions. Children exhibiting these behaviors are typically assigned diagnoses in the American Psychiatric Association *Diagnostic and Statistical Manual of Mental Disorders–Revised Edition* (1987) such as Attention Deficit-Hyperactivity Disorder or Oppositional/ Defiant Disorder.

One of the dilemmas inherent in working with this population is that the persons presenting the problem are not the ones seeking the treatment. Defiant behavior is almost always more of a problem for the defied than for the defiant. It is certainly a rare occurrence for a youngster to walk into the therapist's office and proclaim, "I'm defiant and I'd like to change." It is far more common for the parents and/or teachers to be the ones demanding the change. Likewise, it is the parent who makes the phone call to the therapist, schedules the appointment, and pays the

Phillip A. Phelps • Child Development Unit, Children's Hospital of Pittsburgh, 3705 Fifth Avenue, Pittsburgh, Pennsylvania 15213.

Casebook of the Brief Psychotherapies, edited by Richard A. Wells and Vincent J. Giannetti. Plenum Press, New York, 1993.

bill. The parent is the person who fervently explains to the therapist what the child's problems are and how *he* (it is usually a boy) needs to change. The youngster generally sits quietly, denies the parent report vehemently, or offers countercharges.

This can create a challenge to the therapist. Change of any significance requires a considerable degree of energy and a corresponding degree of will. Change generally entails its own set of consequences, some of which are negative (Papp, 1983). Therefore, motivation to change comes from the belief that the pain of not changing is greater than the perceived risks and consequences of change. There is little reason for the oppositional youngster to believe that giving in to what the parent wants will benefit him. To him, maintaining the status quo means holding on to the power his coercive behavior can command from adults at times.

Thus, when treating this population using a brief treatment model, it seems sensible to enlist the participation of the person who is suffering most from the problem, even if it is not the person with the problem (Fisch et al., 1982). Accurately identifying the complainant as well as enlisting his/her energy and desire for change can be a critical aspect of doing therapy briefly.

In fact, it is not always necessary to include the identified patient in the therapy at all. Sessions can involve the development of behavioral interventions that are based heavily on principles of learning theory. Behavioral change is precipitated by altering behavioral contingencies (Barkley, 1981; Patterson, 1976) and/or by altering coercive family processes (Patterson, 1976).

These interventions presume that, with the proper technology, parents can learn ways to enforce previously unenforceable limits. Treatment generally involves the parents primarily, and it can be extremely effective in relatively brief periods. Parents sometimes quickly learn how to develop their own behavior plans, enabling them to generalize gains far beyond the original presenting behaviors.

Clearly there are times, however, that a strictly behavioral approach is either not helpful or not palatable to the parents. There are other instances when the parents have the skills to enforce limits effectively but are not doing so for a wide variety of reasons. In other words, the problem is sometimes based more on a performance deficit than a skill deficit. The parents also may perceive the problem as residing exclusively within the child and as highly resistant to external manipulation. In these cases, a strictly behavioral approach will be hard to sell.

When such a stalemate occurs, the brief therapist may feel pressures from the parents to have the child seen on an individual basis. In addition, the practitioner may feel a number of other pressures such as to explore pharmacologic interventions or etiologies such as allergies, chemical imbalances, and the like. It is important, of course, to be responsive to these issues, but they are beyond the scope of this chapter. As mentioned above, moving away from work with the complainant can significantly slow the process (if not render it ineffective) yet not being respectful of the parents' underlying message, "We need to do something different" may force them out of treatment. This chapter will examine some alternative responses to such a message.

Wider Versus Longer

There are ways to enlarge the focus of a primarily behavioral approach and still involve the complainants with the most energy for change. One is to weave other aspects of the presenting problems into the picture and to involve other family members. A move of this kind makes sense when it appears there are dynamic/systemic forces operating to block the effectiveness of behavior management strategies and the caretakers' innate parenting skills.

This notion is derived largely from Peggy Papp's (1983) idea of exploring symptoms with an eye toward developing hypotheses. According to Papp, when developing a hypothesis, information is gathered on three different levels: the behavioral, the emotional, and the ideational. Thus, when exploration is at the behavioral level (what people do), the focus is on tracking behavioral sequences. When it is at the emotional level (what people feel), the focus is on the function of the feelings and the form of their expression. When it is on the ideational level (what people think), it is on how the problem is perceived by each family member. At the emotional level, Papp suggests the following consideration:

> The expression of feelings is a powerful tool in influencing other family members. Under what circumstances are feelings aroused and expressed? What counter feelings and reactions do these emotional expressions stir up in others? Just knowing how a family member feels is not particularly helpful, but knowing at what particular moment she chooses to express her sadness, how she expresses it, and how others react to it, indicates its function. (Papp, 1983, p. 22)

Exploration of the ideational level entails a different focus:

> In order to have a clear understanding of this level, it is helpful to gather information concerning each other's family of origin. Since this is where the attitudes, perceptions, beliefs originated, a historical perspective of the extended family often sheds light on current transactions. (Papp, 1983, p. 23)

Exploring the emotional and ideational levels of a presenting problem can be extremely helpful in understanding the context of the behavior and determining where previous attempted solutions have gotten stuck. It allows for the generation of alternative hypotheses that lead to untried interventions. Addressing these levels enables the focus of treatment to broaden while keeping the presenting problems in clear view. It can help avoid the trap of straying too far from the complainant's notion of the problem. Losing the focus of the problem runs the dual risk of lengthening treatment unnecessarily or having the clients terminate prematurely because of the perception it has lost its relevance.

THE CASE OF OPPOSITIONAL COOPERATION

The following case was chosen to illustrate how a behavioral approach was utilized effectively, though temporarily. When the presenting problems recurred a year later, the parents clearly demanded a different approach.

Background Information and Initial Intervention

Jay was initially seen at the age of 6½ years old with presenting concerns of behavior problems at home and hyperactivity in the school environment. He was the second of three children born to James and Katy Boston (ages 37 and 34, respectively). He lived with both parents, a 14-year-old sister (Barbara), and an 8-month-old sister (Kaile). Both parents were college-educated. Mr. Boston owned his own business, and Mrs. Boston was a homemaker at the time they entered treatment.

Jay was described by his parents as difficult to discipline over the previous 2 years and, at the time of evaluation, the difficulties had intruded into the school setting. The initial assessment was performed by a licensed clinical psychologist and a developmental pediatrician. It included a parent interview, a clinical interview with the child, and the administration of a battery of psychological tests, as well as a pediatric physical examination and neurological screening.

The results suggested that Jay was a youngster with superior intellectual functioning and academic performance far below expectancy (though he did not meet educational criterion for placement in a learning-disabled classroom). He was diagnosed with Attention Deficit-Hyperactivity Disorder and Oppositional/Defiant Disorder (American Psychiatric Association, 1985). Recommendations included behavior management training for the parents to learn more effective responses to Jay's problem behavior. Medication was not recommended, and the parents were not interested in pursuing pharmacologic intervention.

The parents came to see me for four sessions focused on behavior management. This treatment was basically a hybrid of the strategies described by Patterson (1976) and Barkley (1981), using time-out as the major cost response in combination with a positive reinforcement schedule for the target behaviors. There was phone consultation with his schoolteacher to discuss his classroom behavior and to establish a behavioral intervention in the classroom.

The parents quickly became invested in the behavioral program, and it was implemented very consistently. Jay seemed motivated by the reinforcers, and he put forth considerable effort toward more positive behavior. At the end of the four sessions, the parents and Jay's teacher were quite pleased with the results. The improvements were reported to have persisted at a 3-month follow-up appointment. The treatment was terminated with the understanding the parents would contact me if any problems resurfaced.

The Family Return to Therapy

There was no further contact with the family for about 13 months. Mrs. Boston then phoned to say that things had deteriorated considerably and they wanted to bring Jay in to see me. An appointment was scheduled for the parents and Jay to come in to see a graduate social work intern and myself to reassess the problem.

The parents appeared for the session quite distressed, with Mrs. Boston seeming almost desperate. She indicated that Jay (now 8 years old) was demonstrating physically aggressive behavior both at home and at school, in addition to obscene language and defiance toward authority. These behavioral symptoms were similar to those that had prompted the initial evaluation. At the same time he was described as having grown "immune" to the discipline techniques that had formerly been effective. The parents acknowledged an extreme sense of frustration, and they felt powerless to manage the current patterns of behavior.

The parents also expressed deep concerns about Jay's emotional well-being. They saw him as "not caring about anything" and showing very little feeling toward others. They talked about hearing Jay make self-denigrating comments and verbalizations such as "I hate myself." Vegetative signs of depression were denied as was any suicidal ideation.

Several events had occurred during the period Jay's behavior problems had escalated. These included the death of the family dog after being struck by a car (1 month prior), his mother's return to work, the family's move to a new home (though the move was only about 500 yards), and the approach of his first confession. The parents reported that Jay seemed quite affected by the death of the dog. They believed he felt responsible because he was the person who opened the door when the dog ran out and he was the one who discovered it lying in the street. They also believed his first confession had affected him because of his firm resistance to this rite of passage.

Jay presented as a bright youngster who had some difficulty expressing feelings, though he was attentive and cooperative throughout the interview. He masked feelings with either appearance of bravado or an "I-don't-care" attitude. It seemed his behavioral outbursts were another means of acting out his feelings.

Developing a New Treatment Contract

Because of the parents' clear need to focus problem exploration on Jay, it was essential to negotiate a contract with the parents that was consistent with their notion of the problem and yet included them as the family members with the most energy for change. This was a critical piece of recontracting with the family. In addition, the parents stated clearly that the former mode of treatment (behavior management training) would not be helpful this time. They wanted Jay to be seen individually.

The parents' perception of the new presentation of Jay's symptoms made sense. Though the type of behaviors Jay was presenting were similar to those a year prior, their focus was now on what it said about his emotional status. In effect, the parents had shifted their concern from "this behavior is a problem" to "we worry what this behavior is communicating about his emotional adjustment."

From the previous sessions a year prior, a fair amount of information was known about the presenting problems from a behavioral perspective. It now appeared time to explore the emotional and ideational aspects of the problem more directly. It seemed clear that the parents had not been maintaining the limits or consequences that had been effective for over a year, and the preliminary operating hypothesis was that there was something inhibiting them from reinstituting what had worked previously. The initial phase of treatment required the exploration of stressors present in other areas of the system and their possible connection with the parents' now ineffective response to Jay's behavior. This information might provide data regarding any positive function Jay's behavior might be serving for the family.

The degree of anger and frustration the parents expressed toward Jay and their exclusive focus on him suggested he was being scapegoated by the rest of the family. This scapegoat role was used to engage the entire family in treatment. They were told it would be helpful to know how the teenage daughter was coping under the stress of Jay's behavior and what her perspective on the problem was.

The parents were quick to accept this notion, and they assured me their now 16-year-old daughter, Barbara, had suffered greatly at the hands of her brother. He constantly pestered her and often hit her with only the slightest provocation. Interestingly, they noted he was very gentle with his now 2-year-old sister, Kaile, and they seldom had to intervene in this regard.

Intervention with the Family

The initial phase of brief family treatment requires a clear understanding of what the goals for therapy are and how progress toward the goal will be recognized (Fisch et al; 1982). Sometimes this process is rather straightforward when the presenting problems are behavioral in nature, but it is still important to check this with the client as a starting point.

This was done in the first family session with the Boston family. All family members were clear about wanting Jay to behave better, and they had no difficulty operationally defining this goal. They decided they wanted Jay to hit less often, have fewer tantrums, and wanted to receive fewer calls/complaints from his teacher. They would spot improvement by keeping track of the frequency of these behaviors. Improvement on an affective level would be experienced as feeling less anger toward him.

Facilitating Jay's expression of what he hoped to get from the process was more of a challenge. He was not able to offer any ideas about how therapy might benefit him. As noted above, change is risky business, and an oppositional youngster is typically holding a lot of cards. If Jay did not see any incentive for change, his cooperation would be quite hard to enlist. He was not pushed to specify a goal but was told to take whatever time he needed to come up with one. This at least communicated to him that he, too, was expected to gain from this process.

After identifying the family's goals for treatment, the next challenge of the first family session was how to defuse the family's anger since it was taking the form of scapegoating Jay. This was a destructive force, and it functioned to empower him even more by putting him solely in charge of whether or not things changed (another reason to determine what the IP is looking for from therapy). I did not put a lot of pressure on myself to diffuse the scapegoating this first session but instead tried to communicate both directly and indirectly that I would not join the family in blaming Jay (nor anyone else in the family).

Finally, there was the task of deciding on the treatment deadline. We agreed to contract for 12 sessions. This allowed time for exploration of the dynamics of the problem, time to develop an intervention, and time to monitor the effectiveness of the intervention. On a more practical level, it allowed enough time to provide involvement through the remainder of the school year.

The family was quick to agree to the contract even though they did not see the need to have an imposed deadline and would have been willing to agree to more than 12 sessions. This is often the case. At the beginning of treatment, clients frequently have little idea of how long the process should last or how quickly or slowly change will take. As the process proceeds, however, the deadline takes on more significance because they know how much longer the therapy will go on, and it provides them a way to gauge the pace of their progress.

At the start of the second session, Mrs. Boston reported that Jay had behaved rather well since the first one. Early in the course of the second session, it became immediately clear that family members were afraid of the mother's anger. This became evident by Barbara's response to her. Barbara was quite verbal and expressive and offered her opinions freely. When she expressed something that her mother seemed to disagree with, however, Barbara would immediately back off her position. It was readily acknowledged that Barbara and father tiptoed around mother's anger while Jay confronted it head on.

This seemed to be a significant clue to how Jay's behavior might be functioning in the family. It was addressed by invoking Peggy Papp's notion of the consequences of change cited above. I explored with them how Jay's courage in "taking on" his parents (particularly his mother) might have some positive aspect to it. The family seemed perplexed by the prospect that Jay's behavior might be helpful to them in some way and that improvement in his behavior might not be all good news. Each person in the family was assigned the task of identifying what the consequences for each member might be if change were to occur.

At the beginning of the third session, the parents again reported Jay's behavior had been quite good since the last session, and they were pleased with the progress. This observation was met with some wonderment as well as skepticism on my part as change is usually mystifying to me. Although I enjoy pontificating about what precipitates change, I don't know how one can truly determine this with any degree of certainty. In my musings, I wondered if change had been precipitated by Jay's being less scapegoated while the family toyed with the idea of his behavior having some positive connotation.

This session was probably the turning point in the therapy, if there is such a thing. The family had followed through poorly on the assignment described above, and this was being discussed with them. During the course of this discussion, Mrs. Boston became angry with Mr. Boston and raised her voice to him. Almost instantaneously, Jay jumped off his chair, stuck his face in hers, and said something obnoxious. She quickly diverted her attention and anger away from her husband and toward her son.

I immediately said to Jay that he must be a very loyal young man to be willing to protect his parents. He was able to get his father off the hook while still enabling his mother to discharge her anger. It enabled both of them to forget about their conflict for a period of time. I added that the way he did it almost instinctively led me to believe he practiced it often.

The family was taken by surprise, and the anger dissipated instantly. The rest of the session focused on how Jay was able to divert anger in the family via his agitation, and the consequences of giving up his protective instincts were discussed. The parents proclaimed their belief that it was not necessary for Jay to "run interference" for them. Using a question borrowed from Olga Silverstein (1987), I wondered aloud about how they might convince Jay of that. The session ended with the family being asked to monitor instances and methods used by Jay to direct members' anger toward himself to shield others.

Returning to Papp's (1983) view on the three levels of hypothesis development earlier, we can see that gaining some understanding of the emotional aspect of the problem brought a new connotation to the behavior. It enabled me to clarify and enrich the working hypothesis that now took the form that the family had difficulty dealing with open expressions of anger, and Jay was doing his best to be the target because of his belief, at some level, that he could handle it. As the anger intensified in the system, his behavior had to escalate in order to keep the system in balance.

It was now being suggested to the family that Jay's behavior was an attempt to solve a dilemma in the family as opposed to being *the* problem, a concept well developed by Fisch, Weakland, and Segal (1982). The parents could not reinstitute an effective behavioral intervention without confronting anger in the system that did not involve Jay.

Looking Back to Go Forward

During the fourth through sixth sessions, the time was right to move to Papp's ideational level of exploration. It seemed appropriate, in this regard, to expand to a trigenerational focus on themes of emotional expression in each parent's family of origin.

Both parents were adult children of alcoholics. Mrs. Boston's father was an alcoholic, and her family's means of emotional expression bordered on the brink of out of control. There were times when it was literally out of control, and she was physically abused.

Mr. Boston's father was also alcoholic. He was a highly respected professional man who was seen by the community as always available, but the family, especially Mr. Boston, experienced him as never available. Mr. Boston described his father as always working or attending social events. His family was quite guarded and emotionally unexpressive, and if Mrs. Boston's family could be characterized as out of control, Mr. Boston's could be characterized as overcontrolled.

Mr. Boston was the oldest, and he never felt able to measure up to expectations. This feeling persisted into the present. When he experienced how highly regarded his father was in the community, he concluded his father did not pay attention to him because he was "not good enough."

During the course of Mr. Boston's presentation of his family history, it became very clear that his family of origin was an issue in this marriage. The way Mr. Boston and the children were treated by his parents was a source of rage to Mrs. Boston. She was easily aroused when the subject was discussed, and she wanted Mr. Boston to stand up for himself and his family when his parents paid more attention to his siblings' families. She stood by the belief that she had resolved the anger and pain connected with her own past and that her husband would be far better off if he would do the same. Mr. Boston responded by weakly defending his family of origin.

Although the content of these sessions were on the parents' backgrounds, the process was centered on the meta-communication that they had issues the two of them needed to attend to and that did not involve Jay. Much of my work was on challenging Jay's attempts to break the tension between his parents and repeatedly asking the two of them if they needed his help. After a while, Jay began to excuse himself from the room (drinks, bathroom, etc.) when his parents heated up rather than intervene. This began to occur shortly after the parents began taking over my role of challenging Jay's intervention into their conflict.

Jay's older sister, Barbara, then made attempts to take over Jay's job by confronting Mr. Boston on issues in their relationship. These issues clearly needed to be addressed but not at the expense of interfering with the parents' attempts to confront their own issues.

Rediscovering Effective Solutions

The parents decided on their own during the seventh session to make a behavioral management contract with Jay. They selected three target behaviors, success, criterion, and rewards. I expressed some concern about the richness of the incentive ($5.00 per day), but I did not discourage the plan because of their enthusiasm and sense of mutual committment. For the most part, the established contract followed guidelines established during the initial treatment a year before.

After the session, I contacted Jay's teacher, and we established a cost-response system to implement in the classroom. I had chosen to wait to do this because I did not want to shift back to a behavioral focus until the parents communicated some degree of readiness. Their independent move to a behavior plan was a clear sign of readiness.

In Session 8, the family reported the behavior plan during the last session was working very well. The parents noted dramatic improvements in Jay's behavior. It was reported that Barbara was now instigating Jay rather than vice versa, and Barbara expressed how angry and hurt she felt because of feeling neglected by her father. This time it was Mrs. Boston who had to be discouraged from jumping in the middle of Mr. Boston and Barbara. It was agreed that the ninth session would be reserved for the father/daughter dyad.

When the family came together for Session 10, things continued to go well for Jay, and the behavior plan continued to be in effect. Keeping in mind the possible negative consequences of change, I cautioned the family about (1) becoming (unwittingly) more lax in following through with limits and (2) experiencing the need for Jay to act out to give parents something they could agree on.

As the treatment deadline grew closer, Jay's behavior continued to be mainly positive. There was one relapse for a week or so where his behavior deteriorated, and I met with the parents alone for Session 12 to discuss what might be occurring. After reviewing this period with them, it appeared to coincide with a period where Mr. Boston was angry with his wife (due to his relationship with his parents) and was unable to express it.

This session with the marital dyad also focused on facilitating more constructive means of resolving conflict, but the goal was not to resolve their conflict. It was for them to explore together where they typically became stuck and how they might use Jay's behavior as a barometer of when they needed to sit down as a couple to address their issues.

A final session was added to allow for one exclusively devoted to termination. Things continued to go better at home, and the teacher also reported marked improvement. The parents commented on Jay's development of compassion and emotional expression. The family's sense of the process of therapy was reviewed, and the session ended with plans for a checkup 6 months later.

Follow up at 6 months, 12 months, and 2 years found the family doing well. Jay continued to behave well at school, and his academic performance was dramatically improved. At the 1-year follow-up, there was some family stress apparently precipitated by Barbara's preparation to leave for college. She had taken up some of the slack for Jay and had interfered with the parents' conflict about the paternal extended family by reinitiating conflict with her father. I pointed this out and suggested she consult with Jay to learn how to resign the position so she could go off to college and discover her own problems. She apparently did so.

Clinical Issues and Overall Evaluation

The preceding case illustrates one approach to the treatment of behavior problems within a brief therapy model. To review, the treatment started with a direct focus on the presenting problems via a behavioral intervention, but later involved a much more systemic focus. Beginning in this manner did not assume there were no systemic forces/dynamics maintaining the behavior, nor did it presume there were no biological/tempermental contributions to the problem. Further, it did not presume that the parents' management skills were the *cause* of the presenting problems. Rather, it started from the hope that teaching the parents effective discipline strategies would be enough to solve the problem and sought to involve the people most distressed by it. This progression from behavioral to systemic, and back again to behavioral, raises a number of clinical issues that merit further discussion.

Going Shorter Is Not Always Going Faster

When doing brief therapy, it is generally helpful to start the journey by taking the simplest and most direct route. I never cease to be amazed how quickly therapy can proceed when I am able to avoid making things any more complicated than they need to be. However, this case, like many, required additional tools and when starting with a behavioral model, it is always important that you prepare the parents for the possibility other interventions may be needed. Then if the focus needs to be broadened, it communicates a sense of moving on rather than starting over.

The practitioner must keep in mind that there are a number of reasons behavioral interventions can fall short. They can fail, for example, because of parent factors such as parental depression, fatigue, or low self-esteem (Barkley, 1981), and similar factors in the child can produce the same result. The obstacle this case illustrated is one found commonly in the treatment of pediatric behavior disorders (Barkley, 1981). Defiant youngsters can easily become the focal point of the parents' time and energy while increasing stress between them. Thus, even if the etiology of the behavior is not marital conflict, marital issues take a back seat for the couple because there is only time and energy to argue about the problem child. If the child suddenly begins improving his behavior, the parents must be ready for the onslaught of their own issues that have been placed on the back burner. If they are not, the child's behavior generally slides back in and overshadows things again.

When the behavioral approach proved insufficient in this case, the next step was to gather additional information in order to generate a new hypothesis that might explain the blockage. This was done by enlarging the perspective to include dynamic issues pertinent to the maintenance of the problem behaviors. This line of inquiry resulted in an observation leading to the critical event of the therapy.

As mentioned earlier, the critical moment was when I noticed Jay interrupt and deflect the parents' conflict. It was as if the observation momentarily froze time for everyone in the room. Although such moments in therapy are precious and rare, this one became a reference point countless times in later sessions, and it generated the hypothesis that guided the remainder of the process.

Staying the Course

Once the hypothesis was revised to account for the emotional aspects of the problem, the line of inquiry switched to the ideational level. This exploration uncovered pertinent issues in the parents' families of origin, issues that were impacting Jay's presenting problems.

It is always difficult to discern what historical information can be used to guide the process rather than distract it. From the work of Olga Silverstein (1987), I learned the utility of gathering trigenerational information only when tracking a specific theme. Tracking with a narrow focus increases the chances of being able to utilize the data without becoming lost in its richness. With the Boston case, for example, I tried to track issues of family limit setting and conflict resolution as these seemed to be the themes most relevant to the working hypothesis. They revealed salient historical information, including how the families of origin directly stirred conflict in the present generation.

This middle phase was the most difficult part of the therapy for me. I was so tempted to branch off and expand the work, and it would have been easy to make the shift to a less systemic focus. There were a lot of good reasons to become focused, for example, on adult-child-of-alcoholics (ACoA) issues with each of the parents, the marital conflicts, or perhaps a hundred other issues the reader sees that I did not. The driving issue for the family remained Jay's behavior problems despite whatever else might have become a driving issue for me.

Of course the parents' backgrounds could not be ignored, nor could the marital conflict, but the presence of the treatment deadline dissuaded me from straying any further from the behavioral symptoms than absolutely necessary. To stay within the contract and time frame it was critical to discern what aspects of these issues were interfering with the parents' (the complainants) ability to effectively manage Jay's behavior. It was also important to keep in mind during the marital session that I had been hired to address Jay's behavior problem, not their marriage. The hypothesis was that Jay's behavior functioned to keep them from confronting the marital issues, but there was no evidence yet to suggest they had to resolve their issues for Jay's behavior to improve or that they could not resolve their issues if Jay's behavior did get better.

When working with behavior problems and with families, it is too often assumed that everything we come across that is out of tune must be a critical part of the presenting problems. We presume that everything related to the problem must be fixed before treatment is terminated. We assume that our intervention is needed in each aspect of the system. These assumptions too often overlook people's ability to independently reorganize around change in a positive way. Challenging these presumptions has helped me adjust my sights regarding what people are looking for when they enter therapy. People are not generally seeking a make over. They are seeking relief from pain. They are seeking it as quickly as possible with as *little change* as possible.

The Boston family eventually determined what action to take in order to hold Jay accountable for his behavior. They decided when they should institute it. They were freed to attempt to resolve their marital differences unimpeded. They apparently did so to their satisfaction. Had they not been able to do so, a new contract could have been negotiated.

How Short Is Short Enough?

The course of therapy could probably have been shorter than it was. Jay's behavior actually improved considerably from the start, and by the time the parents established a new behavior contract with him, things were going very well. It could be argued that the treatment could have terminated by Session 8, whereas others would argue that the work that occurred after the presenting problems had subsided increased the probability that the improvements were stabilized. These kinds of things can never be determined in retrospect. Apparently Mr. and Mrs. Boston believed that it was not time to stop after the eighth session. Another couple might have.

I was concerned that the therapy was ending too soon. I was worried there were too many unresolved issues in the marital system for the parents to stay vigilant with Jay's behavior. I was worried that the ACoA issues would inhibit them from moving forward. There is always unfinished work when people leave therapy, and it's often hard to let go of the felt responsibility to make it all better.

The Essence of Brevity?

It is easy to read case studies about brief treatment and think of all the cases where it can't work. There are, however, plenty of cases where it can. My goal now is to approach cases with the belief they are short-term, unless I am presented with compelling evidence to dissuade that notion.

In this case example, the parents were able to take the behavioral techniques and manage the problem effectively for a year. They were also able to come back and share their need for a different approach. When they returned, the focus of the therapy became what stood in their way of coming up with their own solution or returning to the one they previously found effective. Once the presenting problems lessened, they were able to tackle some significant family issues using their own resources.

I think of this case as illustrative of a number of facets of time-limited work with this population. Doing therapy briefly with youngsters presenting with oppositional behavior generally requires working simultaneously with both static and dynamic elements of the problem. One element involves the application of technology in the form of behavioral interventions. The technology provides a method to the parents, that is to say, a concrete "how-to" guide. The work also requires the art of tracking the process of implementing new technology in an active system, and the actual therapy generally involves weaving back and forth between the technology and the process.

Such an art requires developing the practice of intensely tracking what people are communicating through words and actions. It suggests that one must be vigilant in pursuit of understanding what is going on. I know I have done this well when a critical moment is witnessed and shared with those present. When I first became interested in practicing brief therapy, I perceived a magical element. I thought it was about speeding up an otherwise slow process. I was frightened I could never become a magician. What I have learned through practice is that it is simply a different process.

Brief therapy is about staying focused on the problems presented and on the process. The process of brief therapy requires not pursuing the seemingly endless tributaries that branch off from the presenting problems but of carefully selecting what information to attend and what not to. One can make a cogent argument for following virtually any of these tributaries. One can worry incessantly about whether something important is being overlooked in order to shorten the therapy process. One can quickly get lost when trying to follow all of them.

REFERENCES

American Psychiatric Association. (1987). *Diagnostic and statistical manual of mental disorders* (3rd ed.—revised). Washington, DC: Author.

Barkley, R. (1981). *Hyperactive children: A handbook for diagnosis and treatment*. New York: Guilford.

Fisch, R., Weakland, J., & Segal, L. (1982). *Tactics of change: Doing therapy briefly.* San Francisco: Jossey-Bass.

Papp, P. (1983). *The process of change*. New York: Guilford.

Patterson, G. (1976). The aggressive child: Victim and architect of a coercive system. In E. J. Mash, L. A. Hamerlynck, & L. C. Handy (Eds.), *Behavior modification and families* (pp. 267–316). New York: Brunner/Mazel.

Silverstein, O. (1987). The art of systems therapy: Therapeutic choices of Olga Silverstein. Workshop presentation at Ackerman Institute, New York, NY, October 23 and 24, 1987.

20

Brief Family Therapy with a Low-Socioeconomic Family

Gregory K. Popchak and Richard A. Wells

Introduction

Historically brief family therapy has been one of the most fertile areas in the development of short-term treatment methodology. The seminal contributions of such theorists and practitioners as Jay Haley (1963, 1976), Salvador Minuchin and associates (1967, 1974), and Paul Watzslawick (1967, 1974) have not only influenced and shaped the principles and strategies of brief family therapy, but they have exerted an important effect on therapeutic practice in general. Other significant influences include the work of Alexander and Parsons (1985), Morawetz and Walker (1984), as well as the many publications emanating from the Milwaukee Brief Family Therapy Center (for example, de Shazer, 1985, 1988; O'Hanlon & Weiner-Davis, 1990).

In addition to its immediate emphasis on changing family interactions, brief strategic/structural family therapy, particularly in the work of Minuchin and his colleagues at the Philadelphia Child Guidance Clinic, has been interested in developing therapeutic tactics appropriate for work with poor and disadvantaged client populations. Few other therapies have shown such an interest. This chapter will describe work with a

---

Gregory K. Popchak • Family and Personal Consultation Network, 117 Opal Boulevard, Steubenville, Ohio 43592. Richard A. Wells • School of Social Work, University of Pittsburgh, Pittsburgh, Pennsylvania 15260.

Casebook of the Brief Psychotherapies, edited by Richard A. Wells and Vincent J. Giannetti. Plenum Press, New York, 1993.

low-SES family and will attempt to explicate not only the particular character of their problems but some of the therapeutic strategies most helpful in work with this client population

CASE HISTORY

Presenting Problem

Anthony G. Jr. (little Tony), age 9, was brought to the brief family therapy center of a large urban mental health clinic for assessment after his father, Anthony Sr., had placed a call to the scheduling office. The father stated that the relationship between him and little Tony had reached a head and reported that the youngster lies, steals, swears, and refuses to follow parental authority. The precipitating event was an incident in which the father and mother found more than $80 in a bingo apron under their son's mattress. The parents disagreed as to how to handle the situation, and the mother finally took the money to a local department store to pay off a lay-a-way she had placed there. Though both parents say they know "that probably wasn't right," both also minimized the incident. The mother, for example, denied that Tony knew he was stealing from the church, saying that she believed him when he said someone left it someplace and he found it.

The father reported having difficult with Tony from the time he was 3 years old. Mr. G. responds to these problems by spanking Tony with his hand or with a belt. He also reported that sometimes he feels out of control with his child though further probing determined that this was most likely related to the father's own difficulties with panic disorder than to any question of him physically abusing his son.

The mother disagreed with her husband's style of discipline saying that when there are difficulties with little Tony she prefers to "yell and ground him." On the other hand, she does believe that she is too lenient with him. The mother also reported that Tony has exhibited a series of "obsessions" (her words, NOT a diagnosis) since the age of 3. The first of these was with popular music, his favorite being the hit record "Wooley-Bully." Little Tony would ask his parents to play this number over and over and would also sleep with the record by his side. The next "obsession" was with playing cards, whereas the most recent was with sports and money. It is important to note, however, that these so-called obsessions match the parents' own periodic interests and concerns. For example, Tony's interest in records coincided with the father's former work as a disk jockey at local dances. Likewise, Tony's recent preoccupation with money coincided with the father's placement on Social Security Disability for serious panic attacks and a consequent downturn in the family's financial status.

Family Background

The identified patient, Tony G. Jr., is a 9-year-old white male of Italian-American descent, who shares a room in the family's small and crowded house with his 10-year-old sister Tiffany. His mother is 30 years old, the father is 34, and they have been married for 10 years. The parents volunteered that they married because the mother was pregnant with Tiffany. Further significant information about the immediate family and the parents' respective families of origin was gathered by constructing a genogram during the initial interview.

Gathering data for the genogram was essentially utilized as a joining device, as well as for the historical information revealed. As the latter suggests, there is a considerable history of significant medical and psychiatric problems in Mr. G.'s family of origin. These include an alcoholic father, a mother in treatment for depression, a sister with panic disorder and agrophobia, and another sister with depression. The family shared a number of medical problems including hiatal hernias, high blood pressure, "Mediterranean blood disorder," and a sister with Epstein-Barre syndrome. The father himself had been placed on Social Security Disability in 1985 for panic disorder and, in addition, he had been previously hospitalized for somatization disorder at the same mental health center where the family were now being seen for little Tony's problems.

Within the mother's family of origin, she described an older brother with panic disorder and a younger brother involved in severe drug and alcohol abuse who committed suicide a year ago. Mrs. G. herself was in reasonably good health but is 4 months into an unplanned, unexpected pregnancy. Little Tony had never been in therapy before but suffered from asthma and from allergies to cat hair, dust mites, and down feathers. His sister, Tiffany, on the other hand, had no reported medical or psychiatric history.

The parents described an essentially normal developmental history for Tony. He was walking with assistance at 14 months, spoke his first words at 18 months, and was toilet-trained at approximately 2 years of age. There were no difficulties as he entered school, and Mr. and Mrs. G. stated that his grades were satisfactory, typically Bs, with some As. They reported that he had age-appropriate friendships and usually gets along well with his peers. Likewise the mother and father described

Tony's alleged "obsessions" as abating spontaneously and, as previously noted, directly coinciding with the parents' own interests and worries.

Diagnostic and Assessment Interview

The initial interview began with the father's marked distress over the use of a one-way mirror (and an observing team) in the assessment room. He was not mollified by any proffered explanation until the clinician offered to bring the family behind the mirror to meet the team. Mr. G. decided he did not want to go behind the mirror but only after little Tony decided that *he* would like to do so. (In subsequent sessions the father would typically show some initial concern if observers were present but not to any undue degree.)

Following this initial difficulty, the interview progressed smoothly. The parent's interview revealed much of the current and historical information presented earlier in this chapter. As might be expected, the father was antagonistic and critical toward both his wife and his son. On her part, the mother tended to defer to her husband while, at the same time, interjecting many protective comments about little Tony. Both parents spoke of their frustrations in the marriage, their inability to parent together, and the stress of an unplanned pregnancy that was exacerbating the financial pressures they were already experiencing.

The interview with Tony was also a smooth process as he appeared eager to please and willing to talk. He was very interested in sports and discussed his television viewing habits with the clinician saying, "If nuttin' else is on I'll watch tennis! You know all that stupid stuff." At no point did he appear to be obsessive-compulsive in either his sports interests or in his understandable concerns about money.

In response to questions, he reported being sometimes confused as to what his parents wanted him to do at a given moment. Similarly, he reported being unsure about why he got into trouble when he did, except when it came to him and his sister fighting—this, he knew, was "wrong." He did not deny specific incidents related to him by the clinician, was able to sit still during the interview, and did not exhibit depressed symptomatology nor suicidal or homicidal ideation. Likewise, he denied psychotic episodes, and his parents confirmed this. The clinician asked Tony what three wishes he might have, but he could only think of two: that he could play for the local baseball team in the major-league playoffs and that he would never marry because "girls are fat and ugly and got pimples."

Because of the obvious stressors that could be related to an unplanned pregnancy, the increasingly precarious financial situation of the family, and the apparent increase in tension between the two parents, it was felt that Tony's primary diagnosis on the DSM-III-R would be Adjustment Disorder with Mixed Emotion and Conduct, in addition to Parent–Child Problems (American Psychiatric Association, 1985).

The family agreed with the clinician that family therapy would be an appropriate model for treatment. Further, the assessing clinician promised them that the case would be assigned to him. The family contracted for six sessions of intervention, with an option to continue based upon a review at the end of these six sessions. Despite their agreement to family therapy, the family was somewhat confused about how Tony's behavior could possibly be connected to anything interpersonal. However, they agreed to the notion presented by the therapist that keeping everyone together would be beneficial in that all the family could learn ways to maintain the changes that therapy would bring about in Tony's behavior.

Course of Treatment

Following the framework suggested by Alexander and Parsons (1985) the process of treatment can be seen as falling into three major phases: (1) *assessment*, in which the therapist enters into the family and develops appropriate targets for change; (2) *therapy*, in which therapeutic interventions are initiated and refined; and (3) *education*, in which the family learn specific skills to help them maintain change.

In the early treatment sessions, the family further discussed their apprehension about things ever getting better, a viewpoint that was especially true of the father. The therapist's efforts in these beginning sessions were primarily directed toward moving the discussion away from blaming and toward the solution-oriented question, "How will things be when they are 'better'?" but initially succeeded only in confusing the family further. This was especially the case with Mr. G. who had a much more fixed, negative view than any other family member and, because of his extensive experiences in individual therapy, was unused to the pragmatic, cooperative ambience of family treatment. However, by the third session the family were finally able to list a series of positive goals that were as follows:

1. The parents will learn ways to work together as a team.
2. The children will decrease the bickering between each other.
3. The children will increase compliance to parental directions.

Other goals, such as Tony and Tiffany becoming more interested in engaging in family activities, were discussed and kept as "bonus goals."

That is, their accomplishment would depend upon the completion of the three goals listed above that the family had rated as more important.

During these early sessions, both Mr. and Mrs. G. frequently complained about feeling out of control with their children, and these perceptions were a key area of focus as treatment moved more distinctly into what Alexander and Parsons characterize as the therapy stage. It was apparent that they undermined each other's authority and that, for the mother particularly, being liked was more important than being effective as a parent. Mr. G., for his part, felt he could do nothing as a parent until things got so bad that he simply couldn't stand the way his wife was handling it anymore. At such a point he would then jump in, yell at everyone, occasionally spank the children and send them to their room. Following such an episode the parents would typically argue further about what had happened and whether this was appropriate disciplinary action.

Using relational tracking (Alexander & Parsons, 1985) and reframing (Bandler & Grinder, 1982; Minuchin & Fishman, 1981), the therapist noted that the children tended to bicker to distract the parents and to bring the father into the family interactional system. This pattern was highlighted by the therapist but framed in such a way that the parents were made to see that they had very intelligent and perceptive children and, further, that they (the parents) were their children's teachers. Continuing to use this frame the therapist pointed out that the father and mother can, and indeed *do*, control their children's behavior by the information (i.e., the parental relationship) that they presented to them.

Mr. and Mrs. G. were both heartened and saddened by this reframing, saying that they didn't realize they had such an impact on their children and that it made them feel good to know that they had taught their children many good things. Still, it saddened them to think that they could have taught their children negative things as well. Utilizing Minuchin's strategy of mood manipulation (Minuchin & Fishman, 1981), the therapist agreed with them but heightened their reaction by emphasizing, "And that's what it is to be a parent." He went on to elaborate that all parents give their children their best and worst at times. What made Mr. and Mrs. G., specifically, better than average parents, however, was that they were willing to learn from their mistakes, and that was something to be proud of.

In order to further increase the parent's awareness of the relationship between the children's bickering and their own conflict, a boxing metaphor was presented. This involved the notion of taking off the gloves, giving them to the children, and the parent's assuming referee garb. In relation to this, Mr. and Mrs. G. were assigned the task of monitoring when they themselves fought and the children's reaction to this conflict. Strategically this task was designed both to heighten their awareness of this interactional pattern and—through their assuming the referee role—implicitly suggesting that they could be in charge of their own family.

As the sessions in the therapy stage continued, it also became apparent that fighting served an important function in the family as it was one of the few things they all did together. They agreed to this and added that it was a pretty lousy way of being together. The therapist concurred and gave them a choice—they could decide that they really enjoyed arguing as a family and learn to do it better and more often, or they could come back to the following session with a list of possible activities they could do together instead of fighting.

The family did indeed return to the next interview with a list of things to do. These included taking drives together, going to McDonald's, watching television (especially athletic events), and playing cards and outdoor sports. However, also on the list was arguing, as they felt that it was both important to argue sometime and unrealistic to think that one could extinguish arguing completely. In this latter regard, the family was commended on their insight, especially since the therapist had secretly feared that in the previous session he had given them the impression that they should expect to never argue again. Subsequent sessions then concentrated on making the alternative "being-together" options workable and, at the same time, finding more efficient and productive ways of arguing.

The family was pleased to accept that they could do other things together rather than arguing for its own sake. They could now get on to the business of resolving some of the disputes that, previously and realistically, were the only thing holding them together. In short, the family had formerly believed that if they stopped arguing, they would cease to function as a family and, as a consequence, arguments could not be resolved. Having freed themselves up to engage in other activities as a family, the parents and children could now solve their problems, something that heretofore would have threatened their existence as a family.

Throughout the remainder of the therapy phase both relational tracking and reframing were used to define more specifically the functions served by certain of the problematic behaviors of the family. In this case it was hypothesized, and later confirmed, that the function within the G. family of the arguing behavior was what Alexander and Parsons characterize as "merging." In their terminology, merging is concerned with behaviors that "increase psychological intensity, . . . opportunities for interaction, and . . . strengthen contacts that would otherwise decrease" (Alexander & Parsons, 1985, pp. 18–19). The deciding factor in this analysis was when the therapist attempted to track what the family did together as a family, the members were at a loss to describe a single thing but, in the process, the family erupted in a heated argument.

In other words, the family's frequent arguments served as a method not only to get them in the same room together but also provided an atmosphere in which to share emotionality and psychological intensity. Further, it became evident that the children's bickering served a similar merging function for the parents, who frequently spent time apart from each other even though, due to the father being on disability, they were in the same house all day.

In the final stage of treatment—the education phase—the family addressed new behaviors to fulfill the merging function previously served by arguing. To achieve this, they were taught a method of problem solving that draws from what Bandler and Grinder (1982) and Cameron-Bandler (1985) have called the "six-step reframing" process, a family-oriented version of D'Zurilla and Goldfried's (1971) structured problem solving. In this method, the family members are taught to identify the problem, settle on a goal or function of the problem (i.e., answering the question "What are we trying to do here?"), brainstorm a variety of creative—if not always workable—options, evaluate these options for feasibility and desirability, and, finally, act on an option.

Once learned, the process becomes easily integrated and generalized throughout the family's attempts at problem solving. In this case, the G. family decided that in addition to solving problems instead of arguing about them, they would go out to eat at McDonald's once a week, watch television together in the evenings, talk about the shows and daily events, and take drives on Sundays. It is important to note that this problem-solving method could not be transplanted into the family system until all members had accepted the positive reframes offered in the earlier phase of treatment. This is necessary because, until the reframes are accepted, the family is usually in a "blaming mode" that is counterproductive to problem solving.

Follow-Up

All told, the family had 13 sessions (including the initial interview) with the clinician, as the agreement to recontract at the end of 6 sessions was exercised. Two follow-up visits, spaced a month apart, were utilized to follow their progress. In the follow-up sessions, the parents reported that they felt more in control of themselves and the children and were looking forward to showing the new baby their "new family." Little Tony and Tiffany still bickered, but the tone was different, and the parents were more comfortable in handling this situation together. Likewise, the father still needed "space" and some time to himself but reported that he felt more connected to his family and that he and his wife argued less. Finally, all family members believed that the arguments that did arise solved more problems than they created.

The family was discharged from treatment after the second follow-up session with thanks from the therapist for their hard work and committment. He invited them to call if they ever saw themselves as needing a "booster shot" or if they wanted help in becoming "even better than they already are."

Clinical Issues and Discussion

In work with low-socioeconomic, disorganized families, several key factors must be addressed, at both the point of initial engagement and during the course of therapeutic intervention. These relate to the fact that such families are frequently viewed by the clinician as "resistant" or "unmotivated" and that, on the part of the family, the treating professional is seen as cold, distant, or simply incomprehensible. This suggests that the clinician must utilize a present-oriented framework, explained to the family in clear, nontechnical language that emphasizes the legitimacy and validity of the family's current needs and strengths. In the latter regard, it is essential to look persistently for opportunities to reframe the therapeutic relationship as one in which the family members are the experts and the therapist is a guide or consultant who wants to assist them in utilizing themselves more positively.

Brief family treatment from such a currently focused and competency-based orientation is especially suited to the low-SES family as perhaps their major available resources is themselves and their extended family and friendship network. As the work with the G. family illustrates, an essential portion of the early phase of treatment is devoted to helping the parental figures feel as if they are in control of their family. This is especially important with low-SES families who commonly (and often realistically) perceive themselves as having little or no power over their lives. The currently popular term *empowering* may be nebulous, but specific techniques such as accessing resource states (Cameron-Bandler, 1985) or looking for exceptions (de Shazer, 1985, 1988; O'Hanlon & Weiner-Davis, 1990) offer a means of convincing parents that they can effect and maintain change.

Clinicians can find the volatility and apparent disorganization of these families as an uncomfortable and unsettling context in which to conduct therapy. The early sessions with the G. family, for example, were marked by a great deal of confusion, and heated disputes were common. Yet, as Minuchin and his associates (1967) have repeatedly emphasized, for members of the low-SES family much of their life *is* literally out of their control and their seeming chaos is reflective of this accurate perception. For example, as work began with the G. family, their furniture was repossessed, an event not immediately relevant to the treatment but one that undoubtedly impacted on their perception of an arbitrary and uncertain world. The power such families do have they are often afraid to exercise, or exercise only in an all-or-nothing manner—fluctuating between periods of passive confusion and attempts at rigid control.

The reader will also note that an integral aspect of treatment with the G. family was the persistent and pervasive use of reframing, a technique that has been developed to the state of a fine art in brief family therapy. In a perhaps apocryphal story, Virginia Satir was said to have been working with a family who reported a quarrel in which the husband chased the wife with knife in hand but did not catch her; Satir reframed this incident as indicative of the husband's desire to be closer to his wife. In more recent literature, Beck (1988) makes extensive use of reframing in his adaptation of cognitive therapy to couples and teaches the marital pair to look at the flipside of the behavior of which they are complaining. Couples who learn reframing can then begin to remember that, for example, the procrastination that their spouse practices was originally seen by them as "free-spiritedness." Bandler and Grinder's (1982) volume suggests that reframing is best done by looking for either the positive intention that underlies a behavior or for a context in which the behavior is appropriate.

The earlier description of treatment included many examples of this strategy, but other key reframes with the G. family included helping the father to understand that the mother's "undermining his authority" was her way of asking him to help her parent the children BEFORE she exploded. Thus, it was not a provocation so much as a signal of needing his help. The mother, on the other hand, was able to understand that the father's whining and withdrawal from parenting was actually an attempt to get her to encourage his involvement and his sense of paternal worth. Likewise, the parents were both encouraged to see that the children's bickering was really an attempt to get the parents working together on something.

Another important transaction occurred a few sessions into the therapy phase when the therapist challenged the family to decide whether they wanted to learn how to fight effectively or whether they would develop a list of activities they could engage in rather than fighting. This was intended not only as a paradoxical intervention but, ultimately it was intended to assess the most respectful and ecological solution for the family. If the family chose to continue fighting ("because every family needs to fight," as they had asserted earlier), the therapist would have agreed and then presented more effective ways of fighting. This would be framed as, "You are absolutely correct, it is important to fight, and you would probably agree that since you find it important to do, you want to be good at it—here's how" as a prelude to a move into work on clearer communication and structured problem-solving methods. Whichever of the alternatives chosen by the family, the therapeutic response is the same.

However, we do not want to convey that brief intervention with a low-SES family (or families at any social-status level) is simply a matter of prodding them into action through the artful use of reframing. Reframing is certainly a useful tool in presenting alternative viewpoints to a family, but it must be employed in conjunction with a real sense of respect, on the therapist's part, for the values, beliefs, and style of living integral to the client family. This is especially important with low-SES families, who may have rather different norms about many facets of family life (and radically different living environments) than the typically middle-class clinician. Similarly, Morawetz and Walker (1984), in their work with single-parent families, which are common in the low-SES population, speak of the need to "depathologize" such families so that they are not regarded by clinicians from a negative perspective but are seen as having assets and capability. To adapt and paraphrase one of Morawetz and Walker's key points to the present discussion: The fact that many low-SES families have different beliefs and norms than their higher-SES counterparts does not make them automatically inferior, and a good deal of helpful and positive clinical intervention can be achieved within the context of their lifestyle.

References

Alexander, J., & Parsons, B. (1985). *Functional family therapy.* Monterey, CA: Brooks/Cole.

American Psychiatric Association (1985). *Diagnostic and statistical manual* (3rd ed. revised). Washington, DC: Author.

Bandler, J., & Grinder, B. (1982). *Reframing: Neuro-linguistic programming and the transformation of meaning*. Moab, Utah: Real People Press.

Beck, A. (1988). *Love is never enough.* New York: Harper & Row.

Cameron-Bandler, L. (1985). *Solutions*. San Rafael, CA: Futurepace Inc.

D'Zurilla, T. J., & Goldfried, M. R. (1971). Problem solving and behavior modification. *Journal of Abnormal Psychology, 78*, 107–126.

de Shazer, S. (1985). *Keys to solution in brief therapy.* New York: Norton.

de Shazer, S. (1988). *Clues: Investigating solutions in brief therapy.* New York: Norton.

Haley, J. (1963). *Strategies of psychotherapy.* New York: Grune & Stratton.

Haley, J. (1976). *Problem-solving therapy.* San Francisco: Jossey-Bass.

Minuchin, S. (1974). *Families and family therapy.* Cambridge: Harvard University Press.

Minuchin, S., & Fishman, H. C. (1981). *Family therapy techniques*. Cambridge: Harvard University Press.

Minuchin, S., Montalvo, B., Guerney, B. G., Rosman, B., & Schumer, F. (1967). *Families of the slums*. New York: Basic Books.

Morawetz, A., & Walker, G. (1984). *Brief therapy with single-parent families*. New York: Brunner/Mazel.

O'Hanlon, W. H., & Weiner-Davis, M. (1990). *In search of solutions: A new direction in psychotherapy.* New York: Norton.

Watzslawick, P., Beavin, J. H., & Jackson, D. D. (1967). *Pragmatics of human communication*. New York: Norton.

Watzslawick, P., Weakland, J., & Fisch, R. (1974). *Change: Principles of problem formulation and problem resolution*. New York: Norton.

21

Creating Opportunities for Rapid Change in Marital Therapy

Barry L. Duncan

Introduction

Perhaps solely by virtue of bringing an additional person into the therapeutic context, marital therapy may be the most challenging of clinical practice. The dramatic intensity with which couples may present, the polarization of their viewpoints, and the difficulty inherent in validating each person's perspective without disconfirming the other's can offer a humbling experience to the most seasoned of therapists.

This chapter presents a marital therapy case example from an evolving strategic perspective that eclectically expands the Mental Research Institute (MRI) (Fisch, Weakland, & Segal, 1982; Watzlawick, Weakland, & Fisch, 1974) model by emphasizing the importance of the therapeutic alliance and focusing on meaning and experience revision, as well as behavior change (Duncan, Parks, & Rusk, 1990; Duncan, Solovey, & Rusk, 1992). This brief, technical, eclectic approach attempts to empower common factor effects, as well as direct the parsimonious and selective application of technique from a variety of therapy models (Duncan et al., 1992).

Barry L. Duncan • Dayton Institute for Family Therapy, 65 West Franklin Street, Centerville, Ohio 45459.

Casebook of the Brief Psychotherapies, edited by Richard A. Wells and Vincent J. Giannetti. Plenum Press, New York, 1993.

A "process constructive" theoretical foundation provides the overarching framework for intervention. Process is defined in three ways. A "process"-level system is a meaning-generating system of dynamic social exchange through which individuals accommodate or assimilate ongoing variation in the environment (Buckley, 1967). Marital therapy, then, represents a "system" of interaction involving an exchange of meaning through conversation that inevitably revises as variability or new information is added by the therapist or clients.

A second view of process is provided by the MRI perspective of repetitive solution attempts revolving around the presenting problem; that is, the problem "process." Problems occur as part of a vicious cycle of attempts to adjust or adapt to variation. Based on the individual and shared meanings about the problem or how to solve it, people will try variations on a theme of the same solution pattern over and over again. The solution, in essence, becomes the problem (Watzlawick et al., 1974).

A final definition of process is provided by Held's (1991) content/"process" distinction. Held describes process as the strategies of change; process embodies one's theory of how change occurs (Held, 1991). Content, in contrast, is the object of the change process (Prochaska & DiClemente, 1982). As with other strategically oriented approaches, the current perspective attempts to refrain from imposing explanations predetermined by formal theoretical content and instead attempts to emphasize process, allowing the question of content and the goal of therapy to be determined by each client in each idiosyncratic situation.

A constructivist view (the other component of the theoretical foundation) suggests that reality is invented, not discovered (Watzlawick, 1984) and is evident only through constructed meanings that shape and organize experience. Meaning is generated via the individual's interaction in the social environment and/or its covert rehearsal or internal processing.

The different perspectives of process reflect the flexibility of eclecticism, an emphasis on the interpersonal system of the therapeutic relationship, and a focus on the problem presentation itself. All three descriptions comprise a formal theory that allows for maximum incorporation of the idiosyncratic presentation of the client. Constructivism reinforces a content-free perspective and provides a rationale for the outright primacy of the client's experience, internal frame of reference, and goals in therapy.

The process constructive theoretical foundation permits the acceptance of the frame of reference of the client as hierarchically superior to the formal theory content of the therapist. This process-oriented approach is translated to clinical application by way of three descriptions of how change occurs. One description views strategy as promoting an interruption of the behavioral interaction that constitutes the problem cycle. In MRI terms, strategy entails interdiction of the repetitively misapplied solution attempts of the client and others with whom he or she interacts so that the problem cycle is jammed and a new cycle of behavioral interaction can ensue.

Another description views strategy as promoting meaning revision, either in the interview process or in the client's interactive experience of the problem. Meaning revision in the interview process involves the conversational recreation of the client's experience and the collaborative generation of new or altered meaning. Meaning revision between sessions is encouraged by the therapist's suggestion of competing experiences (interventions, homework assignments).

Still another description views strategy as an extension of the relationship context into the client's social environment. Interventions are explicit therapist behaviors that demonstrate empathy, respect, and genuineness, and validate directly the client's meaning and experience regarding the concern under question. Change occurs as a result of interventions that extend the alliance and the validation context it represents.

CASE IDENTIFICATION AND PRESENTING COMPLAINTS: SETTING THE CONTEXT

Marital therapy offers a variety of options regarding entry points into the couple's problematic experiences. To maximize the opportunities for rapid change, it is helpful to set the context for marital therapy by interviewing the couple together *and* separately. Treatment begins by obtaining an initial problem statement from each individual with the couple together. If there appears to be agreement regarding what the problem is, the therapist may continue gathering information and discussing the marital problems with both individuals present. If there is immediate disagreement regarding the problem or its description, or there appears to be tension between the couple that is preventing an open exchange of views, then it's better to split the couple and proceed with the interview separately.

Regardless of how smoothly the interview is going, it is still important to see each individual separately. Couples usually respond favorably and seem to understand the utility of separate interviews. The therapist simply explains that he or she would like to see each separately and asks which one prefers to go first. This allows the person most distressed to gain "airtime" with the therapist immediately.

Seeing the couple separately has several advantages. It allows the therapist access to an unedited and uncensored description of each individual's perspective regarding the relationship and its problems. Through the presentation of the problem, clients also present their frame of reference, or meaning system to the therapist. Therapeutic awareness of the meanings associated with the problem experience enables the therapist to not only accept those meanings but also to work within the frame of reference of the client. Seeing couples separately also enables the therapist to validate each person's perspective without concern for alienating the other person. Finally, separate interviews allow the opportunity for intervention with both individual's contribution to the marital problem, as well as the ability to address the individual desires of each person.

After the individual interviews, the couple is reunited, and the therapist may share any impressions or suggestions that have arisen from the interview process. It is explained to the couple that each session will contain both individual and couple aspects. Such a therapeutic structure enables three different sets of opportunities to promote rapid change. The marital problems may be altered by virtue of either person initiating a change in the problematic patterns of interaction (Duncan & Rock, 1991), or by the couple acting in concert to address a particular area of concern.

Alice and David were referred to marital therapy by David's company's EAP. The EAP counselor suggested that they needed more in-depth work than the EAP could provide. They were in their early 30s, had been married 7 years, and had two children, ages 1 and 2. The initial problem statement given by David was that he was ambivalent about staying in the marriage and was unsure of his feelings for Alice. Alice reported that she was confused about what David was upset about and wanted to learn how they may communicate more effectively.

Background Information: Describing the Problem and Understanding Its Meaning

The interview is designed to elicit information regarding the vicious cycle of unsuccessful solution attempts surrounding the presenting marital problems. What is first sought is a concrete, action-oriented description specifically addressing the MRI question, "*Who* is doing *what* that presents a problem, to *whom*, and *how* does such a behavior constitute a problem?" (Fisch et al., 1982, p. 70). *How* is particularly important because it directly leads the therapist into the client's experience of the problem and helps define the aspect of the problem that the intervention should address. Additionally, a workable goal is needed. This interactive description (the problem and its solutions) allows for the design of interventions to interrupt the problem process and permit an alternative solution.

Through the detailed pursuit of the presenting problem, the client's attempted solutions, and minimal therapy goals, the content of the problem is thoroughly explored and other descriptions, connections, implications, and distinctions can emerge (Goolishian & Anderson, 1987). Background information is relevant to the degree that it is client-initiated and provides the therapist with the content of what the *client* views as important to the maintenance of the marital problem. The client's presented content identifies the client's idiosyncratic experience of the problem and helps identify the goals for treatment.

The interview itself represents an attempt to construct a frame surrounding the client's presenting problem that allows for problem resolution to occur. Clients unfold the content of their lives, their meaning system that organizes their perceptions and experiences. Therapist questions create a changeable problem definition and facilitate the generation of new meaning.

David volunteered to be interviewed first and said that, from the beginning, he felt as if he was the one who gave more to the relationship. He especially noticed his lack of feeling for Alice after the birth of their second child about a year previously.

Questions aimed at what David's feelings of ambivalence were about and how his marriage was troubled led to David defining the problem as Alice's "inability to communicate about the relationship and her insensitivity to his feelings." According to David, Alice never talked about the relationship. Moreover, she seemed to lack a general sensitivity to David's feelings and was unable to be supportive of him emotionally. David believed that Alice suffered from an emotional deficit resulting from her experiences in her family of origin.

When asked what an indication would be that things were beginning to turn in the right direction, David said that Alice would be willing to discuss the relationship and would openly share her feelings, as well as attempt to understand his feelings. David's attempts to address the lack of communication and insensitivity to his feelings were characterized by open expression of his concerns, followed by criticism of Alice's inadequate response, and finally followed by avoidance of Alice and withdrawal from household and child-care responsibilities.

Alice was resentful of David's persistent discontent and reported that it seemed as if she couldn't do anything right. She didn't understand what David wanted, but hastened to add that it was probably her fault for not figuring it out. In her view, David expected her to handle the kids all day and be waiting for him with open arms *and* legs when he arrived home. Alice noted a communication problem but described the problem as David's attacks and criticisms of her. He often criticized her, calling her an emotionless robot, as well as other accusations of her not being in touch with his or her feelings. Alice said that she was beginning to believe that there was something wrong with her.

Alice reported that David also criticized other things and she felt intimidated by him in conversations because he always seemed to be in control. Alice noted that if David would stop criticizing her and allow her to communicate at her own pace and in her own way, then she would know that things were improving. She also added that if David would help her with the house or kids without being asked, it would also be an indication of improvement. Alice's solutions included telling David that she didn't like being criticized, defending and justifying her behavior, and crying. She had also tried an assertiveness training class with similar results.

Diagnostic and Assessment Interview: Describing the Problem, Revising Its Meaning, and Validating the Client's Experience

The pursuit of an interactional description of the marital concerns was itself part of a process that constructed a frame around the problem that enabled opportunities for the therapist to pursue. The interview with David redefined the problem from a lack of feeling for Alice, to a dissatisfaction with her communication difficulties and emotional insensitivity. Two opportunities arose from the interview: one involved the problem cycle of David's attempts (criticism and withdrawal) to gain communication and support from Alice; The other involved David's view of Alice as emotionally deficient. Two avenues for change also emerged from the interview with Alice: one pertaining to the problem cycle of Alice's attempts (defending, justifying, etc.) to decrease David's criticisms; the other involving Alice's view that she didn't and couldn't understand what David wanted from her.

The interview, however, is more than eliciting information or the quest for meaning revision opportunities. The first interview is the principal medium through which the therapist defines the nature of the relationship as one that is empathic, respectful, and genuine as perceived by the client. The relationship is also defined as one in which an inherent therapeutic goal is to validate the client's experience and replace the invalidation that sometimes accompanies clients to therapy.

Recall Alice's belief that she should have figured out what David wanted and her own invalidating comment that maybe David was right about her incapability of real emotion. The therapist highlighted all the ways that Alice had tried to provide what David wanted and how her attempts were largely met with rejection and withdrawal. The therapist commented that no wonder Alice was at a loss for what to do. If she did attempt to communicate, it was not done the right way; if she did not attempt to communicate, then David criticized her for not communicating enough. Alice was literally damned if she did and damned if she did not.

The therapist offered validation of her experience with David that replaced the invalidation of David's perspective (emotionless robot), as well as her own invalidation (I should have figured this out; maybe he is right). Replacing an invalidating experience opens the possibility for rapid change.

The therapist reunited the couple and complimented their willingness and courage to try marital therapy. He also normalized their difficulties, given the length of their marriage and the trials and tribulations that young children place on a marriage. The therapist then solicited the couple's willingness to engage in an experiment to address their marital problems. Following their approval, David was asked to do something that involved household chores or child care without commenting about it to Alice. David was to observe their interaction thereafter to see if his good deed had any effect on the relationship. Alice was asked to initiate a conversation about anything, as long as it involved the expression of one feeling and she inquired about David's feelings on the topic under concern. Alice was also not to make comment on her initiated conversation, but was to observe the results on subsequent interaction between them.

The homework assignment, or competing experience, was designed to interrupt the current solution attempts of both Alice and David by initiating behaviors appreciably different from David's criticism and avoidance, and Alice's defending. Alice and David's indications of improvement provided useful information for designing the assignment. The assignment was based in client-generated content and directly addressed the couple's reasons for entering therapy. From a solution-focused perspective (deShazer, 1985), such an intervention sets the stage for clients to notice exceptions to their problem that can be further amplified by the therapeutic process.

The suggestion "to do something without comment and observe" given to the couple together represented a way to initiate change while simultaneously avoiding the pitfall of disconfirming either person's frame of reference. The suggestion did not judge who was right or wrong but merely provided a face-saving way that Alice and David might try something different without admitting the incorrectness of their positions.

TREATMENT PROCESS

The therapist quickly noticed a difference in the couple's presentation in Session 2. Both were smiling, and the tension that characterized the first session seemed to have diminished. The therapist inquired about the suggested experiment and David reported that he observed Alice initiate conversations that included feelings on two occasions. David added that those evenings seemed to go very well and that he felt hopeful that the marriage might work out. Alice noted that David helped with dinner and bedtime with the kids three times since the last session. She said that she really appreciated David's help because it allowed her to relax in the evening and enjoy his company. The therapist pursued a sequence of questions that encouraged the couple to elaborate the noted changes and continue to ascribe relationship-enhancing meanings to their successes. This interventive process of "empowering client-ascribed meaning" emphasizes the client's own positive self-ascriptions without the therapist assuming a cheerleading role.

After David left, Alice reiterated her belief that things were much better, but that David had criticized her on a few occasions. Alice tried to defend herself and justify why she did things the way she did, but ultimately felt defeated and under David's control. The therapist told Alice that he had a suggestion to make regarding David's criticisms, but that it would undoubtedly sound crazy and may not fit her particular circumstance. The therapist proposed that the criticism cycle appeared to be related to power. David exercised power and control, for whatever reason, over Alice by criticizing her. The therapist suggested that Alice stop defending and justifying her actions, but rather agree with the criticisms and even exaggerate them. The therapist explained that in this strategy it is important not to sound sarcastic. The purpose would be to decrease the criticisms and allow Alice to feel more in control. Alice and the therapist discussed a couple of examples, and she said that she saw how it could help her avoid manipulation and entanglement in David's verbal barrages.

In the interview with David, the therapist pursued the opportunity that arose from the first session regarding Alice's emotional deficiency. David seemed to hold a meaning regarding Alice's behavior that perhaps served as a self-fulfilling prophecy for his emotional needs not being met. David's criticism and demands for emotional intimacy only served to decrease communication and make it harder for Alice to express her emotions. The therapist suggested that while certain family structures predispose individuals to be less prone to emotional expression, it does not necessarily follow that those individuals cannot become more expressive over time, given the right social context. The therapist suggested that it may not be that Alice had an emotional deficit, but rather that she learned a different language to communicate her feelings than David. Alice tended to be practical and demonstrated how she felt through her behaviors. David agreed and cited examples of how Alice usually demonstrated positive feelings by doing things for people.

The therapist concluded that the problem may be that Alice speaks a behavioral language, whereas David speaks a feeling language. The conversation ended with the therapist suggestion that David continue speaking in Alice's language by doing things to help, which may continue to encourage Alice's speaking in David's language. Alice joined David and the therapist, and the original experiment was reassigned.

The couple returned for Session 3 and entered the therapist's office laughing. Each referred to a list of times and events that chronicled their enactment of the suggested experiment. David said that he felt closer to Alice, and Alice reported that she was pleased to have David involved at home once again. The therapist explored the couple's impressions and promoted the elaboration of how and why the changes were occurring.

When separated, Alice indicated that she was also pleased with the agree-and-exaggerate suggestion. On one occasion, David simply stopped his criticisms and changed the subject. On another occasion, he actually countered Alice's agreement with a rebuttal of the original criticism. In that occurrence, David criticized Alice for not noticing that he had a bad day. Alice responded by saying, "You're right, I am like Mr. Spock and I'll probably always be that way. I guess I wonder how long you're going to put up with me." David replied by reminding Alice that things were getting better and that he was overreacting and should have brought it up himself that he was having a bad day. Alice was delighted. She said that it felt good to not be defensive and not to argue. The strategy seemed to allow David to change his view without being compelled to do so.

The therapist reunited the couple, and David commented that given their differences in language, he would like to find some common ground on which he and Alice could communicate about their relationship. Alice agreed and said that she was hoping for the same thing. The therapist responded to the couple's request and suggested a communication exercise called "the marital quid pro quo" (Jackson & Lederer, 1968) for the next session.

In Session 4, the quid pro quo exercise was facilitated by the therapist. The quid pro quo can stimulate a process that is both relationship enhancing and problem solving. It allows a frank discussion of relationship rules, as well as a specific method of negotiation. Briefly, the exercise has four parts: (1) each person says what he or she would like to see more of or less of that would make the marriage more workable; (2) each person repeats the other's list; (3) each person identifies how he or she has negatively contributed to the relationship; and (4) the experience of the exercise itself is discussed.

Alice and David did very well with the exercise. Alice noted that it was more difficult for her to express her own needs, whereas David noted that it was harder for him to share how he had contributed negatively. Both noted a connection between what they wanted from each other and their own negative contributions; that is, the things they wanted the most were the things that they likely sabotaged by their own behavior. The therapist encouraged further discussion and asked the couple to repeat the exercise and prioritize their lists of "more of's" and "less of's."

The therapist planned on negotiating the lists in the next session, but David called and canceled the next appointment. David said that Alice and he had agreed that they would like to try things on their own.

CLINICAL ISSUES

Alice and David illustrate the multiple avenues of change that exist in marital therapy. The therapist intervened with both Alice and David individually as well as with the couple. The interventions with the couple and Alice were competing experiences, or techniques that sought to alter the context of the actual experience of the problem. Clients are asked to do, think, or feel something different. The intervention with David involved the therapist ascription of a different meaning to Alice's difficulties in expressing her feelings.

The problem with intervention is not a dearth of possibilities but rather a lack of a coherent system of designing interventions to meet the unique needs of the couple's situation under concern. The first and foremost criterion for design is addressing the problem that the clients have identified as important. By interviewing separately, the therapist gained access to the idiosyncratic meaning systems of Alice and David. Each intervention chosen specifically addressed the client's view of the marital problem, instead of a predetermined theoretical content imposed by the therapist.

The competing experience suggested to the couple (do something without commenting and observe) interrupted the problem-maintaining solution attempts and enabled a context for both to ascribe new meanings to their interactions. The intervention also explicitly validated both their perspectives about the relationship. The couple returned noting several positive occurrences, the most important of which was David's expression of hope about the marriage.

The competing experience suggested to Alice (agree and exaggerate) interrupted her ineffective solutions; her behaviorally altered interaction with David permitted the ascription of a different meaning. David admitted, for the first time, that he could let Alice know when he was feeling down, rather than expecting her to know automatically. The intervention directly validated Alice's perspective of being criticized, and offered her a way to decrease the criticisms in a relationship-enhancing manner.

The therapist-ascribed meaning of "different languages" represented the culmination of a meaning revising conversation with David about Alice's emotional deficiency. The meaning of deficiency seemed to limit solution alternatives and perpetuate the problem cycle. The therapist offered an alternative meaning in hope of permitting a different solution option. The therapeutic dialogue around the meaning of deficiency led to a different meaning for Alice's communication difficulties; a meaning that resulted in a different solution strategy suggested by David (a common language of communication). The alternative meaning validated David's view that Alice communicated less verbally than he preferred, and at the same time offered a more benign perspective that led to different remedial action.

TERMINATION AND FOLLOW-UP

During the phone call with David in which he canceled their next appointment, the therapist commented on the amazing turnaround of the couple and complimented David on his hard work. David said that he realized that Alice would never live up to his ideal, but that he loved her anyway. The therapist asked permission to follow-up in 6 months to see how they were doing.

On follow-up, Alice reported that everything was still going OK and that, although there had been some rocky times, they seemed better able to deal with the bad times. Alice said that they still used the format of the quid pro quo and that she continued to use the agree-and-exaggerate strategy. Alice added that not feeling manipulated and controlled allowed her to step back and see how she could initiate more feeling-oriented conversation with David.

Overall Evaluation

Alice and David provide an excellent example of the incredible propensity that people have to make rapid, meaningful changes with minimal therapeutic intervention. Recall that the couple was referred for marital therapy after an assessment was made that the problem could not be addressed in the time permitted by the EAP. It is interesting to note that David did not only solve the original dilemma about staying in the relationship, but the couple also made a number of changes in the confines of just four sessions. This is not a testament to the approach or the therapist, but rather is a confirmation of the irrepressible capacity of individuals to access their inherent strengths in remarkably short periods of time. If one holds the assumption that meaningful change cannot occur rapidly, then that assumption will quite likely prove accurate.

Intervention only offers opportunities for change that promote the utilization of the client's inherent capacities for growth; interventions depend on the client's resources. Empowering opportunities for change occurs by (1) placing the client's meaning system in a superior position to theoretical orientations or personal values; (2) accepting, working within, and validating the client's meaning system both in session and out of session via the interventions themselves; and (3) recognizing that client variables and common factors are far more important to outcome than orientation (specific technique) factors (Duncan, 1992; Lambert, 1986).

References

Buckley, W. (1967). *Sociology and modern systems theory.* Englewood Cliffs, NJ: Prentice-Hall.

deShazer, S. (1985). *Keys to solutions in brief therapy.* New York: W. W. Norton.

Duncan, B. L. (1992). Strategic therapy, eclecticism, and the therapeutic relationship. *Journal of Marital and Family Therapy, 18,* 17–23.

Duncan, B. L., & Rock, J. W. (1991). *Overcoming relationship impasses: Ways to initiate change when your partner won't help.* New York: Plenum Press.

Duncan, B. L., Parks, M. B., & Rusk, G. (1990). Strategic eclecticism: A technical alternative for eclectic psychotherapy. *Psychotherapy, 27,* 568–577.

Duncan, B. L., Solovey, A., & Rusk, G. (1992). *Changing the rules: A client-directed approach to therapy.* New York: Guilford Press.

Fisch, R., Weakland, J., & Segal, L. (1982). *The tactics of change: Doing therapy briefly.* San Francisco: Jossey-Bass.

Goolishian, G., & Anderson, H. (1987). Language systems and therapy: An evolving idea. *Psychotherapy, 24,* 529–538.

Held, B. S. (1991). The process content distinction in psychotherapy revisited. *Psychotherapy, 28,* 207–217.

Jackson, D., & Lederer, W. (1968). *The mirages of marriage.* New York: W. W. Norton.

Lambert, M. (1986). Implications of psychotherapy outcome research for eclectic psychotherapy. In J. B. Norcross (Ed.), *Handbook of eclectic psychotherapy* (pp. 436–462). New York: Brunner/Mazel.

Prochaska, J. O., & DiClemente, C. C. (1982). Trans-theoretical therapy: Toward a more integrative model of change. *Psychotherapy, 19,* 276–288.

Watzlawick, P. (1984). *The invented reality.* New York: W. W. Norton.

Watzlawick, P., Weakland, J., & Fisch, R. (1974). *Change: Principles of problem formation and problem resolution.* New York: W. W. Norton.

22

Brief Treatment of Vaginismus

CATHRYN G. PRIDAL AND JOSEPH LOPICCOLO

INTRODUCTION

Sex therapy, which can be considered a form of brief cognitive/behavioral therapy, is often dated from the 1970 publication of Masters and Johnson's *Human Sexual Inadequacy,* although elements of the sex therapy treatment programs had been used by behavioral and rational-emotive therapists for many years previously. In contrast to psychodynamic or other "depth" therapy approaches, sex therapy focuses on anxiety reduction, skill training, and specific behavioral procedures to eliminate the target problem (LoPiccolo, 1990).

Vaginismus, the focus of this case study, refers to involuntary spastic contractions of the muscles that surround the vagina (Leiblum, Pervin, & Campbell, 1980). In severe cases, intercourse cannot be accomplished, and although penetration may be possible in less severe cases, the pain experienced prevents sexual arousal or pleasure. Vaginismus can be considered a type of phobic response, as it is the fear that penetration will be painful and traumatic that causes the involuntary contractions. However, a simple fear-reduction or systematic-desensitization approach to vaginismus is often unsuccessful, as using only behavioral

CATHRYN G. PRIDAL • Department of Psychology, University of Missouri, Columbia, Missouri 65211 JOSEPH LOPICCOLO • Department of Psychology, University of Missouri, Columbia, Missouri 65211.

Casebook of the Brief Psychotherapies, edited by Richard A. Wells and Vincent J. Giannetti. Plenum Press, New York, 1993.

anxiety-reduction procedures will not deal with the client's emotions and cognitions about what it means to have the penis in the vagina. For example, rape or incest survivors may experience vaginismus because sexual activity triggers traumatic memories of the sexual assault. For other women, penetration may raise issues of emotional vulnerability, dependence, or unresolved sexual-value conflicts that lead to the vaginismic spasm. The challenge in treating vaginismus in a brief therapy format is to integrate these cognitive and emotional issues into the behavioral treatment program that directly focuses on the vaginismic spasms.

CASE IDENTIFICATION AND PRESENTING COMPLAINTS

Rebecca, a 24-year-old engaged woman, was referred by a OB/GYN resident at the University Clinic because she was experiencing vaginal pain such that sexual intercourse was impossible. The gynecologic examination was quite uncomfortable for her, although the physician was able to complete the exam. The physician reported that there was no physical abnormality that would account for the pain, with the possible exception of a somewhat reduced level of vaginal lubrication. Rebecca and her fiancé, Henry, aged 32, had been sexually active together for about 1 year and were to be married in less than 3 months.

Both members of the couple were given the Locke-Wallace Marital Satisfaction Inventory (Locke & Wallace, 1959), in addition to the Sexual Interaction Inventory (LoPiccolo & Steger, 1974) and the Sexual History Questionnaire (Schover, Friedman, Weiler, Heiman, & LoPiccolo, 1982). Their responses on the Locke-Wallace indicated that their relationship was basically sound, with no areas of major difficulty except for their inability to have sexual intercourse. Their responses to the questions on the Sexual Interaction Inventory and Sexual History Questionnaire indicated that their sexual relationship was quite disordered because of the pain Rebecca experienced when they attempted intercourse. The fear of pain permeated all of their physical interactions, such that they both were reluctant to initiate any sexual interactions, or even to be affectionate because affection could be misinterpreted as a lead-in to sexual relations. Compounding their problem was Henry's profession as a minister and his strong fear of pregnancy. He was so afraid of the stigma of Rebecca becoming pregnant before they were married that when they attempted intercourse, he used two condoms, even though she was also taking birth control pills.

Henry and Rebecca began to have sexual intercourse nearly 1 year after they began seriously dating. However, after about 1 month of pleasurable sexual relations, Rebecca developed a severe vaginal infection that took several months to cure. They attempted to have sexual intercourse a few times while she was being treated for the infection, but Rebecca found it too painful to continue. After the infection was finally cured, she continued to experience pain such that intercourse was not possible.

Rebecca and Henry gave similar descriptions of their current attempts at intercourse. Henry would suggest that they "try again," and Rebecca would agree because she felt guilty about not satisfying Henry, and because she remembered the pleasurable orgasms she had before the problems began. Henry would put on the condoms, and they would try to insert his penis with Rebecca lying on her back and Henry above her. Rebecca reported that, "It seems to go in a little way, although it feels scratchy, and then it simply won't go in any further." Rebecca experienced a lot of pain when attempting to insert Henry's penis further into her vagina. They had tried to ease the penis in slowly, or to push it in vigorously, but neither method had succeeded.

Background Information

Some of the background information was elicited by the assessment devices mentioned previously, some of it was elicited during the initial interview, and some was revealed as the therapy sessions progressed. The paper-and-pencil assessment devices (Locke-Wallace, Sexual Interaction Inventory, and Sexual History Questionnaire) used are especially valuable in the context of brief psychotherapy, to reduce the amount of in-session time devoted to history taking.

Rebecca felt that there was little physical affection displayed in her family of origin, so she felt somewhat uncomfortable with public displays of affection. When questioned about relationships with friends, Rebecca described relationships that were companionable, but not interpersonally intimate.

Rebecca had never masturbated and began sexual activity in high school when she experimented with some petting with a boyfriend. Early in her college career, she met a young man who was more sexually experienced than she and had intercourse for the first time with him. She was able to experience intercourse, but found it somewhat uncomfortable because her partner did not engage in much foreplay, and she did not become well lubricated. Despite the discomfort, Rebecca was orgasmic and found herself enjoying sex so much that she felt very dependent upon the relationship. Her male partner took advantage of her dependence and became quite selfish and self-centered in his dealings with her. He finally ended their relationship, and she was devastated. Rebecca had several other dating relationships but did not have sexual intercourse again until well into her current relationship with Henry.

Henry's sexual history was fairly unremarkable. He had masturbated normally as an adolescent and continued to do so as an adult when he did not have a sexual partner. He had been involved in several serious relationships prior to meeting Rebecca and had engaged in sexual intercourse with three previous partners. He had found sex pleasurable and reported that his level of desire for intercourse was about three or four times per week when he was in a serious relationship. Henry had not had any casual sexual encounters because he felt that love was a necessary component of sexual pleasure. He reported that he enjoyed foreplay and using different positions for intercourse. His only concern had always been the fear that his female partner might become pregnant, and this fear did somewhat interfere with his enjoyment of sexual intercourse. Henry was quite distressed with their current problem, was baffled about why they were having these difficulties, and was annoyed with Rebecca for not seeking help sooner.

Diagnostic and Assessment Interview

In a brief psychotherapy format, each therapist–client interaction must be utilized to its fullest extent, and the initial telephone contact with Rebecca was no exception. After obtaining a brief description of the presenting complaint, the format for psychotherapy was discussed. Because of the time constraint of their wedding being scheduled for less than 3 months in the future, a brief psychotherapy format of 10 to 15 sessions was offered with the understanding that, upon further assessment, this format might need to be extended. The clients accepted this offer, so an appointment for the initial therapy session was set for approximately 2 weeks from the telephone consultation date. During this interval, the paper-and-pencil assessment instruments were mailed to Rebecca and Henry, and they completed and returned them several days prior to the initial appointment date. An option regarding the length of the initial therapy session was also discussed during the telephone contact—the choice being to have an extended session, or a regular length session. With one extended assessment session, the therapeutic treatment can begin immediately, whereas with a regular length first session, treatment usually cannot commence until after the second session, when all essential assessment formation is finally gathered. The disadvantage of an extended initial therapy session is that many insurance companies do not reimburse for more than 1 hour per week. Rebecca chose the extended session because she was unwilling to let issues of insurance coverage delay her treatment. She and Henry felt under time pressure because they wished to be able to have intercourse on their honeymoon. The other decision made during the initial telephone contact concerned whether Rebecca and Henry would both attend all of the therapy sessions. After some discussion about their feelings and schedules, it was decided the Rebecca would attend therapy sessions alone at the beginning of therapy and Henry would join her whenever it seemed necessary. Again, this decision was made with the condition of possible alteration after assessment in the first session, or later as therapy progressed.

The first session began with the usual explanation and discussion of the mechanics of therapy—confidentiality, billing, insurance reimbursement, session duration, emergency procedures, and so forth. Next, the therapist obtained a brief history of Rebecca's sexual experiences and her relationship with Henry. The questions asked at this time were guided by Rebecca's responses to the paper-and-pencil assessment forms that she had completed and returned prior to the initial therapy session. In this way, maximum information was obtained with minimal use of therapy time, because questioning was concentrated on the areas of difficulty. In Rebecca's case, for example, both she and her partner's assessment forms indicated that he had no erection difficulties or ejaculation problems, so these topics did not require much in-session time. Instead, in-session assessment thoroughly explored Rebecca's experience of pain during attempted intercourse. She was asked to describe the location of the pain, the intensity of the pain, the quality of the pain, the circumstances that produced the pain, and any activities that eased or exacerbated the pain. For example, the effects of different positions of intercourse, angles of entry of the penis, and depth and rate of insertion were explored in detail. Additionally, Rebecca was asked about all of her experiences with sex in her life up until the point of entering therapy. This topic is especially important to assess with vaginismic clients because this condition can be a result of having been sexually abused as a child, raped as an adult, or having experienced other forms of sexual assault. In Rebecca's case, there was no history of sexual assault. The direct cause of her vaginismus was the pain she experienced during intercourse when she had the vaginal infection. In addition, it seemed likely that she had some unresolved fear and ambivalence about her own sexual desires, resulting from the familial messages about sex she received and from her emotionally disastrous first relationship that included sexual intercourse. These cognitive and emotional issues probably account for the failure of the vaginismus to spontaneously resolve once her vaginal infection was cured.

Since the physician's examination, the paper-and-pencil-assessments and the in-session history supported the diagnosis of vaginismus not caused by any current organic problem, it was decided that Rebecca would follow the treatment program developed for psychogenic vaginismus. The next portion of the initial session was therefore devoted to a thorough explanation of the various components of the vaginismus treatment program. It was explained to Rebecca that basically the treatment program consists of four elements. The first element is deep-muscle-relaxation training, to reduce muscle tension associated with fear and anxiety. The second element is learning to voluntarily control the muscles around the vagina, so that they can be tensed and relaxed at will. The third element involves the patient, in the privacy of her own home, inserting a series of size-graduated dilators, to accustom the vagina to the sensation of painless containment of an object. The smallest of these dilators is only about one-quarter of an inch in diameter, and two inches long. This small size insures that when the client does general body relaxation and then contracts and relaxes the vaginal musculature, insertion will not be uncomfortable. The fourth element is introduced after the largest dilator can be inserted with no discomfort. In this phase of treatment, the male lies motionless on his back, while the woman kneels astride him and gradually, over a few sessions, inserts his penis into her vagina. When penile insertion can be accomplished with no difficulty, the couple begins to experiment with pelvic movements, and then, normal intercourse. While explaining the standard treatment program for vaginismus, the therapist was very careful to stress that progress through the steps of the program would be at Rebecca's pace and under her control. The "deadline" of her wedding date was discussed, and it was suggested that she disregard that date as a short-term goal but rather focus on the idea that successful treatment would ultimately lead to long-term sexual satisfaction in her marriage.

After the treatment program was explained, the therapist introduced progressive muscle relaxation. Rebecca followed the relaxation instructions while the therapist spoke into a tape recorder, thus producing a tape that Rebecca could use to practice relaxation at home. It typically takes 15 to 20 minutes to make a progressive muscle-relaxation tape, and it is a good use of therapy time to make a relaxation tape, rather than simply sending the client home with a standard prerecorded tape, for several reasons. First, while making the tape the therapist can observe the client's reactions and deal with any difficulties at once. A second reason is that the tape can be tailored to the individual client. For example, if the client was raped while walking along a quiet beach, using the imagery of lying on a beach would obviously not be relaxing for that client. Third, hearing her own therapist's voice on the tape encourages the client to recall relaxing in the "safe" environment of the therapy office, and so fosters relaxation at home.

After making the tape, Rebecca was given the opportunity to ask questions and discuss her reactions to the session thus far. She was comfortable with the outlined treatment plan and felt ready to begin. Rebecca was given the homework assignment of daily practice with the relaxation tape, with the suggestion that she also use the relaxation techniques in other situations which made her tense. Additionally, a contract was made that she and Henry would not make any attempts at sexual intercourse. It was explained that each attempt just retraumatized her and reinforced the involuntary vaginismic contractions. Alternate methods of sexual pleasuring, including mutual manual and oral genital caressing, were described and Rebecca expressed her comfort with engaging in these activities. She felt sure that Henry would abide by this contract, as he enjoyed these alternative activities, was interested in her therapeutic progress, and had pretty much given up trying to accomplish intercourse anyway. The therapist also informed Rebecca that they must discontinue the use of condoms, when they resumed intercourse, as condoms are contraindicated in cases of vaginismus because they make entry more difficult to accomplish. Additionally, it was explained that when they resumed intercourse it would not be in their usual male superior position, but instead would, at least initially, be in the female superior position so that Rebecca could control the rate of entry more easily.

Treatment Process

The second therapy session began with a discussion of Rebecca's progress in learning to relax by using the tape made in the initial session. Rebecca had used the tape daily and was confident in her ability to relax. She also had found herself using the relaxation techniques at work and when driving, to relax tense muscles. Rebecca then watched a 30-minute, commercially produced patient-education film entitled *Treating Vaginismus* (LoPiccolo, 1984). This film demonstrates the entire treatment program for vaginismus in a stepwise fashion, with the actress actually inserting the various dilators into a pelvic model and into her own vagina. The film *Treating Vaginismus* is especially useful in a brief psychotherapy format, as the client is able to get an overall picture of the treatment plan without extensive amounts of therapy time being used to present detailed descriptions and explanations. Another benefit of viewing the film is that the client is able to actually see how the dilators should be used and becomes somewhat "desensitized" to the idea of inserting something into her own vagina. The actress in the film presents a coping model, in that she struggles a good deal with some of the treatment steps but is ultimately successful.

Some therapists who do a lot of sex therapy have their own complete set of dilators and access to sterilization equipment, but most therapists do not. If the therapist does not have a set of dilators to lend the client, the referring physician may be asked to prescribe a set of dilators for the client to purchase. However, a set of dilators is quite expensive (around $300), so another option is for the physician to lend the client a set of dilators that can be returned and sterilized after the completion of therapy. The therapist treating Rebecca owns the two smallest dilators, which can be sterilized by boiling, and lends them to clients to get started, until they can obtain larger dilators used later in therapy.

After watching and discussing the film, Rebecca felt comfortable with the idea of proceeding with the smallest dilator. She practiced inserting this dilator into the pelvic model in the therapist's office, and was then given the first dilator to take home. Kegel (1952) exercises, in which the vaginal muscles are voluntarily contracted and relaxed, were described, with the rationale that she could learn to control the contraction of her vaginal muscles through these exercises. Her daily assignment for the next week was to relax (with or without the tape), do three Kegel exercises, relax again, and insert the lubricated dilator into her vagina for a minute or so.

The third therapy session began with a discussion of Rebecca's homework assignment. She reported that she "could not find the time" to use the dilator every day and actually only tried it twice during the preceding week. When she did try to insert the dilator, she experienced some discomfort and so withdrew it immediately. Upon questioning about her failure to do the homework as assigned, Rebecca reported that she was feeling resentful about the pressure she was receiving from Henry to "get better," so they could have intercourse. He had asked her for a word-by-word account of her therapy sessions and had "nagged" her about doing the dilation homework so much that she found herself feeling resentful of him, instead of motivated to have sexual intercourse with him. The therapist supported Rebecca's need for therapy to belong to her and not to share any more of the content of the sessions than she wanted to with Henry. The therapist suggested that perhaps Henry was worried that he was being blamed for Rebecca's pain or was being discussed negatively in the therapy session. Rebecca agreed that these concerns were at least part of what was motivating Henry's behavior, so she accepted a suggestion to reassure him about these issues without revealing session contents that she wished to keep private. The possibility of inviting Henry to attend therapy sessions with Rebecca to deal with these issues was discussed, but she wanted to maintain control of her progress, and felt more able to do so if he was not attending sessions with her at this time.

Rebecca was ready to reengage in the therapeutic process, so she was given the self-help book *Becoming Orgasmic* (Heiman & LoPiccolo, 1988) to begin reading, in addition to her daily dilation assignment. Her homework assignment for the next week was to read the first two chapters of *Becoming Orgasmic,* do the exercises included in these chapters, and continue with daily dilation using the same dilator, but with more relaxation prior to insertion and using more of the lubricant jelly. Rebecca was asked to read *Becoming Orgasmic,* even though she was orgasmic prior to developing vaginismus, because the book leads the reader through a thorough self-exploration of her ideas about sexuality and her physical reactions to pleasurable stimulation.

Rebecca was pleased to report at the beginning of the fourth therapy session that her dilation homework had gone very well, and she felt ready to move on to the next size dilator. Most of this session was devoted to a discussion of her discoveries after reading the first two chapters in *Becoming Orgasmic.* Rebecca's mother had never spoken to her directly about sexuality but had left Rebecca with the impression that it was something women really did not enjoy too much. Instead, her mother implied that sex was the only thing that men really wanted from women, and therefore Rebecca should remain a virgin until marriage, to be sure that someone would marry her. Rebecca also recalled hearing several "horror" stories about painful experiences with first intercourse and with childbirth. On a rational level, she did not believe any of these messages about sex but had come to realize that on an emotional level they were still powerful for her, because she had begun to cry while answering the questions in the book that asked about these family-of-origin messages. The therapist led Rebecca through a reworking of the sexual messages that she had received as a child and teenager, following which, for the first time in months, Rebecca felt excited about the prospect of resuming sexual intercourse with Henry.

The homework assignment for the next week was to read Chapters

3 and 4 in *Becoming Orgasmic,* which involve body exploration. She was also assigned to use the next size larger dilator in her daily dilation sessions. Rebecca was reminded to contact the referring OB/GYN physician to obtain larger dilators to be used during her future dilation sessions.

The fifth session began with a discussion of Rebecca's progress in completing her homework. The dilation homework had gone very well; she had experienced no difficulty with inserting the dilator and had enjoyed the body exploration exercises in *Becoming Orgasmic.* However, she was unable to reach her referring physician to obtain larger dilators. She agreed to use the same dilator for the next week's homework assignment and to have it remain in her vagina for 5 minutes. She was also to ask Henry to read the first four chapters of *Becoming Orgasmic* and discuss them together. Rebecca was pleased that Henry would now be involved with the treatment process under her direction. Alternative objects that many sex therapists use as dilators were discussed, in case she was still unable to connect with her physician. Candles and the plastic barrels from syringes appealed to Rebecca as reasonable alternatives, but she planned to first try to obtain the larger dilators from her physician.

Rebecca began the sixth session by stating that she was going to have to use alternative objects for dilators. She had been able to talk to her physician, only to discover that he did not have a set of graduated diameter dilators, only a set in graduated lengths. Rebecca had talked with Henry, and they felt that they simply could not afford to purchase a set of dilators, given the expenses of their upcoming wedding. Rebecca had discussed the possible alternative dilators with her physician and obtained his approval for their use. She had found three candles that seemed appropriate to her in terms of increasing sizes from the dilators she had already used and showed them to the therapist. The therapist agreed with Rebecca's opinion and assigned dilation with the next two sizes during the next week. Rebecca was to use the next size for the first few days, leaving the dilator in place for at least 5 minutes. Then, if she had no difficulties, she could move on to the next size.

Rebecca and Henry had discussed the first four chapters of *Becoming Orgasmic* as well, and the reading material had provided a framework for talking about their whole sexual and emotional relationship. Rebecca asked if Henry could attend the next therapy session with her, as he had some questions that she wanted the therapist to answer for him. She also seemed ready to let Henry be involved in her therapy, as the control issue had receded in importance after their frank discussion of their feelings about their sexual relationship.

Henry attended the next three sessions (seven, eight, and nine) and volunteered to help Rebecca find dilators to use after the third and largest candle. She was pleased at his desire to *help* her rather than simply do it himself and present her with the results. After some looking, they found plastic syringe barrels at a veterinary supply shop that were available in a range of graduated sizes. The therapist suggested that they purchase a range, with the largest being somewhat larger than Henry's erect penis. Rebecca then could feel confident that, after completing the dilation program, she could comfortably contain Henry's penis in her vagina. Rebecca's dilation homework continued to go well—she had a few minor difficulties but overcame them with relaxation and more lubrication. She also progressed to leaving the dilators in place for 15 minutes while she watched television or read, and felt very comfortable doing so. As Rebecca was feeling so comfortable with the dilation exercises, Henry began to participate in them as well. Initially, he simply observed her relaxing and inserting the dilator, then he put his hand on hers while she inserted the dilator, and finally, he inserted the dilator under her guidance.

The ninth session was 2 weeks prior to their wedding date, and although Rebecca was making good progress, it seemed unlikely that she would complete the dilation program prior to their wedding. She had more difficulty with her homework that week. She felt she needed to hurry through the dilation program to be finished by their wedding date and was feeling tense as a result. Henry stated quite baldly that he wanted their honeymoon to be a "real" honeymoon, as he had fantasized about that sort of honeymoon for his whole life and did not want to be disappointed. Rebecca became quite upset when Henry said this and began to cry openly. The therapist suggested that Henry's fantasy was a common one, but clearly was not helping Rebecca to make therapeutic progress. The couple was planning to go to Jamaica for 4 days after their wedding, so a discussion of enjoyable activities on the island of Jamaica was initiated by the therapist. After they had each identified four or five activities, the therapist suggested that their honeymoon could focus on enjoying each other's company while engaging in those activities, instead of on intercourse. The alternative methods of sexual pleasuring were again presented, and Henry agreed that he could enjoy his honeymoon on those terms.

As there were only 11 days remaining before their wedding, it was decided that the tenth session would be scheduled for after their return from Jamaica. Rebecca felt she simply did not have time for another session before the wedding. For homework, Rebecca was assigned to maintain the level of dilation she was currently doing, on a daily basis, if possible. Her mother was staying in her apartment to help with the wedding, and Rebecca felt she might not be able to find 15 to 20 minutes alone, each day, to do dilation. Permission was given for her to do the dilation exercises every other day, if daily was not feasible. Henry and Rebecca agreed that they would not attempt intercourse while on their honeymoon. Henry told Rebecca that he was satisfied with that agreement, knowing that their future sexual relationship was more important than the few days of their honeymoon. The therapist suggested that they could consider having a "mini-honeymoon" as a celebration after they had completed the treatment program and were able to have intercourse. Both Henry and Rebecca thought that idea was a good one and were looking forward to that time.

Rebecca attended the tenth session alone and reported that they had really enjoyed their trip to Jamaica. They had experienced mutual orgasms using the alternative methods of sexual pleasuring discussed in the ninth therapy session, and had been tempted to try intercourse. They had refrained from doing so because they knew that they would have to "report back" to the therapist, and wanted to be "good clients." Rebecca had not been able to do much dilation during the intervening 2 weeks, so her assignment was to continue with the dilator she had been using for another week. At this point, they had the two largest dilators left to use before beginning the transition to inserting Henry's penis instead of dilators.

Both Henry and Rebecca attended the eleventh therapy session and were embarrassed to admit that they had engaged in sexual intercourse once during the past week. They had both really enjoyed it, and Rebecca had had no difficulties whatsoever. The therapist firmly reminded them about the contract not to attempt intercourse because of the risk of retraumatizing the vaginal muscles such that the involuntary spasms would recur. Both Henry and Rebecca acknowledged their awareness of this risk and repeated their intention not to attempt intercourse again until instructed to do so by the therapist. The homework assignment for the next week was for Rebecca and Henry to use the next-to-largest dilator in daily dilation sessions, for both of them to complete their reading of *Becoming Orgasmic,* and to talk about the book.

The twelfth session was attended by both Henry and Rebecca, and they came in smiling. They had engaged in intercourse four times during the past week, again with no problems. Henry had been reluctant to try intercourse again, but Rebecca had urged him to do so because she had enjoyed it so much the week before. She had not done any of the dilation homework, because they had intercourse immediately after their last therapy session. She felt that, since intercourse was working so well, she no longer needed to do the dilation exercises. At this point the therapist agreed that there was no need to continue the dilation as they were clearly cured, and a final session was scheduled in 2 weeks.

Clinical Issues

The major clinical issue that arose in the treatment of this case concerned Rebecca's noncompliance with therapeutic instructions. In the early phases of therapy, resistance to working directly on the vaginismus was manifested by Rebecca. Rather than responding negatively to this resistance, the therapist used her noncompliance as an entry to some restructuring of Rebecca's thinking about her sexuality, and, most importantly, to her taking a more assertive role in her relationship with Henry. In brief therapy, with a specific, symptom-focused goal, there is often a temptation to avoid opening up such complex issues. However, current broad-spectrum approaches to sex therapy (LoPiccolo, 1992) emphasize that patient "resistance" to behavioral procedures actually indicates that the therapist is making the error of not helping the client find alternative, adaptive methods of dealing with unresolved family-of-origin, individual-dynamic, or couple-relationship issues that partially maintain the target symptom. In Rebecca's case, her vaginismus caused her much distress, but it also had adaptive value for her in dealing with unresolved sexual issues, and her relationship with Henry. Once these issues were addressed directly in therapy, she was able to resume the behavioral treatment of vaginismus. In general, when treating cases of vaginismus, it is critical that the client feel she is in control of the entire therapeutic process. Otherwise, therapy will be perceived as being forced upon her, just as attempts at intercourse have been forced upon her in the past.

Termination and Follow-Up

During the final therapy session, the therapist and client couple engaged in a discussion of the gains made in therapy and the pitfalls to watch for in the future. It was clear that Rebecca had regained voluntary control of her vaginal muscles, through the relaxation and dilation program that she had followed. Additionally, Rebecca felt more able to discuss her needs with Henry as she now had confidence that he would listen to her and respect her ideas. Henry felt more able to count on Rebecca to get things done and to be responsible for herself. They both felt that their sexual relationship had been enhanced by 2 months of engaging in alternative methods of sexual pleasuring without any expectation of intercourse. They planned to spend a weekend in a nearby city, at a nice hotel, to celebrate their therapeutic gains, and to augment their "honeymoon memories."

A relapse-prevention program was outlined to deal with Rebecca's fear that she could have a recurrence of the involuntary vaginal spasms. In about 6 months she was to use the dilators daily for 2 weeks, beginning with the smallest one, and progressing through the largest one she had used prior to the termination of therapy. The description of the treatment element that involves the transition from dilators to the penis was repeated, as a reminder that a system exists for that transition, in case they had trouble with that aspect of their sexual relationship in the future.

As planned, a telephone call was made 3 months later as a follow-up contact. Rebecca and Henry assured the therapist that their sexual relationship continued to be very satisfactory. They were having intercourse several times per week, and they were not experiencing any other relationship difficulties. Their mini-honeymoon had been very enjoyable—they basically stayed in bed for the weekend, making love, talking, and ordering room service when they were hungry. The couple again completed the Sexual Interaction Inventory (LoPiccolo & Steger, 1974) as a posttreatment assessment measure, and all scales were well within the normal range, indicating a high degree of sexual satisfaction for both of them.

OVERALL EVALUATION

The progress of therapy in this case was typical for most cases of vaginismus. Although many clients do make the transition from insertion of the dilators to insertion of the penis nearly as easily as Rebecca and Henry, there are other clients for whom this transition is inordinately difficult. In some cases, the client or her partner can easily insert a dilator that is much larger than his erect penis, but any attempt to insert the penis, no matter how slowly and gently, triggers vaginismic spasms. In these cases, the therapist should explore fully with the client just what accomplishing intercourse (consummating the marriage, in most such cases) means emotionally to the client. Often, there is major ambivalence about the relationship, or about becoming a fully sexually functioning woman. In other such cases, long-repressed memories of childhood sexual abuse or incest may emerge in response to this exploration. Obviously, in all these cases, more intensive psychotherapy will be indicated. However, when such complicating emotional factors are not present and the vaginismic spasm still occurs in response to the penis but not with the largest dilator, a simple procedure is usually successful. In this procedure, a hollow tube larger than the erect penis is used as a dilator (for example, a large syringe barrel). When the client can insert this tubular dilator easily, the partner inserts his penis into the tube while it is in the patient's vagina. In this way, penile entry is accomplished, and the couple is usually able to discontinue use of the tube, and easily insert the penis alone, in only one or two sessions.

Traditional clinical lore suggests that women who suffer from vaginismus are also inorgasmic, do not enjoy sex, and have a low sex drive. This symptom pattern is typical of many vaginismic clients, especially those who were molested as children. However, it is the authors' experience that approximately one-third of vaginismic clients are orgasmic, enjoy sex, and have a normal sex drive, with their sexual problem being focally restricted to vaginismus. Rebecca's case lies somewhere between these extremes. She was orgasmic and had previously enjoyed sex. However, she had significant ambivalence about her sexuality, based on unresolved family of origin and life-history issues, and her sex drive was situationally reduced by some conflicts in her relationship with Henry. In treating vaginismic clients who have never had an orgasm, or who have other sexual difficulties, these problems can be addressed contemporaneously with the vaginismus. The book and film *Becoming Orgasmic* (Heiman & LoPiccolo, 1988) are especially useful in brief therapy with such clients, as research has shown that this self-help program is very effective when combined with a minimal number of psychotherapy sessions (Morokoff & LoPiccolo, 1986). Although the presence of additional sexual problems may sometimes prolong the duration of therapy for vaginismic clients, the probability of treatment success does not seem to be reduced in such cases.

In the early days of sex therapy, a major tenet was the use of a dual sex co-therapy team, with both members of the client couple attending all of the therapy sessions. The financial constraints of private practice and insurance reimbursement rules make the use of a dual sex cotherapy team impractical for all but the wealthiest clients. Fortunately, research has shown that an individual therapist is just as effective as a cotherapy team, even when the therapist is of the opposite sex to the client with the sexual problem (LoPiccolo, Heiman, Hogan, & Roberts, 1985). Similarly, the standard sex therapy format of both members of the client couple attending all therapy sessions is often not practical in these days of dual-career families, nor is such a format always optimal. The authors prefer to conduct a thorough assessment of the couple's relationship and the presenting sexual problem prior to beginning therapy and then make a decision about the format of therapy that will work best for each particular case. In this case, Rebecca felt some resentment toward Henry regarding a power imbalance in their relationship, which added to her difficulties in dealing with the vaginismus. She progressed more quickly through the initial steps of therapy by attending sessions by herself, and Henry was included only when she felt he would be an equal partner in the therapeutic process.

As a final cautionary note, the therapist must insist that the client undergo a gynecologic exam prior to beginning the treatment described in this chapter. There are several physical conditions, such as an imperforate hymen, or a vaginal tumor, that mimic exactly the symptoms of vaginismus, so a physical exam is crucial (Fordney, 1978; Lamont, 1978). Some vaginismic clients also experience vaginismus in the gynecologist's office, such that the exam cannot be completed. In these cases, the exam can be done under light sedation, which eliminates the patient's distress and fear of the examination, and prevents the vaginismus from occurring.

REFERENCES

Fordney, D. (1978). Dyspareunia and vaginismus. *Clinical Obstetrics and Gynecology, 21*(1), 205–221.

Heiman, J. R., & LoPiccolo, J. (1988). *Becoming orgasmic: A personal and sexual growth program for women.* Englewood Cliffs, NJ: Prentice-Hall.

Kegel, A. (1952). Sexual functions of the pubococcygeus muscle. *Western Journal of Surgical Obstetrics and Gynecology, 60,* 521–526.

Lamont, J. (1978). Vaginismus. *American Journal of Obstetrics and Gynecology, 131,* 632–636.

Leiblum, S. R., Pervin, L., & Campbell, E. (1980). The treatment of vaginismus: Success and failure. In S. R. Leiblum & L. Pervin (Eds.), *Principles and practice of sex therapy* (pp. 167–192). New York: Guilford Press.

Locke, H. J., & Wallace, K. M. (1959). Short marital adjustment and prediction tests: Their reliability and validity. *Marriage and Family Living, 21,* 252–255.

LoPiccolo, J. (1984). *Treating vaginismus* (film). Huntington Station, NY: Focus International.

LoPiccolo, J. (1990). Treatment of sexual dysfunction. In A. S. Bellack, M. Hersen, & A. E. Kazdin (Eds.), *International handbook of behavior modification and therapy* (2nd ed.) (pp. 547–564). New York: Plenum Press.

LoPiccolo, J. (1992). Post modern sex therapy for erectile failure. In R. C. Rosen & S. R. Leiblum (Eds.), *Erectile failure: Assessment and treatment* (pp. 171–197). New York: Guilford Press.

LoPiccolo, J., & Steger, J. C. (1974). The Sexual Interaction Inventory: A new instrument for assessment of sexual dysfunction. *Archives of Sexual Behavior, 3*(6), 585–596.

LoPiccolo, J., Heiman, J. R., Hogan, D. R., & Roberts, C. W. (1985). Effectiveness of single therapists versus co-therapy teams in sex therapy. *Journal of Consulting and Clinical Psychology, 53*(3), 287–294.

Masters, W. H., & Johnson, V. E. (1970). *Human sexual inadequacy.* Boston: Little, Brown.

Morokoff, P. J., & LoPiccolo, J. (1986). A comparative evaluation of minimal therapist contact and fifteen session treatment for female orgasmic dysfunction. *Journal of Consulting and Clinical Psychology, 54*(3), 294–300.

Schover, L. R., Friedman, J., Weiler, S., Heiman, J. R., & LoPiccolo, J. (1982). A multiaxial diagnostic system for sexual dysfunctions: An alternative to DSM-III. *Archives of General Psychiatry, 39,* 614–619.

IV

Group Treatment

23

Short-Term Group Therapy with a Chronic Pain Patient

KAREN SUBRAMANIAN AND ELIZABETH SIEGEL

INTRODUCTION

Pain is a multidimensional concept, influenced by psychological, social, and cultural variables as well as the physiological experience. In chronic pain patients, usually defined as patients who experience pain for 6 months or longer, the impact of conditioned factors quite often outweighs the role of sensory damage. This puts the chronic pain patient at risk for long-term psychosocial complications affecting marital and family issues, occupational roles, and emotions (Roy, 1984).

Melzack and Wall's (1983) theory of pain, which demonstrated how pain perception and response result from the interaction of sensory–discriminative, motivational–affective, and cognitive–evaluative components, opened the door to the development of multidimensional treatment programs for chronic pain patients. As treatment strategies to target the psychosocial components of pain were developed and researched, studies reported increasingly effective results. Treatment strategies have primarily focused on cognitive restructuring and relaxation training (Fordyce, 1976; Turner, 1982; Turk, Meichenbaum, & Genest, 1983). Social skills training (specifically assertiveness skills) and its

KAREN SUBRAMANIAN • School of Social Work, University of Southern California, Los Angeles, California 90089-0411. ELIZABETH SIEGEL • New Directions, 837 South Fair Oaks, Suite 201, Pasadena, California 91105.

Casebook of the Brief Psychotherapies, edited by Richard A. Wells and Vincent J. Giannetti. Plenum Press, New York, 1993.

application to chronic pain patients has not been as thoroughly researched (Heinrich, Cohen, & Naliboff, 1982).

Comprehensive pain centers now encompass not only the medical care that patients seek but also address the social and psychological components of pain. For patients who do not have access to these pain centers, short-term psychosocial treatments can be delivered at outpatient clinics while patients continue to receive regular medical services from their physicians. For example, the 8-week (2 hours per week) pain management program presented in this case study teaches the skills of cognitive restructuring, relaxation training, and assertiveness training. The goal is to improve the coping skills of patients with chronic pain, whether or not there are improvements in their medical condition.

The treatment is presented within a group setting that reduces the isolation of the chronic pain patient and enhances their skills acquisition by providing structured interaction and reinforcement. The group is a time-limited structured model in which the group leader is viewed as a facilitator rather than a therapist. Prominent features of this type of group include a predetermined focus and agenda for each session as well as minilectures, home assignments, and structured exercises. Findings from both a pilot study and a controlled experiment indicate that this group treatment is effective in reducing physical and psychosocial dysfunction and negative mood states in adult chronic pain patients of varying ages (Subramanian, 1991).

Case Identification and Presenting Complaints

Mrs. M., a 75-year-old married Caucasian woman, requested the services of the pain management group after reading an announcement in the local newspaper. She had been experiencing pain in both legs for the past 4 years due to a combination of ailments: claudication pains in her legs (cramping pains due to inadequate blood flow) and pain due to arteriosclerosis in the popliteal arteries (just below the knees). Mrs. M. was not able to walk more than one-half a block without pain and spent about 6 hours a day sitting and resting. Her most severe pain occurred at night, quite often resulting in a loss of sleep. Her request for psychosocial treatment followed a year of disappointing surgeries; within a 9-month span, she had had five surgeries that attempted to bypass her failed arteries. Three of the surgeries failed, and the results of the other two were moderate and tenuous. Mrs. M. was taking four prescription medications for her pain condition.

Besides a clinical interview, pretreatment assessment included Mrs. M.'s self-ratings on the Sickness Impact Profile (SIP), a behavioral measure of sickness-related physical and psychosocial dysfunction in 12 areas of life (Bergner, Bobbitt, & Pollard, 1976), and the Profile of Mood States that measures six transient negative moods (McNair, Lorr, & Droppleman, 1971). Pain severity was measured by a numerical scale. When assessed at her first interview, Mrs. M.'s scores on the SIP indicated that she was most dysfunctional in the areas of recreation, home management, ambulation, and problems with sleep and rest. Her highest levels of negative mood states were in the areas of depression and confusion. On a scale of 0 ("no pain") to 10 ("pain as bad as you can imagine"), she reported her worst pain to be a "9" and her average pain to be a "7."

BACKGROUND INFORMATION

Mrs. M. and her husband are retired and have four grown children with whom they are very close. In retirement, she continues to be an active person who participates enthusiastically in family, church, and community activities. These resources also provide her with a strong social network. Before the advent of her pain condition, Mrs. M. and her husband had participated in all church and community activities together; in particular, she and her husband had sung in the church choir for many years. Gradually, her husband was adapting to her changed physical status by occasionally going out by himself, producing a very new pattern in their lives and increasing Mrs. M.'s distress.

The past 4 years had been characterized by a gradual reduction in Mrs. M.'s participation in activities in the home, the church, and the community. Family celebrations, which used to be times of joy, now produced too much pain and took too much effort and energy. As Mrs. M. became more and more incapacitated by her pain, her husband had willingly and without complaint taken over the housekeeping chores and was very attentive and supportive to her during her recent surgeries. At times, however, his caring attitude and behavior slipped into overprotection. Then, when Mrs. M. might feel better and want to perform her customary chores, she had to struggle to get them back. The only other major change in Mrs. M.'s marital relationship was a slowdown in their sexual life, which she attributed more to her pain condition than normal changes due to aging.

Mrs. M.'s relationships with her children are good, and they live near enough to be actively supportive. She is able to accept their love and support, but this acceptance is tempered by feelings of guilt that she is a burden and that her condition takes too much of her family's time.

DIAGNOSTIC AND ASSESSMENT INTERVIEW

At the assessment interview, Mrs. M. gave the impression of being a very vital person. She was neat, well-groomed in modern clothes, positive, compliant, articulate, soft-spoken, honest, and straightforward. Her ability to develop healthy relationships was reflected in her family and community support systems. Except for the current disruption of her life caused by her pain, she appeared to be a very high-functioning woman.

Mrs. M. was obviously not a complainer and took responsibility for her own well-being, as demonstrated by active involvement in her medical treatments and knowledge about her condition. She appeared to have a high internal locus of control and did what she could to help herself and minimize her discomfort. Thus, this treatment program that included "scientific consultation" (her words) by a medical professional and that focused on giving her a way to take back control of her life was well-suited to her personality style.

Her coping patterns focused on being as self-sufficient as possible. Although she often felt very sad and hopeless about her pain condition and frequently cried when she felt overwhelmed by her sad feelings, she avoided sharing these distressing feelings with her family. Much of the time she attempted to cope with her pain and distress through "keeping busy" or by keeping in contact with friends over the telephone or by letter. She wrote one letter to a friend or family member somewhere in the country every day of the week, and she allowed herself to express in her letters those same feelings that she believed she should not reveal to her family. This use of the telephone and correspondence allowed her to reach out to others beyond the bounds of her home to which she had become physically constrained.

Although control and suppression appeared to be her primary modes of coping, she had recently begun to allow herself more free expression of feelings and said she was even beginning to learn to "cuss!" She also used cognitions to help herself cope, by thinking "positively" and using social comparison. She also tried to be realistic by reminding herself that she was 75 and "no spring chicken." Her request for this pain management program marked the first time she had ever sought psychosocial treatment.

A clinical assessment was made that due to her recent surgery failures (the last one occurring 4 months before coming for treatment), she was psychosocially vulnerable which might subsequently exacerbate the severity of her pain. She told of how high her hopes had been before each of the surgeries and how extremely disappointed she was at each failure. She felt helpless but did not know what to do with her feelings of sadness and severe disappointment. Mrs. M. was very guarded in her emotions, masking any strong anger or despair and defending against these feelings by being too cheerful, too optimistic, and too cooperative.

She was a woman "in charge" whose appeal as a client was based in part on this strong motivation to help herself. She seemed well-suited for this particular treatment that requires a partnership between the patient and the group leader, with the patient taking responsibility for learning, practicing, and incorporating the skills into his/her own life.

TREATMENT PROCESS

Session 1

During the first session, Mrs. M. found that she was one of the oldest of six women, whose ages ranged from 58 to 85. The session consisted of introductions, exploration of a canned case study, and a minilecture presenting a rationale for using cognitive/behavioral treatment methods to help patients control their reactions to the pain experience. During the introductions, Mrs. M. discovered that other pain conditions represented in the group (with several patients having more than one condition) included degenerating discs in the lower back, spinal stenosis, lumbar stenosis, neck and shoulder pain from a car injury, TMJ pain, migraine headaches, arthritis, and fibrocytis. She learned that she was not alone in her suffering or her desire to learn to cope more effectively with her pain condition.

The prepared case study is used to facilitate group cohesiveness through member self-disclosure about family support, negative emotions, and coping strengths. Mrs. M., although initially expressing a resistance to examining her feelings too deeply, found that hearing other members disclose gave her some degree of permission to feel and have needs. She spoke about feelings of sadness and depression, extreme fatigue from restless nights, and her need to readjust her levels of activity and participation with family and community.

Mrs. M. found that the combination of minilecture and self-disclosure exercises addressed her dual needs of having a "scientific treatment" aimed at helping her regain control of her life and sharing her anguish with someone other than her family. Her expectations of the program at the end of this session were so high that she was reminded that the group was not a cure for her pain and that in order to thoroughly learn the skills, she would have to continue to practice long after the group ended.

Session 2

The home assignment after the first session helps group members become aware of the feelings and thoughts they have during particularly stressful or painful episodes. Half of the second session then focuses on practice in defining and recognizing self-defeating and self-enhancing thoughts and half focuses on the introduction and initial practice of autogenic relaxation (Shulte & Luthe, 1969).

Although Mrs. M. was initially reticent about discussing deeper and more distressing emotions, she now spoke freely about waking with pain in the middle of the night and thinking: "If I could only have one night free—I never will!" She recognized and was able to verbalize feelings of "despair" and "grief" that if her legs got worse, her feet might also become affected, limiting her mobility even more. This self-disclosure, combined with listening to other members' confidences, appeared to serve an important function for Mrs. M., who now felt she had a safe place in which she could share her extremely personal concerns about her pain. As a result, she felt even closer to other group members by the end of the session.

Although Mrs. M. did not report using any form of formal relaxation before the group treatment began, she did use music to relax at night when she would awaken with leg pains. She found the autogenic relaxation to be comforting and was given a relaxation tape of the exercise in order to practice at home. With her customary need for control and strong motivation to cope, she promised to practice relaxation all 7 days of the week.

Session 3

In Session 3, group members practice using cognitive restructuring and reinforce their practice of autogenic relaxation. Mrs. M. reported to the group that during the previous week, she had awakened in the night with severe pain. She correctly identified her self-defeating thought: "Just when I think the pain may be lessening, I have a setback!" With gentle probing by the group leader, it was revealed that the self-defeating thought she initially expressed was defending against a more fearful thought: "It's never going to get better!" Mrs. M. understood that she tends to minimize the level of distress she is experiencing.

When she tried to change her self defeating thought to a self-enhancing one, she said: "The pain is still so severe and yet I suppose it is too soon to expect anything different." This statement was identified by the group leader as wishful thinking rather than a self-enhancing thought. A self-enhancing or coping thought is partly defined as a realistic cognition (not overly optimistic) that is able to guide a set of positive behaviors. Mrs. M.'s mistake was not unexpected because in her clinical interview she spoke of using "positive thoughts" as a coping strategy. When Mrs. M. called the cognitions "positive thoughts," she was accurately expressing her view of them, and this made it continually difficult for her to successfully utilize this particular strategy.

When asked to present a situation for the practice of thought-switching statements, Mrs. M. spoke of pain during her daily walks. She recognized a common self-defeating thought as: "Walking is such a struggle. The future looks so grim—it can only get worse." At that point she chose to experiment with the thought-switching statement "and now to the positive." This focus on "positive" instead of "coping" resulted in a poor attempt at expressing a subsequent self-enhancing thought: "Walking is so difficult—but maybe it will get better—or I will get used to it. Perhaps some auxiliary vessels will develop, or the ones I have will expand and let more blood through." With the assistance of the other members and the group leader, she was able to accept an improved coping statement: "Walking helps me a little bit; at least it's different, and the pain comes and goes."

As she had promised, Mrs. M. did practice autogenic relaxation every day and reported effective results. She said that when the pain got so severe that it woke her at night, she would go to the living-room sofa so as not to wake her husband and, with the use of the relaxation tape, would find the pain easing and herself relaxing into sleep.

Session 4

Session 4 introduces the assertiveness skills of requests, refusals, and expressions of feeling. One of Mrs. M.'s most troubling problems was that her participation in social and recreational activities with friends and family had diminished and she felt isolated and alone. The fact that her husband was beginning to socialize without her only exacerbated these feelings. She described a situation in which her husband had accepted an invitation to an open house without consulting her.

Although she actually wanted to go, she felt she would be out of place sitting alone while others were talking and mingling while standing. Mrs. M. felt that she aggressively responded to her husband by becoming angry and saying that he should know she could not attend that type of affair. Working in the group, she developed her first attempt at an assertive reply: "It would be nice to see our friends again, but I'll see how well I'm functioning when the day arrives."

Session 5

Mrs. M. was one of the first group members to volunteer for a cognitive/behavioral rehearsal, introduced during this session. Mrs. M.'s examples of cognitive and behavioral situations that she wanted to work on revealed her need to be compliant and to please others—even at the expense of her own physical and psychological well-being. She described a situation in which she had just returned from a walk when a troubled friend called. The friend proceeded to talk at length while Mrs. M. began to feel exhausted and in pain. She did not say: "Oh, please cut it short today!" (which was what she really wanted to do) or use her new assertiveness skills to ask to call her friend back later. Instead, she wanted to practice cognitive restructuring in order to convince herself to continue talking to this friend. She restructured her thoughts to focus on the fact that her friend needed her and that she would be able to manage her pain and fatigue throughout the phone call.

Session 6

When a stressful or painful episode is divided into coping stages, individuals are better able to keep each part of the situation manageable and feel less overwhelmed. These stages, introduced in Session 5, have been identified as preparation, confrontation, critical moments, and positive self-evaluation. Mrs. M. reported to the group that she had practiced this form of coping while receiving an arteriogram (her sixth arteriogram in 7 months). She prepared herself for this painful procedure by remembering that she would have her favorite radiologist and that she really knew what to expect from the procedure. She attempted to distract herself from worrying about the pain by thinking about houseguests she was going to have the following week. When confronting the actual arteriogram, she thought: "I will relax as I breathe deeply; I will expand all my vessels," and "this too will pass." Four times critical moments arose that were extremely painful, and she coped with these by counting how long each pain lasted.

Although she used these coping stages successfully, she found the last stage of self-congratulations impossible to accomplish. However, she appeared to be able to handle the coping stages better than the self-enhancing thoughts as she still continued to call them "positive thoughts" and use examples such as "and now to be positive" (thought-stopping phrase) and "maybe I'll get used to it" (self-enhancing).

Mrs. M. found the concept of imagery, which was introduced during this session, as successful as she had the autogenic relaxation. The image that she focused on appeared as a result of listening to tapes she had made of her children singing when they were very young, resulting in a wonderful image of "cascading, pleasant memories."

Session 7

With only two sessions left in the program, Mrs. M. was encouraged to rehearse and refine any of the skills she wished. She presented three situations in which she had practiced the various skills. First, she had attempted cognitive restructuring after taking one of her walks. Her legs began feeling extremely heavy, and she felt she could hardly lift them. She thought: "I just know I'm going to be stuck with this heaviness even when postsurgery pain has subsided" (self-defeating). She then quickly visualized a lighted hand signal indicating "STOP" to initiate thought switching. Then she thought: "Who knows—who can predict what will happen. Perhaps it will be better than I envision" (self-enhancing, although still focusing on a positive phrase).

Second, she described returning merchandise to a store a year and a half later without a sales slip and successfully employed an assertive request to ask for her money back. Although this situation did not involve pain, experience with this treatment program verifies that assertiveness skills generalize to diverse interpersonal situations quicker than the other skills. Third, she again described using relaxation successfully to get back to sleep in the middle of the night.

Session 8

This session had two goals: to have each member review all of the skills they had learned and to assist members with developing a plan for maintaining their skills in the future. Mrs. M. stated that she liked the skill of relaxation best and found both self-enhancing thoughts and assertiveness most difficult to put into practice. Because assertiveness was the last skill introduced, she did not have much time to practice it during the course of treatment. She was also hindered in its use by previous socialization that had taught her to care for her family first and herself second. She stated that she planned to continue the relaxation skills regularly and to try to incorporate the other skills into her life as best she could. She was forewarned about possible setbacks and encouraged to occasionally review the manual of minilectures and exercises she had received from the group leader. She did not have any other plans for maintaining contact with other members, obtaining additional psychosocial assistance, or for joining any other support groups.

CLINICAL ISSUES

Although group support is essential to this treatment, the basis of the short-term group is structured education and practice in coping skills. The group is most appropriate for individuals who, for reasons of personality, situation, and/or cultural background, are not looking for in-depth self-analysis or personality changes. Mrs. M. guarded her emotions carefully, but her pain was excruciating, and she was finding it difficult to regain her equilibrium. This type of group was helpful because it offered her coping skills without probing her defenses too deeply. Other than learning improved coping skills, Mrs. M. did not want to change her life in any drastic way. At her age, she had made an accommodation to life that was satisfactory to her and her environment; changing too much would mean reevaluating her entire life.

Group process, although less evident than in other types of groups, is still essential to successful group treatment. The concept of universality was important in this group, and most group members agreed that no one could comprehend the pain that they experienced as well as others with a chronic pain condition. Mrs. M. regularly participated at a high level in the group and rapidly developed a cohesive bond with the other group members. In spite of this, she remained a very private person who shared what was appropriate and necessary for learning the skills within the group but did not otherwise share a lot of her personal life. When presented with an opportunity to have a member of her choosing be a "phone buddy" for her between group sessions, she politely refused, saying that she had many telephone contacts.

Chronic pain patients who enter this treatment have already been forced to make the difficult transition from the hierarchial medical model of treatment to the reality that they must make their own decisions and choices about how to cope with their pain condition. Resistance is minimal as members are participants in educationally focused structured activities throughout the group sessions and are given control over the selection and practice of skills.

This group treatment will not be successful for all patients. If a person had fairly good self esteem before the appearance of their pain condition, the group can help them regain that lost self-esteem. However, if their self-esteem was low even before the pain condition, that fact might impede their ability to learn and practice the skills. This treatment requires a degree of acceptance of responsibility for one's attitude and behavior. Thus, characterologically angry, demanding, or dependent individuals may find it frustrating and may be disruptive to group functioning. Because the group moves very quickly, there is no time to work on personality problems that might provide obstacles to a person's integrating the coping skills.

In addition, the skills might not be as useful for those persons who live alone. Although the skills theoretically should help a person reenter a community from which he or she might have become isolated, there is not enough time to reinforce that integration. This places a burden on group leaders who feel that as the group ends, there are no other resources for these isolated individuals.

Termination and Follow-Up

Immediately after the group program, Mrs. M. reported less overall dysfunction in her life, most dramatically in the areas of recreation, home management, and emotional behavior. Mrs. M.'s negative moods also decreased after treatment, most notably in the areas of depression and confusion with a corresponding increase in her sense of vigor.

Six months later, Mrs. M. reported feeling discouraged about her physical condition, finally having come to the realization that there was nothing more medical science could do for her. An overall increase in dysfunction was now observed, although she maintained her improvements in emotional behavior, negative mood states, and vigor.

She felt that the skills training and the group support had both been extremely helpful. To a certain extent, she saw the skills as a distraction from her pain, realizing that she could not focus on her pain and on the coping skills at the same time. She stated "that even though the pain might not go away, there are methods one can learn to cope with it." She was still struggling with assertiveness, finding that free and honest expression of her feelings did not come easily for her. She did believe she was improving, however. While her children encouraged and enjoyed her new assertiveness, she thought her husband appeared confused—either acting surprised or mistaking the assertiveness for anger. At the beginning of this program, Mrs. M. found it important to please others; she had now made a step to "start doing things that I want to do and say things that I want to say."

One year later, Mrs. M. again showed a decrease in her overall dysfunctional status. Her emotional behavior was no longer dysfunctional at all, and improvements in home management were maintained. However, interestingly enough, she had regressed in the area of recreation. Negative moods had increased, although they were still 30% reduced from pretreatment levels, and improvements in vigor were maintained.

Although Mrs. M.'s pain condition, medical interventions, and self-reported pain levels did not change appreciably during this year, she was no longer using any prescription or over-the-counter pain medications. She reported using assertiveness to say "no" to activities she was unable to participate in because of pain, and she stated that it had become easier to express deep feelings such as sadness. When she had self-defeating thoughts, she would think through and proceed with an activity that would be self-enhancing and distract her from the pain. Although her cognitions did lead her to a coping behavior, she was not able to verbalize her self-enhancing thoughts. Relaxation was still a successful coping strategy for her. She expressed a greater acceptance of herself and her physical limitations and was proceeding with living her life as fully as possible. The continued effectiveness of treatment after 1 year indicates that the group experience supported Mrs. M.'s premorbid style of control over her life and helped her to use that control in a more rewarding way.

Overall Evaluation

In this time of modern medical miracles, there are millions living with chronic pain and disabling medical conditions that medical technology cannot cure. Since the relationship between pain and coping is not linear, research results from the study of this program suggest that chronic pain patients can often learn to cope better with their lives whether or not their medical condition has changed. Psychosocial treatment models may be an answer to assisting chronic pain patients with quality-of-life concerns.

References

Bergner, M., Bobbitt, R., & Pollard, W. (1976). The Sickness Impact Profile: Development and final revision of a health status measure. *Medical Care, 19,* 787–805.

Fordyce, W. E. (1976). *Behavioral methods for chronic pain and illness.* St. Louis, MO: C. V. Mosby Co.

Heinrich, R. L., Cohen, M. J., & Naliboff, B. D. (1982). Rehabilitation of pain patients: Coping in interpersonal contexts. In J. Barber & C. Adrian (Eds.), *Psychological approaches to the management of pain* (pp. 118–136). New York: Brunner/Mazel.

McNair, D. M., Lorr, N., & Droppleman, L. F. (1971). *Profile of mood states.* San Diego, CA: Educational and Industrial Testing Service.

Melzack, R., & Wall, P. D. (1983). *The challenge of pain.* New York: Basic Books.

Roy, R. (1984). Chronic pain: A family perspective. *International Journal of Family Therapy, 6,* 31–43.

Schulte, J. H., & Luthe, W. (1969). *Autogenic therapy: Vol. I. Autogenic methods.* New York: Grune & Stratton.

Subramanian, K. (1991). Structured group work for the management of chronic pain: An experimental investigation. *Research on Social Work Practice, 1,* 32–45.

Turner, J. (1982). Comparison of group progressive-relaxation and cognitive-behavioral group therapy for chronic low back pain. *Journal of Consulting and Clinical Psychology, 50,* 757–765.

Turk, D. C., Meichenbaum, D., & Genest, M. (1983). *Pain and behavioral medicine.* New York: Guilford Press.

24

A Short-Term Group Intervention in the Context of Ongoing Individual Psychotherapy

CAROL J. GOLDEN-SCADUTO AND HAROLD S. BERNARD

INTRODUCTION

During the spring of 1989, while the senior author was a psychology intern at a large medical center in New York City, she co-led a short-term, insight-oriented psychotherapy group for patients who had contracted genital herpes. Her co-leader was a male psychology intern. The second author was their supervisor in his capacity as Chief of the Group Psychotherapy Program at the same medical center.

The present chapter will focus on one patient in this short-term group. This patient was a long-term individual psychotherapy patient of the senior author. She saw her for 3 years prior to the group, throughout the duration of the group, and she continues to see her as this chapter is

CAROL J. GOLDEN-SCADUTO • Department of Psychiatry, New York University Medical Center and Bellevue Hospital Center, New York, New York 10016. HAROLD S. BERNARD • Department of Psychiatry and Group Psychotherapy Program, Psychology Service, New York University Medical Center, New York, New York 10016.

Casebook of the Brief Psychotherapies, edited by Richard A. Wells and Vincent J. Giannetti. Plenum Press, New York, 1993.

being written. It is the aim of the authors to describe how the introduction of a short-term group intervention affected this particular patient's overall treatment experience and to draw inferences about combining individual and group interventions in clinical practice.

THE PATIENT

Description

Natasha is a 39-year-old, divorced, European-born woman who emigrated to this country approximately 11 years ago. She is of above-average intelligence, attractive, and speaks fluent English. Her parents live in her native country, and her one sibling, an older brother, lives in another European country. Contact with her parents is regular and frequent, while with her sibling it is only sporadic.

The patient has recently become self-employed in the same personal service business she was in when she began psychotherapy with the senior author 6 years ago. At that time, she expressed her reasons for seeking treatment as the need "to find out where I'm going in life" and "to understand my past and present." She sought treatment at the university clinic where the senior author was a graduate student. A summary of her presenting problems included poor and unstable relationships, feelings of low self-esteem and self-worth, depression and anxiety, loneliness, and a tendency toward impulsive behavior.

Natasha's psychopathology manifested itself at an early age within the context of an extremely dysfunctional family. She reported little knowledge of her parents' early lives, although she was aware that they, and their immediate families, were generally isolated from other family members, partly by choice and partly because of geographical distance. She initially described her father as "intelligent, talented, very dynamic, and appealing—above all to women—the kind of man I would like to marry." Her mother was, and still is, described as "depressed and ineffective," never knowing what was going on around her, and never having assimilated into the life of her adopted country. The patient depicted her family life as characterized by her father's frequent and overt adultery with family friends and acquaintances and, ultimately, with her own friends. She described an overly eroticized relationship with her father throughout her childhood and adolescence. She often felt uncomfortable in her father's presence, indicating that he frequently stared at her in a "sexual" way. However, although his behavior was clearly inappropriate, there was no evidence of actual incest. Apparently her mother acquiesced in her husband's affairs, but Natasha remembered her as constantly crying and not functioning very well. There was a taboo against talking about what was happening in the family, so Natasha was never able to discuss her feelings with anyone.

Natasha's performance in school was poor. She had difficulty concentrating, and her parents were completely unavailable to supply support of any kind. She was constantly told that she was not bright enough to learn anything, and her father made it clear that, in his view, her physical appearance was her most important asset. Extrafamilial relationships were equally poor. The patient had few friends as a child and adolescent, and heterosexual relationships were described as unrequited crushes or one-night stands. She became sexually promiscuous, related to men only on this level, and contracted genital herpes. A major social difficulty, persisting through the first 3 to 4 years of therapy, was Natasha's inability to sustain a conversation and to be comfortable in the presence of others. She described herself as "unable to think of anything to say" and fearing that "I will be thought of as stupid."

Natasha's work history was also marginal. She did odd jobs for short periods of time until she met her husband and came to the United States with him. Although she wanted to work and study, her husband insisted that she stay at home to do the telephone work that his business required. They were married for about 3 years before she left him and began to train for the work she is currently doing.

Formulation

Natasha began psychotherapy with a diagnosis of Borderline Personality Disorder. Underlying depression was masked by impulsive behavior and hypomanic tendencies. Ego weaknesses were manifested by chronic, diffuse, free-floating anxiety and dissociative reactions. The latter were first experienced in childhood and described as "blackouts" in her recounting of these occurrences. They continued throughout the beginning phase of treatment in a form that might be characterized as "twilight" or "reduced consciousness" states and subsequent failure to remember details of events or conversations that were particularly unpleasant or painful for her. In addition, Natasha manifested both addictive and impulsive behaviors. Although never a chronic substance abuser, she did use alcohol, cocaine, and marijuana in social situations that had the potential for becoming anxiety-provoking—even when she was aware that this was not in her best interest. She was unable to tolerate frustration and acted out sexually in order to rid herself of tension.

Finally, Natasha had a poorly integrated concept of self, accompanied by chronic feelings of emptiness and counteracted by hypomanic defenses of keeping busy and convincing herself that she was "popular." Consistent with Kernberg's (1975) formulation of borderline personality disorder, Natasha gave evidence of relying prominently on primitive defensive operations such as denial, splitting, devaluation, externalization, and projective identification.

COURSE OF THERAPY PRIOR TO GROUP INTERVENTION

Natasha originally presented with poor insight and judgment, as well as with difficulty in maintaining directed thought. She was clearly motivated to seek help due to persistent unhappiness and frustration, but she was largely unable/unwilling to look inside herself in an effort to effect changes in her life situation. She was, initially, guarded and somewhat suspicious in her relationship with the therapist. She tended to talk about the people in her life and what they had done to her rather than to examine her own thoughts, feelings, and behavior. In fact, it was at least 6 months before she began to reveal some of the more intimate details of her life. Her style at the time, which was also the major manifestation of her resistance, was one that could be characterized as a "hit-and-run" approach. She would present material in a fast, disorganized "spilling" of events, with selective inattention to the details that could have helped to clarify her behavior and thereby have led to an awareness of unconscious motivations. Although the therapist consistently attempted to help Natasha begin to cultivate some perspective about her life in order to help develop an observing ego, she maintained an extremely unreflective stance and almost always balked at attempts at clarification. She thus remained unaware of her own part in the unfolding events of her life for much of the first two years of treatment.

Toward the end of the second year, Natasha began to show signs of being less resistant to clarification and more receptive to confrontation. Interpretations began to be offered occasionally by the patient herself, and she began to present clinical material with a desire to explore her underlying motivation. She clearly became more organized in her presentation and was able to maintain directed thought without the structure previously required from the therapist.

Early in the therapeutic work, Natasha described her interpersonal life as full of disappointments. She had a new romantic interest every few months. Invariably, the men she met were initially described as "someone I could fall in love with," but eventually she would report, "He's not for me." She would immediately have sex with these men and then, just as quickly, regret it. Although she complained often that men used her only as a sex object, it took 2 years of therapy before she was able to recognize that she did a great deal to provoke such treatment.

Because of Natasha's frequent sexual contacts, the issue of her genital herpes came up often, although it was never a focal point of the treatment. Initially, she gave no thought to the consequences of not telling her partners that she was infected and saw no need to do so. As the treatment progressed and she developed not only an observing ego but a more defined superego as well, she began to see that her behavior was problematic, and she started to change. Although still a long way from being able to tell her partners about the herpes, she was much more careful as to the timing of her sexual activity, and she expressed both the need and the desire to be able to be honest about her condition with the men with whom she became involved.

Originally, the therapist was quite obviously seen as the idealized "all-good" mother. This representation then alternated with a devalued image of the therapist that contained Natasha's attempt to deal with her envy and jealousy as well as with her feelings of low self-worth. Again, toward the end of the first 2 years in therapy, the patient began to establish a more integrated view of the therapist as someone who was a companion and an aide in the effort to understand herself. She was able to accept the premise that the relationship had to exist within clear boundaries and that the previously desired friendship was not feasible.

The most significant countertransferential feelings emerged early in treatment and continued throughout much of the first 2 years. These were, clearly, grounded in the patient's use of projective identification. The therapist frequently found herself feeling angry, left out, and controlled as a result of Natasha's "hit-and-run" style. She was able to use these feelings to understand both Natasha's feelings in the presence of others and the feelings of others in Natasha's presence. The foregoing is an overview of the patient and her treatment during the first 3 years and prior to the introduction of the idea of a short-term group intervention.

SHORT-TERM GROUP INTERVENTION

Impact on Individual Treatment Prior to Beginning Group

During the fall of 1988, Natasha began a relationship with a man that lasted approximately 3 months and seemed to be her most appropriate heterosexual relationship to date. She began to explore issues of intimacy and to work on skills that would enable her to communicate her feelings and needs more clearly. When the relationship ended, Natasha took appropriate responsibility for her conduct and seemed able to integrate the experience.

The issue of herpes came up more and more frequently in her sessions, and, in November 1988, the therapist suggested the possibility of her joining a 15-week time-limited group for people with genital herpes. Natasha was both eager and afraid to join the group. She mentioned that her recent lover had contracted herpes from her and, at one point, said, "That's his problem." When the therapist confronted her about this, Natasha became very angry; this opened the way to processing possible feelings she would have if the members of the herpes group were also confrontative with her. The processing of other issues related to joining the group also began at this time. These included exploring what it meant to her to be part of a group, being the only member in individual treatment with one of the co-therapists (since all the other patients referred to the group were unknown to the two prospective therapists), working with a second therapist, sharing her therapist with other patients, and watching her therapist work with other patients. During this time, she also met the co-therapist.

From the initial decision to join the group until the group intervention began a number of months later, Natasha and her therapist focused on transference issues. Her fantasies about being a "privileged" patient because of her relationship with the therapist and her expectations of being protected were explored. She became anxious and confused when asked if she would be able to share these feelings with the group. As the starting date of the group approached, Natasha became more anxious in individual treatment and more angry and sensitive both to attempts at clarification as well as to confrontation by the therapist. She began to complain about her difficulties getting to the therapist's office (something she had never before mentioned) and her anticipation that it would be very inconvenient when she would have to come twice a week (to group as well as to her individual sessions). She also began to miss appointments. When the issue of a fee for the group was brought up, she became enraged that she would have to pay a higher fee for group than for individual sessions. (This was due to the fact that she was earning much more money than when she had begun individual treatment, and her individual therapy fee had never been adjusted because of an administrative policy peculiar to the clinic in which she was being seen.) As attempts were made to process these issues, she threatened to leave therapy entirely. However, the work progressed and she seemed prepared to enter the group on schedule.

Description of Group

The group ran for 15 consecutive weeks and met for 1 hour and 15 minutes per session. In addition to Natasha, one patient was referred by a staff psychologist of the medical center, and the others were recruited through a genital herpes support network. Only three men were considered for the group, and none was deemed appropriate; thus, the group was composed of women only.

The group began with 10 members. However, one member dropped out prior to the first session, a second stopped attending after the third session, and a third dropped out after the tenth session. The other seven members completed the 15-week course of treatment.

The aim of the group intervention was to help members understand their responses to their condition in the context of their overall adaptation in life. Because the literature on sufferers of genital herpes has made it clear that these patients often use herpes as a way of not focusing on other, more deeply rooted problems (Drob & Bernard, 1985), this was understood to be a formidable challenge. In attempting to clarify some of the ways in which herpes may have exacerbated (but not caused) difficulties that were primarily interpersonal in nature, attention to the here-and-now of the group interaction was emphasized, and members were encouraged to give one another open and honest feedback. Even though this approach was made explicit to the members prior to the beginning of the group, there was initially a great deal of resistance to it that took the form of members trying to focus only on their concrete, herpes-related concerns. Nevertheless, and in the face of often severe opposition by the members, the co-leaders were able to shape the group into an insight-oriented entity. At the end of the 15 weeks, it was felt by both co-leaders and the supervisor that the aim of the intervention had been met and that the group had been successful for most of the members.

Course of Combined Treatment

Natasha did not attend the first group meeting or the individual session on that same evening. (The therapist had been able to arrange to see her individually on the night of the group.) She also did not call to cancel, which is something she had never done before. When the therapist called her, she refused to talk and she did not return subsequent phone calls. Finally, on the day prior to the second group meeting, Natasha agreed to talk to the therapist over the phone. The therapist attempted to recapitulate recent events, recognizing Natasha's anger over the issue of payment. More important, however, an interpretation was offered to her, suggesting that her rage and acting out were her attempts at defending against the possibility of "losing" the therapist and their exclusive relationship. This appeared to have an immediately calming effect on Natasha, and she agreed to come to both sessions the next day.

For the next several weeks, Natasha came regularly to group sessions, albeit often late, but she missed three consecutive individual sessions. Her requests to talk on the phone were denied, and boundaries were firmly drawn. She was reminded that attendance at group therapy was contingent upon remaining in individual treatment, as previously contracted. When she did arrive for her first individual session after several weeks, she immediately presented the therapist with the required forms and a check for the group sessions, saying, "Maybe I need someone to keep after me." She then became argumentative in an attempt to justify her missed appointments. The therapist made several interpretations of her behavior: (1) she continued to be terrified at the possibility of losing their exclusive relationship; (2) she was, in essence, asking for preferential treatment by the therapist; (3) she was attempting to "leave" the therapist before the therapist could leave her; and (4) her behavior had the unconscious motivation of wanting the therapist to feel angry with her so that she would "abandon" her and thereby prove that people are not to be trusted. The therapist related her unconsciously motivated behaviors to her relationships with people in her everyday world, especially to her parents who were, in fact, never available and not trustworthy. She admitted to having some awareness of these feelings, and she added that she realized that holding them in was causing her to act aggressively toward the therapist as well as toward the people in her life outside treatment. She also acknowledged that she was aware of holding back her feelings in the group. This session was clearly a positive turning point in the work with Natasha in both treatment modalities.

As mentioned, Natasha began coming regularly to the group after missing the initial session, although she continued to be late most of the time. She was completely silent for the first five sessions she attended. However, a change became obvious after the individual session described above; she began to talk about her sexual behavior and the fact that she does not tell partners about her condition. Members of the group were adamant in their expression of anger and disapproval of her behavior. During the next individual session, Natasha expressed unhappiness about the previous group session; she felt that she had not honestly expressed her feelings when the group had attacked her. During the individual session, she came to recognize how anxious she had become during the group session and how it had resulted in her mind going blank. She expressed mixed feelings toward the therapist; she was unhappy that she had not "rescued" her from the group attack, but she also stated that she felt the therapist was "there" for her.

During the next group session, Natasha remained silent, saying only that she was tired and had not wanted to come to group. However, in her next individual session, she acknowledged being annoyed with herself for not participating. Although she had things to say, she felt threatened by others in the group, and she was uncomfortable with her individual therapist. She suggested that she felt the impulse "to perform for 'mother' as the oldest 'child' in the group."

During the next group session, Natasha was encouraged by the co-therapist to express her feelings about the fact that many group members were missing. Although she declined to do so, she was able to respond to encouragement to express other feelings not previously shared. She (appropriately) confronted the co-therapist with her resentment at what she perceived as condescension when she did not understand a word he had used. After she received some support for this sentiment, she expressed direct feelings to a group member who, she felt, had made a distracting comment.

In the individual session that followed, Natasha spoke of being proud of herself for what she had been able to say in the group. However, she also said that she did not like being "applauded" for her behavior because it made her feel like a child. Through exploration, she came to realize that what was bothersome to her was not the praise itself, but rather her need for praise. She also talked about her anger at absent group members and at herself for being chronically late.

Over the next several sessions, Natasha continued in her attempts to speak in the group and to express what she felt toward other members. When she became anxious and confused, she was able to express these feelings in the group as well. Her experiences in the group were continually processed in her individual sessions, and she began to express a desire for a long-term group experience. She began to report how she was expressing (seemingly appropriately) negative feelings toward her roommate in an attempt to make her living situation more viable. She voiced a desire for feedback from the group, but also a fear that she would hear how far she still had to go in her development. She decided she would not ask the group for feedback at this juncture.

During the thirteenth group session, Natasha expressed admiration and envy toward another member of the group because of her ability to take care of herself. She continued to speak, telling the group that she wished that, in her 20s, she could have been where she feels she is now in her emotional development. When another member asked how a person could begin to feel better about herself, her therapist suggested that Natasha could speak to the question. She responded by speaking of her 4-year treatment, indicating how it had helped her to get in touch with her feelings, but also admitting that she had various difficulties which she saw as unresolved.

At the fifteenth and final session of the group, Natasha reported that she had revealed the fact of her herpes to some female friends. She felt that this was a great triumph for her, but she continued to wrestle with whether she could acknowledge her condition to a man whom she had been dating sporadically over a 6-year period. Although the group members encouraged her to do so, she was terrified that it might risk the relationship because she had been dishonest with him for so long. It was on this note that the group ended.

Course of Individual Treatment Following Termination of Group

During her next individual session, Natasha reviewed her 4-year course of therapy. She stated that she was thrilled with what was happening to her and indicated that she saw the therapist as "the caring and protective mother I never had." She disclosed that she had come to view her "crisis" before entering the group as a turning point. For her, this meant that she was able to understand, and now clearly say, how past events and relationships with important people in her life still influenced her behavior in the present. She was also able to begin to separate reactions to those people from reactions to people who currently populated her life (specifically the therapist).

Individual treatment continued for another 16 months. During the final phase of treatment, Natasha focused her attention on her relationship with, and feelings toward, her parents—especially her father. She began to talk more about her sexual behavior and fantasy life and the kinds of men to whom she was attracted. She also began to identify patterns in her relationships with men. Specifically, she was beginning to understand that she felt most comfortable and most uninhibited sexually with men whom she did not respect or even like. Concomitantly, she realized that she was anxious and uncomfortable around those men with whom she would like to begin a relationship and who, she felt, would be possibilities for a serious, long-lasting commitment. In general, Natasha became more self-observing and self-critical about her behavior.

Natasha initiated discussion of termination at about the beginning of the fifth year of treatment, and this was an ongoing topic for exploration for an entire year before termination actually occurred. She clearly understood that there were important areas of her life that remained unresolved, but she (and the therapist) believed that she had made excellent progress in all areas of functioning. The therapist ultimately indicated that she would be comfortable with either a decision to terminate or a decision to continue with therapy at that time. Thus, Natasha truly made the final decision "to test her wings." She left knowing that she would be free to contact the therapist again at any time in the future.

Approximately 7 months after termination, Natasha contacted the therapist and resumed treatment. At the time this chapter is being written, she has been back in once-weekly individual psychotherapy for 3 months, working on the various issues that had been explored to some degree in her initial course of treatment.

Conclusion: Impact of Group Intervention on Ongoing Treatment

It seems clear that the introduction of a short-term group experience into this long-term treatment had a significant impact on the overall treatment experience. It certainly had an important effect on the exploration of transference material. Natasha had the opportunity to observe her individual therapist at work in the group setting and thereby to "share" her with other patients. Because her individual therapist worked with a colleague in leading the group, she also had the opportunity to experience working with another therapist and to compare and contrast the two. All this gave rise to a range of feelings and reactions, both while the group was going on and thereafter, that ultimately helped Natasha understand more fully the nature and origin of her complicated relationship with her individual therapist (Wong, 1983).

We believe the concurrent treatment experiences Natasha had during the 15 weeks she was in the group were mutually reinforcing. There were times when she was able to use her individual sessions to form strategies for how to make the group work for her and thus to resolve certain impasses she had reached as a group member. Even when things were going well in the group, her individual sessions helped to enrich her perspective about what was occurring, thereby making the experience a more valuable one for her.

At the same time, the group experience enriched her individual work. Specifically, it provided a wealth of data about how Natasha reacted to, and interacted with, a range of other people, which constituted significant "grist for the mill." Both she and her therapist agreed that the group contributed significantly to the value of the work they were doing at the time she participated in the group and, to a lesser degree, thereafter. In conclusion, it is our view that combined individual and group treatment is often the richest way to work with patients who present for outpatient psychotherapy.

REFERENCES

Drob, S., & Bernard, H. (1985). Two models of brief group psychotherapy for herpes sufferers. *Group, 9*(3), 14–20.

Kernberg, O. (1975). *Borderline conditions and pathological narcissism.* New York: Jason Aronson.

Wong, N. (1983). Combined individual and group psychotherapy. In H. I. Kaplan & B. J. Sadock, (Eds.), *Comprehensive group psychotherapy* (2nd ed., pp. 73–83). Baltimore: Williams & Wilkins.

25

Short-Term Group Therapy with Depressed Adolescents

STUART FINE AND MERVYN GILBERT

INTRODUCTION

Group therapy has frequently been recommended as a treatment modality for adolescents. This is because peers are so important in determining adolescent values, behaviors, and perceptions, all of which facilitate successful separation from the family and the achievement of an autonomous identity. In recent years there have been descriptions of this form of therapy including systematic reviews of the literature (Azima & Richmond, 1989) and empirical investigations of treatment efficacy (Kolvin et al., 1981; Plienis et al., 1987; Reynolds & Coats, 1986). There have also been discussions of the indications for short-term group therapy (Klein, 1985; Poey, 1985). Garvin (1990) has suggested that brief therapy may encourage a more intensive effort on the part of the client but requires a more active role and broader repertoire on the part of the therapist.

Our research for the last several years has evaluated the effectiveness of short-term group therapy with a clinical sample of adolescents (Fine et al., 1989; Fine, Forth, Gilbert, & Haley, 1991). This interest grew out of our prior experience with more conventional adolescent group therapy (Fine, Knight-Webb, & Breau, 1976). More specifically, we have

STUART FINE • Division of Child Psychiatry, University of British Columbia, Vancouver, British Columbia, Canada V5Z 1M9. MERVYN GILBERT • Department of Psychology, Vancouver General Hospital, Vancouver, British Columbia, Canada V5Z 1M9.

Casebook of the Brief Psychotherapies, edited by Richard A. Wells and Vincent J. Giannetti. Plenum Press, New York, 1993.

compared a social skills training approach with a therapeutic discussion approach to brief group therapy with depressed teenagers. Our choice of therapeutic modalities was predicated on various theoretical, empirical, and practical considerations. Although therapeutic discussion reflects experiential and insight-oriented traditions (e.g., Yalom, 1985), social skills training stems from behavioral and cognitive/behavioral research and practice (e.g., Rotheram, 1980). Both dynamic support groups (Poey, 1985) and social skills training programs (Lewinsohn et al., 1990) have demonstrated improvement of symptoms. The goal of the former is to encourage cohesion, universality, catharsis, and interpersonal learning (Corder, Whiteside, & Haizlip, 1981), whereas the latter is aimed at learning and practicing various interpersonal, behavioral, and cognitive skills (Michelson, Sugai, Wood, & Kazdin, 1983).

In this chapter, we will discuss our clinical experience and observations in using these two contrasting group approaches. Rather than discussing a "case" per se, we will concentrate on detailed description of the structure, process, and interpersonal dynamics of the approaches utilized. In effect, the group itself will be the "case," as we believe this will best enable other clinicians to adapt either of the modalities to their particular practice setting. Our focus will be on practical and clinical issues; however, it is worth briefly describing our research as this influenced our clinical approach. More detailed information about specific research findings is available elsewhere (Fine et al., 1991).

All of the adolescents in these groups had been referred to our outpatient program because of depressive symptomatology. The majority (64%) satisfied DSM-III criteria for Major Depressive Disorder, assessed by clinical interview and by a semistructured interview with adolescents and their parents. Self-report ratings of depression, cognitive distortions, and self-image were also gathered. Measures were readministered immediately after the group therapy and at a 9-month follow-up.

Adolescents were assigned to either a 12-session social skills group or to a 12-session therapeutic support group. At posttreatment the depressed subjects did better in the therapeutic support group than in the social skills training; however, at follow-up, those in the social skills groups caught up and showed equal improvement.

Group Formation and Initial Process

Prior to the group sessions, each patient and his or her family were interviewed by one or both of the co-therapists to explain the nature of the group, identify areas of difficulty, and to address concerns. Initial membership consisted of between 8 and 12 adolescents. Most were depressed; however, we deliberately included several adolescents with other diagnoses, as we had previously found that a diagnostic mixture, including the possibility of volunteer adolescents served to activate group participation (Fine et al., 1976).

The groups were held on a weekly basis lasting for an hour and a half at the end of the afternoon. All sessions included the provision of a snack, consumed during a brief break. This proved to be rich in therapeutic opportunities, as participants took part in deciding what they would like for a snack that gave them safe opportunities for leadership and decision making. During subsequent sessions, early arrivals frequently assisted the group leaders in preparing food, and members often brought extra food for their peers. Groups were conducted in a large room where participants sat around a table and there was access to a blackboard and videotape equipment.

There were a number of other common elements to the two group approaches. For instance, all groups were conducted by two co-therapists. Although their professional training, theoretical orientation, and group experience varied, there was always at least one therapist who had previously led a group with teenagers. Although it is possible for a group of this size to be conducted by one group leader, we felt that two had several advantages. Their presence made it easier to deal with certain individuals who, for example, showed overactive or disruptive behavior. Such group members responded to the proximity of one of the co-therapists who could subtly redirect their activities. There were occasions where participants became upset and left the group, and it was important to have a therapist to attend to them because of concerns about safety. Group members frequently displayed a preference for one or the other group leader, probably because of their varying projections of parental roles. Indeed, there were some instances where it was assumed that groups leaders were married. It was important for group leaders to be sensitive to efforts to "split" them or form individual coalitions, while at the same time remaining aware of their own individual preferences or countertransferences. This was enhanced by a comfortable relationship between the group leaders and ample time for discussion of the content and process prior to and following each session. With some planning, group leaders were often able to use aspects of their relationship within the group itself, for example, by discussing or role playing how they had resolved a problem between themselves.

There were similar goals for both modalities in the initial session: determining expectations for subsequent sessions; meeting and learning about the participants; and beginning to establish a therapeutic milieu.

The group typically began with a brief round of introductions that included name, age, and grade. It was acknowledged that participants were likely to be feeling somewhat confused and possibly nervous about what the group would be like. They were asked to attend at least three sessions before making a decision about leaving. The importance of promptness, consistent attendance, and letting the group leaders know if they would not be able to attend a session were stressed because the presence of each individual was important to the group. They were assured as to the confidentiality of information discussed in the group. Finally, members were asked to decide about the timing of the break, smoking policy, the nature of snacks, and other procedural concerns.

Description of Therapeutic Discussion Group

The rationale underlying the therapeutic discussion group is that a supportive adolescent milieu provides a unique opportunity for teenagers to interact in a context free of the preconceived demands experienced in their school, family, or social group. The role of the group leaders is primarily to encourage members to experience, express, and critically examine their feelings and beliefs in a secure setting. This is only possible if there is an atmosphere of respect for each participant and for his or her contribution to the group. This is most likely to be accomplished, according to Hurst, Stein, Korchin, and Soskin (1978), with a high level of caring combined with self-expression.

In the initial session, participants were given an opportunity to get to know each other better. The "warm-up" exercise we found the most useful was to ask participants to spend a few minutes to pair up and "interview" one another with respect to family background, personal interests, and related information. Following this, each member provided a brief introduction of his/her partner. Inevitably this process revealed common characteristics such as school, musical preferences, or extracurricular activities. Because every member was requested to both actively present a peer and to be presented, there was an environment of mutual engagement with minimal threat. The first session closed with a clarification of any questions that might have arisen and an expression of appreciation for the presence and contribution of all participants.

The second session was aimed at building cohesion and identifying therapeutic issues. Participants were told that the purpose of the group was to help people deal with difficult experiences in their lives and that those who were most sensitive to the problems of a teenager were other teenagers. Structured activities were often introduced such as drawing a diagram describing family constellation and other important people in their lives, or making a list of "topics." Presentation of these encouraged self-disclosure and inevitably emphasized commonalities among group members. They were then asked to attempt to identify specific aspects of their lives that they wanted to explore. As far as possible, these should involve current circumstances over which they had some control. This was not to deny the relevance of prior traumatic experiences or uncontrollable events but rather to focus on the here-and-now and realistic expectations. Several members usually volunteered to present their particular issues. Further discussion involved gathering information, providing support, and specifying goals or alternate coping strategies.

Subsequent sessions followed a similar pattern. In the following weeks, there were specific queries as to how an individual was doing in understanding and resolving identified concerns. Over the course of the group, there were a number of changes in its process. Initially, group leaders were very active in encouraging participation, requesting information, and orchestrating conversation. As the group evolved, leaders were less directive and more facilitative and reflective. Teenagers took a greater responsibility for initiating discussion, requesting clarification, and making specific suggestions. There was a similar shift from a primary focus on individual issues and external events to consideration of the group as a whole. This was most apparent in expression of concern for the well-being of both present and absent members, reduced deference or opposition to group leaders, and awareness of impending termination. Although the tone was primarily supportive throughout the group, there was some confrontation, particularly in the latter sessions. This was monitored carefully by the group leaders, positively reframed, and addressed as part of the group process.

In the last session, the goal was to support individual change and to help members deal with the anxiety of termination. This required increased structure on the part of the group leaders. Participants were asked to state the degree to which goals had been met, and reports of success were met with praise and encouragement. Although some individuals felt that they had made limited progress, very deliberate efforts were made to comment positively, if only to commend a participant for being able to identify and tackle a challenging issue. They were asked for feedback about their group experience, both positive and negative. This proved useful to get members to view themselves as seasoned graduates who were now prepared to move on. Participants typically ended the session by exchanging phone numbers and planning a reunion. Although there may have been subsequent individual contacts, reunions did not occur in our experience. This suggests that this was simply a ritualistic means for dealing with separation and loss.

Typical Session in the Therapeutic Discussion Group: Week 5[1]

Eight of the original 10 members arrived for group. One had dropped out, and another had called in sick. After informing the group of this, participants were asked about major events over the last week. Tricia, who had been vying for group leadership in an aggressive and provocative manner, opened by rather glibly describing her mother's decision to move to a distant city. She then claimed that she was going to move in with her 21-year-old boyfriend. Despite some rather skeptical queries from both participants and leaders, she maintained a buoyant presentation with a marked reluctance to acknowledge the issues that this raised. This was particularly evident as Tricia had identified an improved relationship with her mother as her personal goal. This was pointed out, but she dismissed it with the claim that "We'll probably get along better if she's somewhere else."

This set the tone as subsequent participants described their week in a rather superficial way, partially because they were still somewhat insecure with one another but also because of Tricia's inconsistent and confusing disclosure. The situation changed when Catherine stated that she had had a bad day as a result of a friend accusing her of making a prior suicidal gesture for attention. This friend suggested, "Next time you try and kill yourself, try to do the job right." This elicited shocked but consistent support from her fellow group members, several of whom described related experiences with peers and family members. Catherine was visibly upset, and one of the group leaders did a spontaneous role play with her in order to help her to deal with such occurrences while expressing her feelings of hurt, anger, and betrayal.

Subsequent discussion about assertion and risk taking with peers stemmed from this incident. Although some members claimed very open and trusting relationships, others were much less willing to take risks. Further discourse revealed that, despite claims of intimacy and individuality, all members were strongly influenced by the values, behaviors, and expectations of their particular peer subgroup. It became apparent that this was a reflection of the basic adolescent conflict between the need for affiliation and autonomy. This was not challenged directly, but rather various ways of asserting one's identity while avoid-

[1]In order to protect patient confidentiality, the following description is a *composite* but typical account of a middle session in the therapeutic discussion modality. A similar procedure was employed in describing the social skills group session.

ing alienation were discussed. The group ended with encouragement of individual efforts with particular support and request for an update from Catherine. Tricia's dramatic presentation and inability to deal with issues in group were of concern to the group leaders so they subsequently contacted her individual therapist to clarify the situation and to ensure that there was immediate support available.

DESCRIPTION OF THE ADOLESCENT SOCIAL SKILLS GROUP

The adolescent social skills program was based on two overlapping strategies: behavioral skill training and social problem solving. The assumption underlying our social skills group is that many troubled adolescents lack the skills necessary for effective interpersonal encounters. The function of the social skills program is to provide an opportunity for participants to learn, practice, and receive corrective feedback about their interactional repertoire. Although the focus is on adaptive social behaviors, attention was also given to affective and cognitive factors that interfere with effective interactions. Although the ultimate goal is the application of new skills within the individual's existing social environment, the group is viewed as a controlled and supportive milieu in which participants can discuss, observe, and practice relevant skills. The role of the group leaders is to instruct participants in selected skill areas and to structure the group for opportunities to learn and apply these skills. The program is based on a previously prepared manual that identifies a number of specific skill areas and provides examples and opportunities for discussion, practice, and future application.

In the initial session, the nature of social skills was clarified and a rationale for learning them was provided. Social skills were defined as the ability to get along with others in a way that allowed both parties to express their thoughts, feelings, and opinions in a direct manner while respecting the rights of others to do the same. It was emphasized that social competence varies considerably among people and that we could all learn and help one another improve existing social skills, and therefore feel good about ourselves and our interpersonal relationships. The group ended with some discussion of these ideas and clarification of any questions.

The second session introduced the content of the program and helped individuals identify specific interpersonal goals for themselves. Social skills were divided into six different areas: identifying feelings in oneself and others, assertiveness, conversational skills, giving and receiving positive and negative feedback, social problem solving, and negotiation and conflict resolution. Participants were asked to identify areas of their own lives where they experienced interpersonal difficulties. The remainder of the session was spent discussing and specifying individual social goals.

In subsequent sessions, the group leaders defined and provided a rationale for each particular skill area. The skill was then broken down into components or steps. The group leaders role played a positive and negative example of these skills that were then discussed. Participants were asked to provide examples of related situations to be role played. This was a critical aspect of each session and was frequently augmented by reversing roles or introducing complications to otherwise successful applications. Feedback was encouraged with an emphasis on humor and support. The intent was to promote generalization of the particular skill to situations beyond the group. Each session closed with an opportunity for home practice, which was referred to as "the real thing," given the potentially negative connotations of "homework." This typically included a handout summarizing the topic area and a corresponding task for the participant to attempt. Although group members were not discouraged from tackling difficult examples, easier ones were also provided as these were less threatening and more likely to lead to success. These frequently required cooperation of parents or friends that provided further support for the teenager. These assignments were discussed in the following week's session.

Over the course of the group, participants did take an increasingly active role in initiating activities. Although successful application of skills was certainly encouraged, the emphasis was on an individual's sense of satisfaction with his or her efforts, as some family and peer situations were exceptionally complex and less amenable to change. Also, nascent skills might be rather awkward when initially attempted, and it took time and practice for the individual to fully integrate them into his or her repertoire. The final session was conceptualized as a "graduation," in order to emphasize the fact that participants had mastered a curriculum and to help them deal with termination anxiety. The topic areas were briefly reviewed and discussed and participants were asked about meeting their particular interpersonal goals. Abundant support and encouragement was provided for all members regardless of their degree of success. The group ended with a solicitation of suggestions for future programs.

Typical Session in the Social Skills Group: Week 5

Seven of the original nine members arrived for the group. One had dropped out, and one was on vacation with her parents. Participants were asked about their success with the "real thing" of the preceding week. This involved giving and receiving compliments. Several members reported being the recipients of positive feedback at home and school, including Betty, who admitted to being rather surprised at having been praised by her father for her report card. Lisa proudly recounted the fact that she accepted a compliment from her best friend without dismissing it and putting herself down as she was wont to do.

The topic for the session was how to give effective criticism. This skill was presented as important as it was indicative of reciprocal respect and honesty between people and was likely to lead to a change in behavior if done properly. The skill was broken down into appropriate timing and nonverbal communication, personal rather than accusatory statements, specific requests for alternative behaviors, and receptiveness to discussion. The group leaders then role played a situation in which one chided the other for being chronically late. This was done in a sarcastic fashion and soon led to an escalation of insults and accusations over past irrelevant grievances. Participants gleefully provided feedback that was incorporated into a more successful role play.

Group members were then asked for examples from their own lives. Brad proffered the opinion that he would "feel like a goof" if he talked to his friends in the manner that the group leaders did. This was discussed, and it was stressed that people had to use the idiomatic language and style that was appropriate for themselves and their social context. Heather brought up the wish to tell her mother that she felt she was inattentive to her needs for support and attention that was in keeping with her personal goal of improving her communications within her family. She became tearful when discussing this and discussion revealed a difficult situation where all family members took great pains not to "upset" her mother who seemingly had her own emotional difficulties. This was greeted with considerable support from her peers, and various suggestions were offered. These were implemented with Heather playing the role of both herself and her mother. Although the success of these strategies varied, Heather expressed some confidence in her ability to voice her concerns while accepting that her mother might not be able, or wish, to change her behavior.

The group ended with the distribution of handouts summarizing the skill area and the assignment of "the real thing." Participants were asked to seek their parents' help by deciding on something on which they could practice giving negative feedback. Although this could be a real situation, various, deliberately absurd alternatives were provided such as criticizing the color of their father's socks. They were asked to practice the skill and be prepared to discuss this the following week.

SPECIFIC ISSUES IN BRIEF GROUP THERAPY WITH ADOLESCENTS

Although there are a number of issues that are common to other forms of group therapies, some tend to be much more salient and potentially disruptive in brief therapy, as there is less time for remediation through structural changes or self-correction via the group process.

The first issue involves those who drop out of the group. Some attrition is inevitable. Indeed, Lothstein (1978) has pointed out that exclusion of some participants is an aspect of the formation of cohesion. Nevertheless, the loss of group members, particularly in the later sessions, can be detrimental to the morale of the remaining participants. We have been able to reduce the frequency and negative impact of dropouts by emphasizing voluntary participation without undue parental or therapist pressure. In the first session of the group, we acknowledge that the adolescent may feel ambivalent or anxious about group. Our request that they commit themselves to three sessions before making any final decisions increases the likelihood of continuation while respecting their right to terminate. When dropouts do occur, we contact the adolescent to ensure their well-being and the availability of alternate care, if needed. The loss of a member is also raised with the group and discussed in a nonblaming manner.

A second issue pertains to the degree of homogeneity among participants (Garfield, 1986). Although our primary interest was in the treatment of depressed adolescents, we included teenagers with a variety of diagnoses in order to provide greater diversity. The possibility of using volunteer adolescents or "alumni" from prior groups may also be considered to provide positive role models and encourage participation. In our work we have excluded teenagers suffering from a psychotic disorder, significant neurological impairment, or a serious conduct disorder. Although a diversity of backgrounds and issues is beneficial, we have found that it is important to be sensitive to excessive disparity in intellectual, social, and emotional development. Although we felt that our age range of 13 to 17 was sufficiently narrow, it was apparent during the course of several groups that the conceptual abilities and interests of our older, brighter, and more autonomous members were clearly beyond that of their younger counterparts. This was typically resolved by steering the level of the group to the mean level but at the risk of befuddling or boring some participants. Awareness of this issue during the pregroup interviews and selection of members will mitigate its occurrence.

Given the brief and closed nature of the groups, it was necessary to expedite group engagement and cohesion and encourage a willingness to disclose and address personal issues. This was partially accomplished by the interviews with candidates and their families prior to the group, where we were able to explain the nature and intent of the program and identify relevant concerns, thus reducing anxiety and setting the stage for participation. Once the group began, the use of various warm-up exercises was very helpful for participants to get to know one another and share in a safe and structured form of self-disclosure. Providing group members with some say in determining content and structural components of the program, such as the nature of snacks, helped enhance their feeling of "ownership" and responsibility and thus participation.

Finally, the relative brevity of the groups necessitated a balance between the therapeutic issues and personal needs of individual members versus the evolution and needs of the group as a whole. In both modalities there was an emphasis on the selection of individual concerns and goals. This not only helped to provide a realistic focus for therapeutic efforts but also ensured that there was an opportunity for attention to each participant over the course of the group. A related point is the occurrence of individual crises during the program, such as the disclosure of suicidal risk or emerging thought disorder. When these arose, they had to be directly addressed with respect for both the needs and safety of the individual and the group as a whole. It is for this reason that we insisted on the availability of an individual therapist for every participant who was then contacted to provide more in-depth exploration, support, and, if necessary, hospitalization.

Conclusions and Recommendations

Our experience with brief group therapy with adolescents indicates that two diverse modalities are effective in reducing serious clinical symptomatology. Although there are some notable theoretical and practical differences between these approaches, they also share a number of commonalities in both process and structure. There remains a need to determine the nature and exclusivity of the therapeutic components. In addition, research is necessary to ascertain the appropriate match between the type of group therapy and the clinical, developmental, and personality characteristics of the participants. In the absence of such information, the choice of intervention must depend on the training and orientation of the therapists and the needs of the teenagers.

The approaches that we have used represent only two possible group therapy modalities. There are a number of alternative group modalities that could be implemented, either in isolation or combination. Group treatment can be used together with individual or family work for maximal therapeutic impact. We have certainly found brief group therapy to be a challenging and rewarding venture and would strongly recommend that it be considered by clinicians.

Acknowledgments

The authors gratefully acknowledge the significant contribution of the therapists and patients to the writing of this chapter. In addition, Dr. Rene Weideman of the Department of Psychology, Vancouver General Hospital, made some very useful suggestions for improving an earlier draft.

References

Azima, F. J. C., & Richmond, L. H. (1989). *Adolescent group psychotherapy.* Madison, CT: International Universities Press.

Corder, B. F., Whiteside, L., & Haizlip, T. M. (1981). A study of curative factors. *International Journal of Group Psychotherapy, 31,* 345–354.

Fine, S., Knight-Webb, G., & Breau, K. (1976). Volunteer adolescents in adolescent group therapy. *British Journal of Psychiatry, 129,* 407–413.

Fine, S., Gilbert, M., Schmidt, L., Haley, G., Maxwell, A., & Forth, A. (1989). Short term group therapy with depressed adolescents. *Canadian Journal of Psychiatry, 34,* 97–102.

Fine, S., Forth, A., Gilbert, M., & Haley, G. (1991). Group therapy for adolescent depressive disorder: A comparison of social skills and therapeutic support. *Journal of the American Academy of Child and Adolescent Psychiatry, 30,* 79–85.

Garfield, S. L. (1986). Research on client variables in psychotherapy. In S. L. Garfield & A. E. Bergin (Eds.), *Handbook of psychotherapy and behavior change: An empirical analysis* (3rd ed., pp. 213–256). New York: Wiley.

Garvin, D. G. (1990). Short term group therapy. In R. A. Wells & V. J. Giannetti (Eds.), *Handbook of the brief psychotherapies* (pp. 513–535). New York: Plenum Press.

Hurst, A., Stein, K., Korchin, S., & Soskin, W. (1978). Leadership style determinants of cohesiveness in adolescent groups. *International Journal of Group Psychotherapy, 28,* 263–277.

Klein, R. H. (1985). Some principles of short-term group therapy. *International Journal of Group Psychotherapy, 35,* 309–330.

Kolvin, I., Garside, R. F., Nichol, A. R., MacMillan, A., Wolstenholme, F., & Leitch, I. M. (1981). *Help starts here: The maladjusted child in the ordinary school.* London: Tavistock Publications.

Lewinsohn, P. M., Clarke, G. N., Hops, H., & Andrews, J. (1990). Cognitive-behavioral treatment for depressed adolescents. *Behavior Therapy, 21,* 385–401.

Lothstein, L. M. (1978). The group psychotherapy dropout phenomenon revisited. *American Journal of Psychiatry, 135*(12), 1492–1495.

Michelson, L., Sugai, D., Wood, R., & Kazdin, A. (1983). *Social skills assessment and training with children: An empirically based handbook.* New York: Plenum Press.

Plienis, A., Hansen, D., Ford, F., Smith, S., Stark, L., & Kelly, J. (1987). Behavioral small group training to improve the social skills of emotionally-disordered adolescents. *Behavior Therapy, 18,* 17–32.

Poey, K. (1985). Guidelines for the practice of brief dynamic group therapy. *International Journal of Group Psychotherapy, 35,* 351–354.

Reynolds, W. H., & Coats, K. (1986). A comparison of cognitive-behavioral and relaxation training for the treatment of depressed adolescents. *Journal of Consulting & Clinical Psychology, 54,* 653–660.

Rotheram, M. (1980). Social skills training and programs in elementary and high school classrooms. In D. P. Rathjen & J. P. Foreyt (Eds.), *Social competence: Interventions for children and adults* (pp. 69–112). New York: Pergamon Press.

Yalom, I. (1985). *The theory and practice of group psychotherapy.* New York: Basic Books.

Index